Cardiology in Primary Care

Clive Handler

Consultant Cardiologist
Highgate Hospital, London

Radcliffe Publishing Ltd
18 Marcham Road
Abingdon
Oxon OX14 1AA
United Kingdom

www.radcliffe-oxford.com
Electronic catalogue and worldwide online ordering facility.

British Library Cataloguing in Publication Data

A catalogue record for this book is available from the British Library.

ISBN 1 85775 833 1

Typeset by Advance Typesetting Ltd, Oxford
Printed and bound by TJ International Ltd, Padstow, Cornwall

Contents

Foreword

Cardiovascular disease remains the leading cause of death in the Western world, with over half a million deaths a year in the United States attributable to coronary artery disease alone.

These statistics are challenging to the clinical community, particularly the primary care physician who can fulfil the special role in prevention, education and interventional treatments, thereby resulting in modification of the disease.

The high incidence of cardiovascular disease is compounded by the ageing of our population, with a greater number of patients presenting for invasive procedures and revascularisations.

The author has produced an excellent book specifically written for primary care physicians. He has wisely been very aware of national health targets and the enormous responsibilities in primary care of identifying patients at risk.

Most primary care physicians in the UK will not have received any formal cardiological training, but this book provides simple and yet clear and well-written information that can be used effectively in the management of patients in primary care. There are excellent case studies, advice and treatment on common conditions and, perhaps most refreshingly of all, an explanation of invasive procedures, operative interventions and the care and long-term management of patients with coronary artery disease.

This book is enjoyable to read and, when necessary, can also be used as a quick reference, and should give most primary care physicians the confidence to treat their patients with greater understanding and insight.

Martin Adler
General Practitioner
Middlesex
June 2004

Foreword

In this short book Dr Handler has distilled the essence of cardiology and presented it in an accessible format for those who have other lives. The pace of developments in cardiology over the last ten years has been breathtaking. Many new classes of drugs have been developed and care delivery has been revolutionised by new investigational techniques, improvements in the technical quality of older tests and many new interventional treatments. All of these developments have been underpinned by landmark trials providing an unparalleled evidence base for the new ways of working. The National Service Framework and NICE initiatives, as well as a large array of national and international guidelines, have raised expectations that all healthcare clinicians will understand the place of all these treatments in individual patients. The expectations of patients, managers and lawyers are difficult enough for those who work full time in cardiology to meet, for those in primary care remaining abreast of the current thinking has become a near impossible challenge. *Cardiology in Primary Care* meets this challenge and more, by bringing the reader up to date with how all these advances apply in practice. The structure of the book allows one to take any clinical problem (the overweight patient, the dizzy patient, etc) and understand in a few moments how the problem should be investigated and treated, as well as indicating at what point referral to hospital is appropriate. In addition, what will happen in secondary care is explained, as well as the likely outcome for the patient. Difficult concepts such as numbers needed to treat (NNT) and relative versus absolute benefit are dealt with simply and in a consistent fashion, making such ideas part of the natural thinking of the reader. This puts the primary care physician firmly in charge, knowing how the patient should be managed from first presentation through to discharge or long-term follow up.

Each chapter starts with clinical vignettes dealing with typical 'heart sink' situations and explaining in a few sentences how to proceed in each instance. An overview of the subject follows, then the role of the primary care team in diagnosing, investigating and managing each problem is dealt with. At the end of each chapter is a list detailing the most important points that need to be covered in discussions with the patient.

This book is essential reading for all primary care physicians and specialist nurses working with cardiac patients, and also meets the needs of today's medical students as well as healthcare managers.

Gerry Coghlan
Consultant Cardiologist
The Royal Free Hospital
London
June 2004

Preface

GPs and practice nurses have always been actively involved in the management of patients with cardiovascular disorders, but are now expected to provide a more specialised service.

Recent advances and changes in emphasis in the management of common cardiovascular conditions present primary care clinicians with major challenges. Cardiovascular disease prevention, the diagnosis and management of heart failure, coronary artery disease, suspected myocardial infarction, hypertension and arrhythmias and, less frequently, the management of valve abnormalities and occasionally congenital heart disease are daily challenges. New methods of diagnosis and treatment necessitate an understanding of the value, limitations and, in some cases, risks of these techniques.

Our patients are better informed than ever before and, understandably and justifiably, they expect high-quality care. Information published by the media and on the Internet may both inform and concern patients. Patients expect GPs to know about recent medical advances and provide guidance on the often confusing and conflicting new information in cardiology.

The use of evidence-based guidelines on disease management is not always straightforward in deciding optimum management for individual patients who have complex comorbidity and whose clinical profile does not fit precisely with the guideline criteria. Patients' views on how they wish to be treated must also be considered, and this is particularly relevant with regard to the management of cardiovascular risk factors.

The increasing availability of 'open-access' facilities for cardiac investigations has made it easier for GPs to obtain diagnostic information, but effective and appropriate use of cardiac investigations, the interpretation of test results and their implications for clinical management often present difficulties. Patients expect GPs to provide information about the need for and implications of the results of investigations, and may need further explanation of what they have been told by hospital staff. These tasks present significant workload pressures and challenges, and demand high-quality communication skills of primary care clinicians.

The impetus for writing this book derived from the enjoyable and educational experiences I have had over a period of several years providing cardiology outreach services in primary care, and talking with and learning from a large number of my colleagues who tell me about the clinical problems that commonly confront them in their daily work.

I have tried to provide comprehensive and relevant background information and clinical management guidance on common cardiological problems that present to primary care practitioners. I am conscious that some of the information provided may be out of date by the time this book is published, but it is these rapid advances in cardiology that make it so interesting and lively. I hope that my colleagues in primary care find the book useful, and that they will let me know how the next edition may be improved.

Clive Handler
June 2004

Acknowledgements

I am very grateful to the following people who have in various ways helped me with this project: the staff at Sheepcot Medical Centre, Heathfielde Medical Centre, Belmont Health Centre and the Keats Group Practice with whom I have provided outreach services, and the many other GP colleagues with whom I work; Lionel Kopelowitz, who introduced me to Radcliffe Publishing, and to my excellent editorial director, Gillian Nineham; Stanley Curry, David Myers, Amina Karim, Lynne Turner-Stokes and Lawrence Cohen; my colleagues at St Mary's Hospital – Brian Glenville, Rodney Foale, Wyn Davies, Nick Peters, Jamil Mayet and Iqbal Malik; my colleagues at University College Hospital – Malcolm Walker, Howard Swanton and Derek Yellon. I would also like to thank Dr Gerry Coghlan for his meticulous and constructive criticism of the manuscript.

About the author

Clive Handler BSc, MD, MRCP, FACC, FESC, qualified from Guy's Hospital Medical School and trained in general medicine and cardiology in London and the USA. After working as a consultant cardiologist at Northwick Park and St Mary's hospitals, he entered independent clinical practice in London. He is a Fellow of the American College of Cardiology and the European Society of Cardiology. He is the editor of *Guy's Hospital – 250 Years* and co-editor, with Dr Michael Cleman of Yale University, of *Classic Papers in Coronary Angioplasty* (to be published in 2004). He is the author of original research papers on general cardiology and the diagnosis and management of coronary artery disease. His clinical interests are in the prevention and management of coronary artery disease, hypertension and heart failure.

He is married with three children, and lives in Highgate.

This book is dedicated to Caroline, Charlotte, Sophie, Julius and Sylvia, and to my patients.

CHAPTER 1

The patient and primary care

Primary care clinicians and their role in treating cardiovascular disease

More patients with cardiovascular disease are being diagnosed, investigated, treated and followed up in primary care for a number of reasons. These include National Health Service (NHS) policies and targets placing a greater responsibility for cardiovascular disease prevention on primary care physicians and nurses, and changes in the thresholds for treating cardiovascular risk factors. For example, more aggressive lipid lowering and treatment of hypertension are recommended for diabetics, and are 'health targets' for primary care. Obesity and smoking are common and important cardiovascular risk factors, and the primary care team is expected to play a major role in reducing all components of cardiovascular risk.

The changing face of primary care

The GP surgery has changed in character over the last decade and will continue to evolve, even though its main purpose will be to offer a diagnostic and management service for patients. Purpose-built multi-disciplinary health centres that provide modern, preventive and diagnostic facilities are steadily replacing single-handed doctors, who continue to provide high-quality care.

Primary care cardiovascular physicians

A logical consequence of the increasingly prominent role of primary care physicians in managing patients with cardiovascular problems is the growing number of GPs with an interest in cardiovascular medicine. They have established themselves as a large, active and academic group with a special interest group and membership of the British Cardiac Society (BCS). Diploma courses, conferences and postgraduate education abound, and are part of continuing professional development (CPD). GPs and specialists working together both in hospital clinics and in primary care will produce a large number of interested GPs with enhanced training and experience in cardiology, who are able to provide an increasingly refined and broad specialist service.

Although some patients use the Internet as a medical information source and may ask friends and family about medical matters, most generally prefer to seek advice from their primary care team, whom they know and trust. It is important, therefore, that all advice given is clear, accurate, up to date, understandable, non-alarmist and reassuring when appropriate.

Present and potential future tasks for primary care physicians

- Identify patients who require referral to a cardiologist for diagnosis and management advice and, where necessary, long-term joint care.
- Provide the specialist with the appropriate documentation and information concerning the patient's history.
- Identify patients with acute cardiac conditions, including acute coronary syndromes, acute myocardial infarction, acute heart failure and haemodynamically important arrhythmias, and refer them immediately to hospital in such a way that they are managed quickly.
- Estimate the absolute cardiovascular risk for patients and then decide whether it is appropriate to treat and monitor risk factors, and how best to do this.
- In patients with suspected or known coronary heart disease, estimate the patient's absolute cardiovascular risk. With an understanding of Bayes' theorem and an appreciation of the value and limitations of exercise testing and other non-invasive tests, assess the probability of coronary heart disease, decide whether further testing is appropriate, and if it is, choose the most appropriate test to use.
- Educate patients about cardiovascular risk factor modification, and involve them as the key players in reducing their own risk.
- If the GP disagrees with certain aspects of the management recommended by the cardiologist (or any specialist), then the GP should discuss this with the specialist.
- Consult and discuss cases with relevant specialists with regard to individual clinical problems and also improving the quality of clinical services and the development of investigations, access to specialist opinions and provision of community cardiac services.
- Seek advice and support in varied and novel ways for medical education, professional development and other postgraduate activities in order to remain well informed and acquire the knowledge necessary to remain critical of new medical and drug information, literature or politically driven initiatives.
- The primary care team must try to remain clinically interested, intellectually and physically fit and fresh, good humoured and dedicated to providing their patients with the best possible advice. Their job is stressful and demanding.
- Explain to patients the reasons for investigations, what the tests involve and why a particular treatment has been chosen.
- Ensure that patients understand why medication has been prescribed, and try to improve their compliance with intelligent, skilful prescribing.
- Consider cost-effectiveness in all aspects of clinical management.
- Reflect upon and audit current practice.

Outreach clinics

Over the last few years, some GPs have established cardiology outreach clinics. A consultant cardiologist works with the GP in the surgery, providing a joint consultation service. This has several advantages. Patients prefer to see the specialist in their GP surgery rather than attend a hospital. It is unusual for patients to see the same doctor at each hospital outpatient visit, and test results and records are often not available. However, some hospital cardiac departments are establishing interlinked databases between the consultation room, the various investigation facilities and the patient records, and this will have obvious benefits.

Outreach clinics reduce bureaucratic problems and also have other advantages.

- The GP can discuss the patient with the cardiologist face to face, rather than by letter or telephone. GP referral letters to specialists may no longer be necessary, and therefore cannot be mislaid.
- Patients are more likely to attend the outreach appointment, because attending the GP surgery is easier, quicker, cheaper, more personal and less intimidating than attending hospital.
- There may be fewer inappropriate referrals for open-access investigations if cardiologists rather than primary care physicians request cardiac investigations. This should result in more efficient use of resources.
- Combined primary care and specialist clinics provide a two-way learning experience and help to forge solid professional relationships based on an understanding of the problems that each clinician encounters.
- Outreach clinics bring doctors together and provide an opportunity for research and audit, development of protocols for investigation and treatment, and a forum for informed and sensible discussion of how healthcare delivery can be developed and refined in the future.

However, there are resource implications. Outreach clinics take a hospital-based specialist away from the hospital for a few hours perhaps once a month, whereas the clinics might be performed by a cardiovascular specialist GP.

The patient's view

This is not known, but most patients want and expect an easily accessed GP to be able to provide advice and help at all times, and a sympathetic expert experienced specialist who is able to give them the best possible advice quickly.

Cardiac investigations in primary care

Patients may need to attend hospital for investigation, although new portable echocardiography machines, ambulatory blood pressure recording, 24-hour ECG monitoring devices and cycle exercise testing are now available. Most of these investigations are already performed in primary care health centres, thus reducing waiting times.

The use of cardiac tests in primary care necessitates an understanding both of their indications and of their value and limitations in different conditions. Test-result interpretation is based on this knowledge and extensive experience.

Patients and primary care clinicians

Primary care is undergoing a revolution. Patients are more interested and knowledgeable and have higher expectations of their doctors and nurses and the health service than ever before.

Patients are also increasingly likely to have a consultation with a nurse rather than a doctor. They may want the answers to specific lifestyle questions, as well as presenting with symptoms. They are more informed, more likely to question the advice given, and less prepared to wait to see a specialist or have an investigation.

Many GPs are now expert in primary and secondary prevention of coronary heart disease, and are being encouraged to develop their interests and skills in cardiology. Some are providing specialist services in hospital cardiac departments. Nurses are also playing an increasingly important diagnostic and therapeutic role in both primary care and hospital care.

The patient's perspective: what do patients want from their GP?

The doctor's interest, time and a quality consultation

Patients want the opportunity and time to explain how they feel and what they are worried about. They want their doctor to listen, understand, care and take them and their concerns seriously. They want reassurance, help, advice and a sympathetic explanation of their symptoms. One of the most important but difficult components of clinical medicine, that requires skill and experience, is explaining treatment and management options and decisions to patients. This ability is not easily obtained from any written source, and there is no substitute for experience, a self-critical stance, and listening to and learning from skilful colleagues.

Providing information about treatment

Patients want a clear explanation of the drugs and other treatment recommended, and what any investigations, procedures and operations involve and their risks. This is usually very difficult and time-consuming, particularly if the patient speaks a different language and has different cultural and religious beliefs. Technical words should be avoided and the information must be tailored to the individual patient.

The most commonly asked questions about drug prescribing centre on why the drug has been prescribed, its side-effects, and how it may interfere with the patient's lifestyle and eating and drinking habits.

The purpose of investigations and what they involve should also be explained simply (*see* Chapter 25).

Although it is most appropriate for the details of cardiac procedures and operations to be discussed by the specialist, primary care clinicians should be able to provide basic information about most cardiac procedures and operations. This is facilitated by clear, prompt communication with specialists. In this context, GPs find regular updates, tutorials and hospital teaching sessions helpful.

It is good practice to involve patients in certain treatment options, particularly where there may be more than one option (e.g. in the treatment of coronary heart disease, or in cardiovascular prevention). Even where there is evidence of a clear treatment benefit (e.g. aortic valve surgery for severe aortic stenosis), it is important for patients to be aware of the potential risks as well as the benefits.

Continuity of care

Several methods have been tried in an attempt to shorten the time patients have to wait in order to see their NHS GP. With a shortage of GPs and an increasing demand from patients and more work to do, it is going to be difficult to shorten waiting times even with the use of practice nurses. Continuity of care is an important aspect of quality of care, and is recognised as a patient priority, but is compromised by different staff seeing the patient. Management protocols reduce the negative aspects of fragmented medical management, but it is difficult in the management of chronic diseases such as angina, or risk factor modification, to ensure a uniform approach, pace and tone to treatment with multiple baton changes.

Speedy appropriate investigations

If investigations or specialist consultations are necessary, the patient will not want to wait a long time. Most patients are aware that delays may be beyond the control of their GP. However, their own anxiety may override their sympathy for the GP, who is expected to deliver prompt, high-quality medical services in the face of prolonged waiting times, ever-changing organisational issues and 'targets', and resource restrictions imposed on both the primary care team and the hospital service. Patients want all aspects of their medical care to be addressed quickly. They may want to see a specialist even when the GP may not consider this necessary. Patients want to feel better quickly.

The Internet and other sources of medical information have led to patients wanting information on the clinical experience and expertise of the cardiologist to whom they are to be referred, the quality and range of diagnostic equipment and treatments available at their local hospital, and whether they would benefit from being sent to a more specialised unit.

What does the primary healthcare team need to do?

The primary healthcare team has a difficult sub-specialist role that includes diagnosis, referring patients to the appropriate specialist, explaining test results and specialist management plans, and they have a major responsibility for prescribing medication approved by their local therapeutics committee. They also have a key role in long-term monitoring and management of chronic conditions (e.g. identifying and reducing cardiovascular risk and managing valve and heart muscle abnormalities). It is important that all members of the team understand the principles of management of the common cardiovascular conditions.

They have to listen to the patient and understand what the patient needs and try to help them. Patients must be treated courteously, with respect, and made to feel at ease and able to ask the clinician questions, which should be answered openly, honestly and sensitively. This is difficult in the short time that is allocated in most busy GP practices. There is a great art in talking to worried patients whose fear, desperation or confusion may transpose to anger. The primary healthcare team needs to have the resources, time, energy, training and ability to cope with patients' demands and increasing expectations. All those involved in the care of patients with cardiovascular problems should have the necessary knowledge and skills.

Some patients have a 'hidden agenda' or secret fears about their health, prompted by the illness of a friend or member of the family, and it is important to elicit this. Their symptoms may be a manifestation of anxiety related to their personal or family life, or work-related worries, and the GP and nurse are usually in an advantageous position to unravel and tease out any underlying problem. This may be all that is required to help the patient.

The nurse practitioner

Nurse practitioners are increasingly important members of the primary healthcare team, and play a prominent role in patient care, performing many parts of the traditional doctor's role. Patients are generally positive about the idea of seeing a nurse in primary care, and trust their professional ability.

Cardiovascular risk assessment and treatment, weight reduction, diet and dietary supplements and personal lifestyle advice, including advice on smoking, alcohol, exercise and sex, are important and commonly encountered aspects of cardiology in primary care. Nurses therefore need to have a sound knowledge of the role of these factors in clinical care. They may also be engaged in clinical evaluation, and so will need to be able to take a cardiac history, examine the patient and make a diagnosis in collaboration with the GP. As well as having an understanding of cardiac tests, they should feel confident about drawing up a management plan, and know which patients need to be referred for a specialist opinion.

Other members of the primary healthcare team

Pharmacists, physiotherapists, dietitians and complementary medical specialists play an increasingly prominent role in primary care, and each has an integrated role in different conditions.

Pharmacists

Pharmacists need to provide advice on possible drug side-effects, which are an important issue with the increasing and desirable intention of effective treatment of heart failure, vascular disease and control of risk factors such as hypertension, diabetes and hyperlipidaemia. Dose adjustments in the elderly and those with renal or liver impairment, and simplification of treatment and dosage regimes to improve compliance, are key areas where a pharmacist can make major improvements to clinical care and lighten the workload for the GP.

Dietitians

Dietitians have expertise in dietary regimes to help patients lose weight and improve diabetic control, hypertension and hyperlipidaemia. Patients may want to know whether new dietary supplements and vitamins are beneficial, and what foods are beneficial or harmful. Alcohol is popular, and patients may be confused about its benefits and dangers with regard to their particular condition, and how much and what type they should drink.

Physiotherapists

Physiotherapists have specialised knowledge and skills in a range of conditions. Their advice and encouragement to patients to exercise regularly, and provision of an exercise prescription as part of primary and secondary prevention of coronary heart disease, treatment of heart failure and after heart surgery, are important and of proven efficacy. These facilities should be available in primary care. Cardiac rehabilitation in primary care could be arranged, and patients would prefer it.

Dental care

Patients with heart valve conditions should have good oral hygiene and access to a dentist who has a knowledge of the evolving indications for antibiotic prophylaxis and dental assessments before valve surgery.

Complementary medicine and practitioners

Complementary practitioners work in some practices in the UK, and for certain conditions they may have a role to play. For example, yoga and meditation have no side-effects and may reduce stress levels and be used as part of the treatment of patients with hypertension, although there is no evidence that they provide any objective benefit.

Acupuncture

A large number of GPs are now offering patients acupuncture, and this is used to treat musculoskeletal problems, smoking addiction and a variety of other conditions.

Non-clinical staff

Non-clinical staff should be aware of their role and the crucially important administrative part they play in the work of the practice and the moral support they provide for the clinical team.

Reviewing cardiac patients in primary care

Subsequent chapters addressing specific cardiac conditions will deal with referral to specialists. Recognising when patients should be referred requires experience, judgement and an understanding of their condition. When patients are referred back to the GP after specialist management, it is important for the primary care team to be aware of when they need to be reviewed by a specialist.

Acute cardiac conditions occurring as either a new problem (e.g. a suspected heart attack) or a change in a previously controlled condition (e.g. heart failure or arrhythmia) pose difficulties in primary care, and are a source of stress and anxiety to all concerned. The common conditions will be dealt with in subsequent chapters. It is important that these conditions are recognised so that appropriate treatment (e.g. oxygen, diuretics and diamorphine for heart failure) can be started in primary care without delay.

References and further reading

- Chambers R, Wakley G and Iqbal Z (2001) *Cardiovascular Disease Matters in Primary Care*. Radcliffe Medical Press, Oxford.
- Iqbal Z, Chambers R and Woodmansey P (2001) *Implementing the National Service Framework for Coronary Heart Disease in Primary Care*. Radcliffe Medical Press, Oxford.
- NHS Executive (2000) *National Service Framework for Coronary Heart Disease*. Department of Health, London.
- Secretary of State for Health (1999) *Saving Lives: our healthier nation*. Department of Health, London.

CHAPTER 2

History

Case studies

1 A 28-year-old woman with chest pain and personal problems was referred to the local hospital cardiology clinic by your practice partner for an exercise test, but she is unwilling to have this done and wants to see you for a second opinion. What would you do?

2 An 85-year-old man with a history of occasional episodes of angina during the last 20 years comes to see you complaining of chest pain while gardening. What would you do?

3 A 43-year-old man, recently discharged from hospital after a myocardial infarct, has angina while lying in bed. What would you do?

4 A 31-year-old woman complains of 'fluttering' in her chest with stress. What would you do?

5 A 60-year-old businessman with a previous history of coronary artery bypass surgery notices increased breathlessness when walking upstairs. What would you do?

History

Why the history is crucial to patient management

Try to obtain as thorough a history as possible from the first consultation. This may provide the diagnosis and save time, confusion and unnecessary investigations.

> The history often provides the diagnosis, is therapeutic and forms the basis for management. It is the foundation of the doctor–patient relationship.

A sympathetic and productive consultation will form the foundation of a long-lasting bond of trust, friendship and respect, which are key components of the doctor–patient relationship. Patients may forgive medical mistakes but do not forget an abrupt, uncaring manner, and this may make them angry and litigious if they or a relative feel that something has gone wrong at any stage.

With the increasing use of protocol-driven, nurse-delivered clinical services in primary care, and the use of open-access investigations, the history will become increasingly important as the basis for clinical management and the justification for complex, costly investigations which may have complications. Readily available investigations are no substitute for a carefully taken, comprehensive, thoughtful history. Management, including the relevant investigations, should be formulated after you have taken the history and made a diagnosis. Treatment should not be based solely on the results of investigations.

What is the patient worried about?

It is very important to understand and record accurately (in the patient's own words when appropriate) the patient's main symptoms and how they affect their life. If the patient uses a medical word, such as 'palpitation', ask them what they mean by this.

Assessing cardiovascular risk

The history provides essential information for assessing cardiovascular risk, the probability of an individual having vascular disease and its prognosis, which in turn determine management. Subsequent chapters will discuss the individual cardiovascular risk factors in more detail. Age, previous cardiovascular events or interventions, smoking, hypertension, hyperlipidaemia, diabetes, a family history of premature coronary heart disease, diet, weight, lifestyle and less well-established risk factors are important components of the history. Establishing their presence or absence aids risk stratification, helping to identify those at high and low risk of having cardiovascular disease. For example, coronary artery disease is unlikely in a young patient with no risk factors, but almost certain in a patient with exertional chest pain and more than one risk factor.

Vascular disease is common. All adult patients should be questioned about risk factors so that they can be given advice to reduce their cardiovascular risk and improve their prognosis.

When can the history provide the diagnosis?

A diagnosis can often be made from the history. For example, the patient may give a clear history of angina. Ectopic beats may be the most likely cause of a patient's unpleasant palpitation, although this diagnosis usually requires ECG confirmation. A diagnosis of heart failure is difficult to make from the history alone, and in this case investigations are required to assess cardiac function and establish the cause.

Symptom severity determines management

It is essential to gain a clear understanding of the frequency and severity of the patient's symptoms, their effect on his or her day-to-day activities and any lifestyle changes the patient has had to make. For example, the management of a patient with unstable angina and rest pain is very different from that of an elderly patient who has occasional episodes of mild angina only with severe exertion. Whereas the young patient should be referred for inpatient assessment and treatment, the patient with infrequent, predictable symptoms may be appropriately treated in primary care with prophylactic glyceryl trinitrate (GTN) and aspirin, and may not need a specialist opinion unless the symptoms become unstable.

If the history is unclear, a diagnosis must be made and investigations will be necessary. Cardiac causes of chest pain, syncope or breathlessness should be excluded first if the patient is at risk from coronary heart disease or there are signs of structural heart disease.

Grading symptoms of angina and breathlessness according to severity, using internationally accepted classifications, is helpful. However, for many patients a clear description of the symptom and how it impacts on the patient's day-to-day activities provides a more memorable, relevant and vivid record of their problem.

Patients with cardiac disorders may have symptoms only when they exert themselves, and may reduce their activities. It is important to document a patient's exercise tolerance. They may not volunteer this information, so they should be asked whether they can exercise or walk quickly on the flat, how far they can walk, whether they can walk upstairs (and if so, how many stairs they can walk), and whether they have had to slow down (and if so, over what time period).

Taking the history

There is no 'best' way to do this.

It is helpful to have details of previous myocardial revascularisation or heart operations. Patients who complain of chest pain should be asked about cardiovascular risk factors.

Pro formas

Structured history pro formas filled in by nurses may be helpful and time saving in recording details of family and personal history, including details of medication and past illnesses. However, on their own they are no substitute for a carefully taken history, and do not have the same therapeutic impact. Patients may not understand the value of pro formas and may feel that their symptoms are not being taken seriously.

The patient's story

Despite time restrictions in general practice, patients should be allowed to talk about their symptoms and concerns. As with formal psychotherapy, they feel better as soon as they start doing this, and feel that they are being helped. Knowing when to interrupt a patient's narrative to ask direct questions or encourage them to expand or contract on part of their history is a difficult art.

The importance of the primary care record

It is crucial that the patient's history is recorded as accurately as possible. It is particularly important in the management of patients with coronary artery disease and other chronic conditions that the dates and sequence of events, all interventions (including drug and surgical treatments) and relevant medical conditions are recorded chronologically.

Patients may present with chest pain or a myocardial infarct, and may have had coronary angioplasty or coronary artery surgery. They may have diabetes and hypertension and be on lipid-lowering treatment. It is important for the GP to provide this information in the referral letter to the cardiologist. Even with modern information technology, hospital medical records are less than perfect, so the primary care records are very important and may be the most complete and readily accessible patient record.

History possibly relevant to the presenting complaint

Angina may occasionally be precipitated by severe anaemia and hypothyroidism. Patients with usually well-controlled heart failure may decompensate as a result of an intercurrent chest infection or myocardial infarction, or due to being unable or forgetting to take their medication, or as a result of an arrhythmia-like atrial fibrillation. Coexisting relevant medical or social conditions should be recorded.

Drug history

Ensure that the patient is taking their prescribed drugs in the prescribed doses at the prescribed times. Ask them whether they take any non-prescription tablets. It is important to be aware of potential side-effects of commonly used cardiac medication. For example, eye drops containing β-blockers are relevant to patients with heart failure, bradycardia, asthma or fatigue. Non-steroidal anti-inflammatory drugs may cause renal failure or anaemia. Homeopathic drugs have a variety of actions, and cocaine and opiates have major cardiovascular side-effects. Young otherwise healthy patients with chest pain or breathlessness should be asked about substance abuse, particularly involving cocaine and other sympathomimetic drugs.

Possible drug-related symptoms

More patients are using more drugs, and patients are often worried that their symptoms are due to drug side-effects. It is sometimes necessary to test this possibility. Suspected drugs may need to be stopped to see whether the symptoms resolve, and then restarted to see whether the symptoms recur.

Cardiovascular risk factors

These should be on the patient's database. Adults need to be checked and monitored for cardiovascular risk factors. Children should be advised to reduce their future risk of developing cardiovascular disease by having a healthy diet, not smoking, and taking regular exercise.

All patients who smoke should be helped as much as possible and strongly advised to stop.

Family history

A patient with a close family relative who had a definite myocardial infarct or had angioplasty or coronary artery surgery when aged under 50 years is at high risk of developing coronary artery disease. Hypertrophic cardiomyopathy also has a genetic and familial basis. Screening the children of affected individuals aged under 50 years should be considered.

The commonest and most important cardiac symptoms are as follows:

- chest pain, tightness or discomfort
- shortness of breath
- palpitation
- loss of consciousness (syncope) or dizziness.

Patients do not usually describe their symptoms in these words.

Related vascular symptoms include the following:

- transient ischaemic attacks
- claudication
- leg swelling.

Chest discomfort, chest pain and breathlessness

This is understandably very worrying for the patient, who may report directly to the hospital emergency department or request urgent advice in the surgery.

Note: The most important cause to consider is angina, myocardial infarction or another form of acute coronary syndrome.

The diagnosis must be made from the history. Physical examination is usually unremarkable, but heart failure, arrhythmia and hypertension should be looked for.

The differential diagnosis of chest pain is shown in Table 2.1.

Table 2.1:   Differential diagnosis of chest pain

Cause	*History*
Angina	Short-lasting, precipitated by exertion or stress, relieved by rest or GTN
Myocardial infarct	Intense, autonomic symptoms, long-lasting
Oesophageal pain	Epigastric, related to food, position or sometimes exertion, nausea, relieved by antacids and H_2-blockers
Pneumonia, pulmonary embolus	Pleuritic pain
Gall-bladder	Nausea, fever, possible obstructive features
Chest wall pain	(Tietze's syndrome) Trauma, localised tenderness, positional, long-lasting
Aortic dissection	Severe localised mid-back pain in a hypertensive patient
Anxiety	Personality, previous history, features not compatible with angina
Acute pericarditis	Sharp, worse with inspiration, positional – relieved by leaning forward, recent flu-like illness
Acute pancreatitis	Epigastric, continuous, fever, abdominal symptoms
Shingles	Skin rash

Angina

The diagnosis of angina is made only from the history, and not from a test result. Patients may have test results indicating coronary artery disease, but may not have angina. A 'positive' exercise test result may indicate ischaemia, but in the absence of symptoms this does not mean that the patient has angina. Patients only have angina if they have compatible symptoms.

Angina is probable if:

- chest discomfort/breathlessness is related to exercise and/or emotion
- symptoms are relieved promptly by rest and/or GTN
- one or more risk factors for coronary artery disease are present.

Character of anginal symptoms

Angina is usually described as chest discomfort, tightness, pressure, burning or breath-lessness lasting for seconds or a few minutes in the chest and radiating to the arms and/or neck. It is often more noticeable in cold weather (which increases blood pressure) or after heavy meals (when blood is diverted to the gut). It may be felt only in the jaw or arms. The location of the symptom is less important diagnostically. Localised 'pin-pricking' pain felt under the left breast is very rarely angina. Patients rarely describe 'pain' unless they are experiencing a heart attack or infarct, when the pain is more intense, lasts longer and is associated with autonomic symptoms of sweating and nausea (see Chapter 15 on myocardial infarction). It is preferable to ask the patient about chest discomfort rather than pain.

Note: It is important to recognise that breathlessness may be the only symptom of coronary artery disease. It is an 'anginal equivalent'. In patients at risk of coronary artery disease, it should always be considered to represent myocardial ischaemia rather than a respiratory symptom.

Angina or indigestion?

This is a common clinical problem. It is often very difficult to distinguish between angina and oesophageal pain, which may also be precipitated by exertion and relieved by GTN. The two conditions are common and may coexist. The important practical management point is to exclude coronary artery disease before investigating a gastro-oesophageal problem in patients with cardiovascular risk factors. Oesophageal pain responds to antacids, H_2-blockers and proton-pump inhibitors, but angina does not.

The Canadian classification of severity of anginal symptoms

Angina is graded according to its severity and impact on the daily activities of the patient. Cardiologists use this classification to describe a patient's symptoms. However, it is equally important to record the patient's description of their symptoms in the notes, and to relay these in a referral letter.

- Grade I – no limitation to ordinary physical activity (e.g. walking and running upstairs, jogging, gardening). Angina only with strenuous physical activity.
- Grade II – slight limitation of ordinary activity. Patients can perform all of the above activities, but may experience angina when exercising in cold weather, after heavy meals, or when performing ordinary activities quickly (e.g. running upstairs).

- Grade III – marked limitation of physical activity (e.g. angina when walking 100 metres, or up one flight of stairs).
- Grade IV – angina with any physical activity, or at rest.

Breathlessness (dyspnoea)

This is an unpleasant and uncomfortable awareness of breathing. It is classified using the New York Heart Association classification. The causes are listed in Table 2.2.

Table 2.2:   Causes of breathlessness

Cause	Clinical and investigative clues
Angina	See above
Heart failure	Myocardial infarct – ECG, echocardiogram
	Cardiomyopathy – echocardiogram
	Valve abnormality – examination, echocardiogram and Doppler
Arrhythmia	ECG, 24-hour ECG
Chronic obstructive airways disease	Bronchitis – productive cough, chest X-ray, peak flow rate
	Emphysema – lung function, chest X-ray
Asthma	Lung function
Pregnancy	Usually after the second trimester
Obesity	Snoring or phasic breathing (sleep apnoea) at night
Pneumothorax	Chest X-ray
Pulmonary emboli	Ventilation:perfusion lung scan, CT pulmonary angiogram
Pleural effusion	Examination, chest X-ray
Severe anaemia	Blood count
Unfit	History and examination, exercise test
Anxiety	History and examination, exercise test

It is important to know:

- how long the patient has been breathless
- what level of activities the patient was able to do and what they are now able to do
- whether it is primarily a heart or lung disorder
- orthopnoea suggests left heart failure
- past medical history – rheumatic heart disease, lung disease
- any associated symptoms:
  - chest pain/discomfort – angina
  - palpitation – arrhythmia, cardiomyopathy
  - cough/wheeze – asthma/chronic obstructive airways disease, angiotensin-converting-enzyme (ACE) inhibitor
  - ankle swelling – congestive heart failure or right heart failure due to chronic obstructive lung disease.

The New York Heart Association classification of dyspnoea

- Class I – no symptoms with ordinary physical activity.

- Class II – slight limitation of physical activity, but no symptoms at rest. Ordinary physical activity results in any or all of the following: fatigue, angina, palpitations, breathlessness.
- Class III – comfortable at rest, but slight physical activity results in symptoms.
- Class IV – discomfort with any physical activity.

Sudden severe breathlessness

Pulmonary oedema
Usually due to left heart failure resulting from myocardial infarction, pulmonary oedema causes breathlessness, cough or wheeze, usually while lying flat, and is relieved after a few minutes when the patient stands or sits up. It can be confused with asthma, and is sometimes confusingly termed 'cardiac asthma'.

Any cause of an elevated pulmonary venous pressure may result in pulmonary oedema (e.g. mitral stenosis and rarely a left atrial myxoma).

Occasionally, a prolonged tachycardia (e.g. atrial fibrillation or ventricular tachycardia) may result in pulmonary oedema in patients with impaired left ventricular function.

'Flash' pulmonary oedema is occasionally seen in patients with bilateral renal artery stenosis.

Palpitation

This is an unpleasant awareness of the heartbeat. The history is important, but the diagnosis is made by recording the electrocardiogram or an ambulatory ECG during symptoms.

Regular palpitation
Sinus tachycardia is very common, and occurs during exercise, during stress or when visiting the surgery.

Patients may describe a fast forceful pounding in the chest. It is important to capture this on the ECG and explain it to the patient so that reassurance can be given, rather than ordering further tests.

Supraventricular tachycardia
This is less common, and may be due to abnormal electrical pathways in:

- the atrioventricular node (atrioventricular node re-entry)
- atrioventricular bypass tracts (Wolff-Parkinson-White's syndrome).

With fast heart rates, patients may feel light-headed or faint, and those with underlying coronary heart disease may experience angina or breathlessness. Both conditions are generally benign and, importantly, can be cured by ablation, and they should be referred to an expert electrophysiologist.

Irregular palpitation
Atrial and ventricular ectopic beats are the commonest cause of irregular palpitation.

Patients often describe 'skipped' or 'missed' beats and worry that their heart might stop. These symptoms are due to the compensatory pause initiated by an ectopic beat occurring after a normal sinus beat. The sinus beat delayed by the compensatory pause may be felt as a forceful thud in the chest.

Patients like to see proof that their symptoms are understood and are being taken seriously. Showing them the ECG recording and explaining it is very effective, and they are usually fully reassured when told that ectopic beats are always benign if the heart muscle and blood supply are normal.

They do not need treatment unless they are very symptomatic despite reassurance and the knowledge that anti-arrhythmic drugs and β-blockers may make the symptoms worse.

Atrial fibrillation

The incidence of atrial fibrillation increases with age, and it is common in patients aged over 60 years. Patients may experience 'flutters' in the chest, although atrial fibrillation may be detected on a 24-hour ECG recording and the patient may be symptom-free.

Syncope

This word derives from the Greek word meaning to 'cut short'. This is a fairly common, sudden and brief loss of consciousness, with spontaneous recovery due to inadequate blood supply to the brain (often called 'a simple faint'). It is usually benign, except in the 10% of cases where it is due to a cardiac condition, which doubles the risk of sudden death.

> Cardiac causes should be investigated first, so patients should initially be referred to a cardiologist.

Cardiac causes of syncope

These are listed in Table 2.3. The presence of coronary artery disease, impaired ventricular function, congestive heart failure and congenital heart disease identifies patients who may have cardiac syncope. Ventricular tachycardia and bradycardia are the commonest causes of cardiac syncope, and usually occur in patients with structural heart disease. These patients have a 6-month mortality rate of more than 10%. Therefore patients with known or suspected cardiovascular or structural heart disease who present with syncope should initially be referred to a cardiologist.

A cardiac cause of syncope should be suspected in patients who have had a myocardial infarction or myocardial revascularisation, or who have left ventricular hypertrophy due to hypertension or aortic valve stenosis. Syncope may be due to pulmonary embolism.

The history should allow you to characterise the symptoms, and it provides the diagnosis in around 40% of cases. Associated palpitation prompts investigations for a cardiac arrhythmia with ambulatory ECG recording. Recording an ECG during an attack is the only certain way to identify or exclude an arrhythmia as the cause of syncope, but this is rarely possible. Most patients have insignificant arrhythmias on ambulatory ECG recordings, but this does not exclude arrhythmic syncope.

Table 2.3:   Causes of syncope

Cause	Diagnosis	Treatment
Arrhythmias		
Complete heart block and asystole	ECG/24-hour ECG	Pacemaker
Ventricular tachycardia and/or		
fibrillation (CHD/DCM/HCM)	ECG/24-hour ECG	Revascularisation
	EPS	Cardioverter
		defibrillator
Mechanical outflow obstruction		
of the left ventricle		
Severe aortic stenosis	Echocardiogram	Valve replacement
Severe obstructive cardiomyopathy	Echocardiogram	Medical with or
		without ICD
Non-cardiac causes		
Cough syncope	History	Avoidance
Postural hypotension	History	Avoidance
Malignant vasovagal syndrome	Tilt test	Pacemaker
Epilepsy	EEG, brain scan	Medical
Metabolic	Blood tests	Refer

ECG, electrocardiogram; 24-hour ECG, 24-hour electrocardiography; CHD, coronary heart disease; DCM, dilated cardiomyopathy; HCM, hypertrophic obstructive cardiomyopathy; ICD, implantable cardiac defibrillator; EPS, electrophysiological study; EEG, electroencephalogram.

Continuous loop event monitoring or an implantable recorder may be used in patients with occasional syncope.

Exertional syncope suggests aortic stenosis, hypertrophic cardiomyopathy or coronary artery disease.

A family history of sudden death suggests the long QT syndrome or the Brugada syndrome. Both of these rare conditions are diagnosed from the ECG. The Brugada syndrome is diagnosed by ST elevation in leads V_1 to V_3, is eight times more common in males, and most commonly presents in adults.

Examination may show hypertension, a heart murmur of aortic or mitral valve disease, or less commonly signs of heart failure. These should be investigated with echocardiography. Look for orthostatic hypotension by measuring the blood pressure 3 minutes after the patient has assumed a standing position following a supine period of 5 minutes.

The ECG may show signs of myocardial infarction, bundle branch block, bradycardia or complete heart block which necessitate urgent pacemaker implantation or a long QT interval. Rarely, arrhythmogenic right ventricular dysplasia may cause syncope, and it is often diagnosed by T-wave inversion in leads V_1, V_2 and V_3. Tall QRS complexes and T-wave inversion suggest hypertrophic cardiomyopathy. These patients should be referred.

Exercise testing is useful for evaluating suspected coronary artery disease and exercise-related syncope (chronotropic incompetence or exertional arrhythmia). Blood tests may show hypo- or hyperkalaemia or hyponatraemia, but are usually normal.

Treatment of cardiac syncope

Patients with suspected arrhythmia should be referred to a cardiologist for investigation, which may include invasive electrophysiological testing. Coronary angiography is indicated for patients with known or suspected ventricular tachycardia. Both myocardial revascularisation and an implantable cardioverter defibrillator may be necessary. Permanent pacing is indicated for patients with complete heart block and symptomatic bradycardia.

Neurally mediated syncope

Around 50% of cases of syncope are neurally mediated. This mechanism accounts for emotional fainting, fainting after prolonged standing, situational syncope (cough, micturition, defaecation syncope), vasovagal syncope, exercise-related syncope in fit individuals and carotid sinus syncope.

> Young patients without structural heart disease who have a history consistent with the presence of vasovagal, orthostatic or medication-induced syncope have a good prognosis.

Investigation of neurally mediated syncope

Tilt testing is used to provoke vasovagal syncope. It has a sensitivity of 66% and a specificity of 90%, and so is useful for excluding neurally mediated syncope. Both false positives and false negatives are common. Patients are tilted head up while their blood pressure and pulse rate are recorded. Patients with neurally mediated syncope have an impaired heart rate and blood pressure response, and may benefit from implantation of a pacemaker.

Treatment of neurally mediated syncope

There is little evidence from trials to guide treatment. No drug has been shown to result in long-term significant benefit.

Dual-chamber pacemaker implantation reduces symptoms by 85% in patients shown by tilt testing to have a significant drop in heart rate associated with symptoms. Patients should be advised to lie down when they feel an attack coming on.

Orthostatic hypotension

Orthostatic hypotension occurs when a person stands up quickly. It is common in patients who are taking hypotensive agents or β-blockers which blunt the compensatory tachycardia of a reduced blood pressure. Orthostatic hypotension may be due to volume depletion, medication (hypotensive drugs and β-blockers) or autonomic dysfunction (Parkinson's disease and diabetes). Treatment includes volume replacement and a detailed review of the patient's drugs.

Around 20% of cases of syncope are due to panic disorders, anxiety, depression or alcohol and substance abuse. The remainder include cardiac arrhythmias and other cardiac conditions, but it is important that these are excluded early in the investigation of syncope.

Differential diagnosis of syncope

Syncope must be distinguished from *vertigo*, which is associated with a sense of motion or rotation. Syncope may be precipitated by pain, exercise, micturition, defaecation or stress, and is associated with nausea and sweating.

Seizures due to epilepsy may be associated with disorientation, an aura, slowness in returning to consciousness after the attack, and tonic and clonic movements.
Unexplained syncope is a diagnosis of exclusion, and except in patients with undiagnosed cardiac syncope, it has a benign prognosis. Patients with unexplained syncope should be advised to stop driving and inform the Driver and Vehicle Licensing Agency (DVLA).

Transient ischaemic attacks

A transient ischaemic attack is defined as an episode of cerebral ischaemia lasting for less than 24 hours and manifested as any one of the following:

* brain dysfunction
* dysphasia or dysarthria
* weakness or sensory disturbance in the face and/or arm and/or leg
* visual disturbance in either one eye or a hemianopia.

Full investigation is required. Transient ischaemic attacks must be distinguished from migraine, other cerebral problems, local eye problems and vascular problems. Patients should be referred to a neurologist or physician with expertise in this field.

Leg pain and leg swelling

Table 2.4:   Causes of leg pain and/or swelling

Causes	Clinical features	Investigations
Claudication	Related to walking, relieved by rest Diminished or absent foot pulses Diabetes	Duplex ultrasound
Cellulitis	Signs of infection of the skin, fever	Exclude deep vein thrombosis, underlying venous problem
	Signs of vascular disease elsewhere	
Deep vein thrombosis	Swelling, tenderness Recent immobility/surgery Obesity, previous DVT, cancer	Duplex ultrasound D-dimer Venography
Nerve root pain	Shock-like pain that is relieved by sitting	MRI scan of spine
Rheumatological	Joint disorders – arthritis	Blood tests X-ray MRI scan Examination of fluid

Table 2.5: Causes of leg swelling

Causes	Clinical features	Investigations
Venous hypertension	Varicose veins	Exclude other causes of venous hypertension
	Phlebitis	
	History of childbirth	
	Prolonged standing	
Deep vein thrombosis	(see above)	(see above)
Heart failure	Right or congestive heart failure (?cause)	ECG
	Raised venous pressure	Chest X-ray
	Liver enlargement	Echocardiogram
	Mitral valve murmur	
	Added heart sounds	
	Arrhythmia	

Answers to case studies

1 Speak to your practice colleague, discuss the case and decide whether it is in the patient's best interests to see you. If you do see her, ask her what she wants, what she feels might be underlying the cause of her chest pain, and why she wanted to see you. Other issues in her life may be relevant to her symptoms. It is highly unlikely that she has coronary artery disease (*see* Chapters 9 and 14 on exercise testing and angina, respectively).

2 Ask the patient how often and under what circumstances he experiences angina, and whether he feels that his condition has deteriorated significantly recently. If not, advise him to continue on his current drug treatment, which should include aspirin and prophylactic GTN. His risk factors should be reviewed. If his symptoms are not adequately controlled, he will need prophylactic anti-anginal tablets. Specialist referral should be considered if his symptoms deteriorate and significantly affect his quality of life.

3 This patient may have unstable post-infarction angina, and should be referred back to hospital as soon as possible for treatment and investigation.

4 A full history and examination should be undertaken. Causes of fluttering include ectopic beats. The patient may need specialist referral and investigation, but can be reassured that it is unlikely she has a dangerous arrhythmia if she has not experienced any other symptoms.

5 We need to find out why this patient is breathless. Is it due to heart failure, recurrent angina or another cause? Ask about symptoms of orthopnoea, nocturnal dyspnoea, chest infection, leg swelling and chest pain. Look for relevant signs on examination. He will need referral and investigation. If you have access to a quick chest X-ray, this would be helpful for investigating possible heart failure, chest infection or pneumonia, which can be treated before waiting for a specialist consultation. An ECG might show a change which suggests ischaemia, infarction or an arrhythmia.

Further reading

The Canadian classification of angina and the New York Heart Association functional classification are both adapted from the following:

- Goldman L, Cook EF and Loscalzo A (1981) Comparative reproducibility and validity of systems for assessing cardiovascular functional class: advantages of a new specific activity scale. *Circulation.* **64**: 1227.
- Kapoor WN (2000) Syncope. *NEJM.* **343**: 1856–62.

CHAPTER 3

Clinical examination

Case studies

1 You hear a murmur in a 23-year-old pregnant woman. What characteristics of the murmur and other findings on examination are important for management?

2 You feel an irregular pulse and hear a heart murmur in a 71-year-old woman who had 'scarlet fever' as a child. What would you do?

3 A 76-year-old man with chronic airways disease and a recent chest infection comes to see you, and you hear lung crackles. What other physical signs would you specifically look for?

4 A fit 38-year-old marathon runner comes for a check-up. You hear a systolic murmur. What other aspects of the murmur would you record and how would you decide whether it is necessary to refer him?

5 A 68-year-old diabetic woman comes to see you with aching legs, tiredness, breathlessness and a history suggestive of a transient ischaemic attack. What physical signs would you look for and why?

Diagnostic benefits of physical examination

Modern cardiac investigations provide important diagnostic and prognostic information, but have not made physical examination redundant. Time limits on consultations may make it difficult to examine patients in primary care, but physical examination remains an essential and diagnostically useful part of the consultation. A gentle and focused systematic physical examination has an incalculable therapeutic effect on patients, who can be reassured that their symptoms have been taken seriously. A thorough examination need not take more than a few minutes, is inexpensive, and contributes to professional satisfaction and education.

The finding of hypertension, an irregular pulse, signs of heart failure, heart murmurs, a dilated pulsating abdominal aorta, absent leg pulses, or femoral artery or carotid artery bruits provides important diagnostic information. Investigations may be requested, treatment can be started and specialist referral considered, depending on the diagnosis, the patient's wishes and the response to treatment.

Requesting investigations

The request should provide relevant clinical details, and pose the clinical question which should be answerable with the test result. Investigations should only be requested if the result would influence management.

Professional benefits of physical examination

An informed and comprehensive clinical evaluation improves the quality of referral letters and the validity of requests for open-access investigations.

Patients without cardiac disease are grateful and reassured when told after the examination that they have nothing to worry about. If abnormalities are found, this can be explained to the patient and further tests and specialist referral arranged if necessary.

Examining patients

Ask the patient's permission to examine them. A chaperone may be required for some patients. Patients should be examined on an examination couch in a good light, and they should be comfortable, warm and relaxed.

Questions to be answered by cardiac examination

- Does the patient look well?
- Is the patient in sinus rhythm?
- Does the patient have a normal heart?
- Is the blood pressure normal?
- Are there any signs of heart failure and if so, what is the cause?
- Are there any signs of peripheral vascular disease or carotid artery disease?
- Does the abdominal aorta feel normal?
- What investigations are necessary?

Useful and reliable physical signs: high predictive accuracy

Several cardiac conditions can be diagnosed in primary care after a systematic physical examination and attention to discriminatory signs (*see* Table 3.1). The cause of each physical sign must be investigated and established.

Table 3.1:   Physical signs, their possible diagnoses and investigations

Sign	Possible diagnosis	Investigations
Xanthelasma	Hyperlipidaemia	Lipid profile
Irregular pulse	Ectopic beats	ECG
	Atrial fibrillation	24-hour ECG if arrhythmia is not captured on ECG
Slow pulse rate (< 40 beats/minute)	Complete heart block	ECG
Raised venous pressure	Right heart failure (?cause)	Echocardiogram Chest X-ray
Systolic waves in venous pulse	Tricuspid regurgitation	Echocardiogram
Visible carotid artery pulsation	Aortic regurgitation Kinked carotid artery	Echocardiogram Carotid ultrasound
Slow carotid upstroke	Aortic stenosis	Echocardiogram
Jerky carotid upstroke	HOCM	Echocardiogram
Dyskinetic apex beat	Left ventricular aneurysm	Echocardiogram
Left ventricular heave	Hypertension Aortic stenosis	Check blood pressure Echocardiogram
Pansystolic murmur (S1 and S2 inaudible)	Mitral regurgitation Ventricular septal defect	Echocardiogram
Mid-systolic click and late systolic murmur	Mitral valve prolapse	Echocardiogram
Ejection murmur	Normal Aortic stenosis Thickened aortic valve HOCM	Echocardiogram
Diastolic murmur	Aortic regurgitation	Echocardiogram
Carotid artery pulsation	Always abnormal	
Loud first heart sound and diastolic murmur	Mitral stenosis Always abnormal	Echocardiogram
Absent or reduced leg/ foot pulses	Peripheral vascular disease	Doppler examination Consider vascular disease elsewhere
Abdominal aortic pulsation	Aortic aneurysm	Ultrasound examination

HOCM = hypertrophic obstructive cardiomyopathy.

Physical signs that should be interpreted with caution

Some physical signs have a low predictive accuracy for diagnosis (*see* Table 3.2) because they are not specific or sensitive for cardiac disease. They may be caused by non-cardiac conditions.

Table 3.2:   Physical signs that should be interpreted with caution

Sign	Implication	Confounder	Test
Splinter haemorrhages	Infective endocarditis	Trauma	Clinical picture Blood tests
Lung crackles	Heart failure	Lung disease Normal	Chest X-ray Lung function
External jugular vein distension	Right heart failure	Kinked vein	Examination Ultrasound
Visible carotid artery pulsation	Aortic regurgitation	Anxiety Hyperthyroidism	History Thyroid function tests Ultrasound
High blood pressure	Hypertension	Anxiety/'white coat' syndrome	24-hour blood pressure
Systolic murmur	Valve disease	Normal	Echocardiogram

Inspection

Occasionally, the possibility of a cardiac abnormality is suggested by the patient's physical appearance (*see* Table 3.3).

Table 3.3:   Abnormal physical features and their possible related cardiac abnormality

Physical feature	Cardiac abnormality
Tall stature Marfan's syndrome	Aortic regurgitation, mitral valve prolapse and regurgitation, aortic dissection
Dwarf, Down's syndrome	Septal defects
Obesity	Hypertension, hyperlipidaemia, diabetes; sleep apnoea in severe obesity
Skin pigmentation Addison's disease	Low blood pressure and fainting
Kyphoscoliosis Depressed sternum	Spurious cardiac enlargement on chest X-ray
Breathless at rest	Heart failure
Chronic airways disease	Right heart failure
Foot and leg oedema	Heart failure
Varicose veins	Venous hypertension, foot oedema, implications for coronary artery bypass surgery and vein harvesting
Earlobe crease	Premature coronary artery disease in a young person
Arcus Xanthomata Xanthelasma	Hyperlipidaemia

Systematic examination of the cardiovascular system

1 The hands

Warm dry hands with a low venous tone (dilated veins) indicate a good peripheral circulation and cardiac output. Cold hands with a high venous tone are a sign of circulatory impairment and low cardiac output. Hand veins may be less prominent in young female patients. Normal people may have cold hands and peripheral cyanosis if they are cold.

2 The pulse

Radial pulse

Measure both rate and rhythm. An 'absent' radial pulse may be truly absent following occlusion of the brachial artery after using the radial or brachial artery for cardiac catheterisation, or it may be aberrant and difficult to feel. An irregular pulse may be due to ectopic beats or atrial fibrillation. A hard artery is a sign of atheroma and hypertension.

Carotid artery pulse

Look for the vigorous outward pulsation of aortic regurgitation. Feel the pulse for its rate of rise and amplitude. A slow rate of rise and amplitude suggests aortic stenosis, whereas a jerky upstroke suggests hypertrophic obstructive cardiomyopathy.

Listen for bruits, which suggest widespread atheroma and the possibility of other risk factors.

Femoral artery pulse

A bruit and decreased amplitude suggest local atheromatous disease. Feel the radial and femoral pulses together. A delay in the femoral pulse suggests coarctation of the aorta, which is a cause of hypertension.

Foot arteries

An absent pulse in the foot arteries indicates peripheral vascular disease. Consider all risk factors and renal artery stenosis.

3 The internal jugular venous pulse

It is worth looking for this, even though it can be difficult. Examine the patient in a good light. The external jugular venous pulse is easier to see, but may not provide accurate information about the right heart filling pressure and right atrial pressure due to kinking of the vessel in the neck fascia. Make sure that the patient is lying at approximately 45° with the neck relaxed and the head turned to one side. Venous pulsation causes an inward movement of the skin, whereas arterial pulsation causes an outward movement. The height of the pulse is measured from the sternal angle.

Normal venous pulse

There should be a softly expansile, compressible 'flicker' above the clavicle which can be compressed by one finger at the base of the neck.

Abnormal venous pulse

The height of the pulse is raised in right and congestive (i.e. right combined with left) heart failure. A raised fixed pulse is found in superior vena caval obstruction due to malignant disease. Large systolic waves are seen in tricuspid regurgitation.

4 Auscultation

Non-specialists may find auscultation difficult and intimidating, and this may relate to medical school experiences, the quality of teaching they have received and lack of practice. Auscultation is difficult, but if it is approached systematically it is possible to glean useful information. Record your findings and differential diagnosis in your referral letter. Your opinion may well be proved correct by investigations! From a personal development and educational point of view, this is important, enjoyable and takes very little extra time.

Echocardiography and Doppler examination have taught us that although auscultation is a useful diagnostic part of the examination, it is imperfect even with the best and most experienced ears.

Objectives of auscultation in primary care

The priority in primary care is to listen and record heart murmurs and added heart sounds, and to refer patients for a specialist opinion and further investigation. The commonly occurring conditions encountered in primary care are listed in Table 3.1.

Characterising a murmur

Evaluation of a cardiac murmur usually includes the location of maximum loudness, radiation, timing (systolic or diastolic), intensity, pitch and duration. Record and report any abnormalities and suggest a diagnosis, and also record normality. The information from a subsequent echocardiogram and Doppler examination will be educational. Try to grade and record the loudness or intensity of the murmur, as this will provide a useful clinical baseline.

Positioning the patient to maximise the murmur

Mitral murmurs are most easily heard with the patient first lying on the left side and then sitting forward to hear aortic murmurs. The pansystolic murmur of mitral regurgitation is heard most easily with the patient lying on the left side.

Tricuspid regurgitation can usually be diagnosed by seeing systolic (V) waves in the venous pulse. The murmur is quiet because the pressure gradients on the right side of the heart are lower than those on the left side.

The ejection systolic murmur of aortic stenosis can be heard all over the chest and radiates to the neck. Diastolic murmurs are quieter. Aortic regurgitation is heard most easily if the patient is sitting forward with their breath held in expiration.

Order of examination for auscultation

It is useful to use a system for auscultation. Listen to the heart sounds separately in order, then listen for added heart sounds, and then for systolic and diastolic murmurs. Concentrating on individual components of the cardiac cycle increases the yield of diagnostic information.

First heart sound: closure of the mitral and tricuspid valves
1   Loud:
   - mitral stenosis
   - tachycardia
   - short PR interval.
2   Quiet:
   - aortic stenosis
   - long PR interval (first-degree heart block).

Second heart sound: closure of the aortic and pulmonary valves
- Loud A2 – hypertension.
- Loud P2 – pulmonary hypertension.
- Quiet A2 – aortic stenosis.
- Quiet P2 – pulmonary stenosis.
- Fixed split of second heart sound – atrial septal defect.

5 Measurement and recording of the blood pressure

6 Diagnosis

Analyse your findings and make a diagnosis and management plan.

Answers to case studies

1   Ejection systolic murmurs are almost universal during pregnancy. It is important to distinguish this benign murmur from previously undiagnosed rheumatic heart disease (consisting of mitral valve stenosis, mitral regurgitation and less commonly aortic valve disease) or the mid-systolic click and late systolic murmur of mitral valve prolapse. Both a pregnancy-related tachycardia and mitral stenosis may cause a loud first heart sound, but an opening snap may be heard with a pliable stenosed mitral valve. A slow carotid upstroke distinguishes the ejection systolic murmur of important aortic valve stenosis from the increased blood flow and turbulence that are heard during pregnancy or tachycardia. Echocardiography is safe during pregnancy, and reassures the patient. She may need referral if there is structural heart disease.

2   One possibility is atrial fibrillation and mitral valve disease. Listen for the loud first heart sound, opening snap and diastolic murmur of mitral stenosis and the pansystolic murmur of mitral regurgitation. Probably more common is the combination of ectopic beats and an aortic ejection murmur. Arrange an

echocardiogram and perform an ECG. Refer the patient if there is significant aortic or mitral valve disease.

3   You would look for signs of heart failure – a raised jugular venous pressure, an enlarged liver and peripheral oedema. Signs of left heart failure include a tachycardia and a third and/or fourth heart sound (if the patient is in sinus rhythm). The lung crackles may be due to his airways disease and chest infection, and less likely may be due to lung fibrosis rather than pulmonary oedema. Arrange a chest X-ray. Request an echocardiogram if the patient is in heart failure.

4   The murmur may be benign, due to an athlete's hypertrophic heart, slow heart rate and increased stroke volume. It could also be due to undiagnosed structural heart disease, including mitral valve prolapse, aortic valve disease or hyper-trophic obstructive cardiomyopathy. Feel the carotid upstroke, which may be 'jerky' in HOCM. An ECG and echocardiogram will provide the diagnosis.

5   This patient may have heart failure and widespread vascular disease. Examine her carotid arteries for bruits, and her leg and feet arteries. Listen over her renal arteries for bruits. She may have a dilated abdominal aorta, too. Look for signs of heart failure and localised chest signs. She will need echocardiography, a chest X-ray and leg Doppler studies. She may also need brain scanning (CT or preferably MRI). Check her renal and thyroid function, glucose and lipid levels and blood count.

CHAPTER 4

Guidelines and risk estimation in clinical management

What is risk and risk assessment?

An understanding of 'risk' is essential to clinical management. The term 'risk' is used in several contexts. These include the 'risk' of developing coronary heart disease, the 'risk' of developing a complication from the disease (e.g. myocardial infarction) and the risk associated with an investigation (e.g. coronary angiography) or with treatment (medical or surgical).

Risk assessment and treatment decisions

Risk assessment in cardiovascular disease is the identification of patients with a high or low probability of developing or having coronary heart disease. Treatment decisions involve a risk assessment of patients, weighing up the benefits and risks of treatment against the risks of non-treatment. Knowledge of the natural history of the condition is essential. These decisions are complex and include logistic and financial considerations. For example, not all patients with atrial fibrillation should receive anticoagulation, because the risks of bleeding might outweigh the reduction in thromboembolism. A raised cholesterol level does not necessarily mean that a patient should be given a statin, because the decision to treat depends on the patient's absolute coronary risk as well as the overall benefit to him or her.

Treatment decisions are more complex when the evidence base from trials does not translate directly to the patient sitting in front of you. Treatment decisions need to be based on trial evidence and treatment guidelines, but interpreted in the context of an individual patient's clinical situation. Management guidelines now exist for a number of procedures and treatments, and clinicians are expected to be familiar with them and to use them. This chapter discusses the use of guidelines and the principles and methods of risk estimation in clinical decision making.

To treat or not to treat?

One of the greatest challenges in clinical medicine is deciding whether or not to initiate 'lifelong' primary prevention treatment for an asymptomatic patient. Patients who have borderline hypertension but whose absolute coronary risk is defined as low may not need medication. However, new evidence may emerge that prompts the production of new guidelines which suggest lowering the treatment threshold. Alternatively, the patient's risk profile may change, which might increase their risk, thus necessitating treatment.

Risk assessment highlights a difficult aspect of clinical decision making. One example is coronary artery surgery for patients with angina. This procedure has greatest prognostic effect in patients at high risk of complications, and is of relatively little prognostic benefit in those at low risk who have a good prognosis.

The prognosis of most cardiovascular conditions depends on a number of factors, some of which can be measured by performing investigations (e.g. the extent of coronary artery disease can be determined by using angiography). Other factors of prognostic importance include the following:

- age
- coexisting medical and cardiovascular conditions. These include the presence or absence of cardiovascular risk factors, coronary anatomy and left ventricular function and renal function. In certain cases (e.g. elderly or frail patients with a poor prognosis due to malignancy), one should carefully consider which investigations are appropriate before embarking on possibly futile treatment which may have adverse effects
- potential drug interactions.

Legal implications of guidelines on clinical management

A guideline may be defined as information designed to aid a practitioner and patient in pursuing the most appropriate healthcare response to specific clinical circumstances. Guidelines are usually based on scientific evidence.

Clinicians may be concerned about the legal implications of deviating from guidelines, and about whether adherence to guidelines protects them from liability.

In UK law:

the mere fact that a protocol or guideline exists for the care of a particular condition does not of itself establish that compliance with it would be reasonable in the circumstances, or that non-compliance would be negligent. As guideline-informed health care increasingly becomes customary, so acting outside the guidance of guidelines could expose doctors to the possibility of being found negligent, unless they can prove a special justification in the circumstances.

Guidelines are guidelines, not law. They have to be applied according to the patient's specific clinical circumstances, taking into account the clinician's considered view, the opinion of his or her colleagues when applicable, the patient's wishes, and logistic, practical and economic factors.

Clinical management guidelines are relatively new, and are being formulated for an increasing number of procedures and conditions. They are consensus statements based on available data from clinical trials with specified, acceptable protocol characteristics, including double-blind treatments, adequate follow-up, randomisation to either active or placebo treatments, appropriate and balanced patient demography, 'hard' end-points relevant to the question asked of the trial, and adequate statistical power. It is important to remember that the interpretation of trial results is based on opinion, and that guidelines are not infallible.

Treatment guidelines for coronary heart disease are based on estimated *absolute coronary heart disease risk*. They are designed to help clinicians, patients and others involved in funding healthcare to make informed and appropriate clinical decisions and to reduce healthcare costs. They have both benefits and drawbacks (*see* Boxes 4.1 and 4.2). Abba Eban, the former Israeli Ambassador to the United Nations, said 'consensus means that lots of people say collectively what no one believes individually'. Nevertheless, guidelines are here to stay and, if used wisely, can enhance, simplify and standardise clinical management. However, they do not remove the need for sound, experienced clinical judgement, and they should not displace a critical and questioning attitude.

Ultimately, the clinician responsible for the care of the patient has to decide whether the guidelines proposed are relevant and should be applied to the patient sitting in the consulting room.

Box 4.1:   Potential benefits of guidelines

- They ensure a minimum quality of care.
- They standardise the management of high-volume, procedure-related activities and common clinical conditions.
- They reduce the use of inappropriate or unproven investigations or treatment.
- They provide comparative procedural outcome data for audit.
- They push up the clinical quality of 'average' institutions to the 'best'.
- They restrict the use of costly procedures or treatments to situations where there is sufficient evidence that they are 'effective'.

Box 4.2:   Potential drawbacks of guidelines

- Interpretation of trial results is based on opinion.
- The guideline writers may not be active clinicians in the relevant field.
- Randomised trials usually include only low-risk individuals, and the results may not be relevant to the patient in the real world, in whom other clinical considerations and their personal wishes demand individualised management.
- They ensure only a minimum quality of care.
- Decisions based on cost and consensus may deprive patients of new treatments.
- There is loss of professional autonomy.
- They stifle creativity and innovation ('cookbook medicine').
- They lead to mediocre rather than high-quality medicine.
- Guidelines may not be applicable to individual patients.
- They may be out of date or redundant.
- There are concerns about litigation.
- The condition or disease may change.

Value, use and limitations of guidelines

Examples of guidelines leading to organisational changes and improved clinical outcomes include a reduction in door-to-needle times and the secondary prevention treatments after myocardial infarction.

Guideline utilisation is increased if the guidelines make clinical sense, are clear, concise and up to date, and apply to the overwhelming majority of patients with the specified condition. One current major problem is the large number of guidelines from a variety of sources (local and national) for the same condition. Clinicians find this both confusing and overwhelming, and this may make them disinclined to use any of them!

Cardiovascular risk management

Cardiovascular risk factor management is one illustration of the recent rapid evolution and reorganisation of healthcare service delivery. There are many political, management, financial, medical and demographic reasons for these changes, which have led to different healthcare professionals providing a variety of different clinical services.

Coronary heart disease: global and national mortality and economic considerations

It is estimated that there will be a doubling in world deaths from coronary heart disease, from 13.1 million in 1990 to 24.8 million in 2020. Because of the importance of coronary heart disease as a global cause of death and morbidity, and the social and economic consequences, risk assessment and management are fundamental to cardiovascular care. Each year coronary heart disease costs the NHS £1.6 billion and the UK economy £10 billion.

Death rates from coronary heart disease in the UK are among the highest in the world. It is the commonest cause of premature death, accounting for one in four male deaths and one in six female deaths, and it caused 125 000 deaths in 2000. The UK has high levels of standard risk factors and, compared with the USA and most European countries, a low level of intervention.

Risk factors for coronary heart disease

Appropriate and effective cardiovascular risk factor management is based on a knowledge of the relative importance of these factors (*see* Table 4.1 and Box 4.3) and the overall or global coronary or preferably (and more comprehensive) *cardiovascular* (including cerebrovascular) risk confronting the individual.

The modifiable and non-modifiable risk factors for coronary heart disease are listed in Table 4.1.

Table 4.1:   Risk factors for coronary heart disease

Modifiable factors	Non-modifiable factors
High LDL cholesterol	Age
High blood pressure	Gender
Smoking	Family history
Low HDL cholesterol	Genetic factors
Diabetes and glucose intolerance	Birth-weight
Lack of exercise	
Left ventricular hypertrophy	
Central obesity	
Homocysteine level	
Clotting factors	
Oral contraceptives	

LDL, low-density lipoprotein; HDL, high-density lipoprotein.

Box 4.3:   Protective factors for coronary heart disease

- Moderate alcohol consumption
- Exercise
- Dietary monounsaturated fat (olive oil, rape seed oil)
- Fruit and vegetables
- High HDL cholesterol
- Fish
- Aspirin

Risk stratification

Appropriate, safe and cost-effective prevention strategies are based on risk stratification. This means identifying patients at different levels of risk and targeting treatments towards those at high risk who have most to gain, while not treating those at low risk who have little if anything to gain and for whom the risks of treatment outweigh the potential benefits.

Cardiovascular risk is influenced to varying degrees by risk factors. It should be remembered and explained to patients that these are risk factors and not causes. Atheromatous vascular disease is only partly explained by the currently established risk factors. The comparative importance of emerging risk factors is at present unclear.

The predictive accuracy of *single* risk factors (e.g. cholesterol or blood pressure) is poor, but it is improved by counting the number of risk factors. Risk estimation using risk equations derived from large prospective epidemiological studies such as the

Framingham study further improves predictive accuracy, and includes risk factors of known prognostic value.

Absolute risk

The *absolute risk* of a patient developing cardiovascular complications from hypertension, for example, and the decision to treat the patient depend not on the level of the blood pressure alone, but on an estimation of the overall or *absolute risk*. Absolute risk also determines the probability of benefit from antihypertensive treatment. Treatment guidelines for hypertension and hyperlipidaemia are based on absolute risk estimation, which is obtained by weighting appropriately all of the major risk factors. Currently available risk-factor tools estimate a patient's *coronary heart disease risk* using the patient's age, gender, smoking status, the presence of diabetes, and whether the patient has known vascular disease and target organ damage. *Cardiovascular disease risk*, which includes the risk of stroke, is calculated by multiplying the coronary heart disease risk by 4/3. Thus a patient with a coronary heart disease risk of 30% has a cardiovascular disease risk of 40%. This conversion is less accurate at the extremes of age.

Absolute risk reduction

Using the example of a randomised, placebo-controlled trial, the *absolute risk reduction* is the difference in the probabilities of an event in the control and treatment groups. If the adverse event rate in the treatment group is less than that in the control group, this indicates a potential benefit from the treatment.

Relative risk

The relative benefit of an active treatment over a control is usually expressed as the *relative risk*, the relative risk reduction or the odds ratio. It is used to characterise the relative effect of a treatment compared with a placebo, in a group of patients and does not involve comparison of individual patients. In a controlled randomised trial, for example, the relative risk of the treatment is the probability of an event in the active treatment group divided by the probability of an event in the control group. Beneficial treatments would have a relative risk of < 1.

The *relative risk reduction* is derived by subtracting the relative risk from 1. Therefore a relative risk of 0 indicates that the treatment results in neither benefit nor harm. Relative risk reduction can also be expressed as the absolute risk reduction divided by the probability of an event in the control arm.

Relative risk reduction does not translate to individual benefit

Hypertension treatment decreases the risk of all cardiovascular complications by around 25%, mainly by reducing stroke by 38% and coronary events by 16%. The *relative risk reduction* associated with antihypertensive treatment is 25% in all groups of patients (male and female patients of all ages, and smokers and non-smokers). However, the likelihood that an individual patient will benefit from antihypertensive treatment depends on their absolute risk of a cardiovascular complication. The estimated relative risk reduction of 25% may apply to those patients at moderate to high risk of a cardiovascular complication but not to patients at low risk, and so the potential toxicity and cost of the treatment may outweigh its small potential benefits.

Absolute risk reduction and the 'number needed to treat'

This is the number of patients a clinician needs to treat with a particular drug in order to expect to prevent one adverse event. It can be expressed as the *reciprocal of the absolute risk reduction*. In clinical decision making, it is useful and meaningful to use the term 'number needed to treat' because this enables clinicians and patients to think of treatment benefits in terms of patients rather than abstract probabilities. It is calculated as the inverse of the absolute risk reduction.

For example, a group of patients with untreated *moderate* hypertension has a 20% *absolute risk* of stroke, but this is reduced to 12% with antihypertensive treatment which confers a *relative risk reduction* of 40%. The *absolute risk reduction* is $0.20 - 0.12 = 0.08$. The reciprocal of this number is 13, which indicates that the clinician would *need to treat around 13 moderately hypertensive patients* for 5 years before one stroke would be prevented by the treatment.

In contrast, consider a group of patients with untreated *mild* hypertension with a 1.5% *absolute risk* of stroke, which is reduced to 0.9% with antihypertensive treatment which confers a *relative risk reduction* of 40%. The absolute risk reduction is $0.015 - 0.009 = 0.006$. The reciprocal of this number is 167. Therefore the clinician would *need to treat 167 patients with mild hypertension* for 5 years before they could expect to prevent one stroke. These examples are useful for clinicians, and can be used to explain management decisions to patients who may be confused about the advice they are given which depends on their absolute risk and the estimated absolute risk reduction.

Table 4.2 provides another example, using 10-year absolute coronary heart disease risk derived from the Joint British Societies risk prediction chart. It can be seen that the absolute benefit of treating these two patients largely depends on their baseline absolute risk. The number of patients needed to be treated for 5 years to prevent one stroke is

Table 4.2:   Number of patients needed to be treated for 5 years to prevent one stroke

	Patient A	Patient B
Blood pressure (mmHg)	165/100	165/100
Gender	Male	Female
Age (years)	60	44
Diabetes	Yes	No
Total: HDL-cholesterol ratio	8	4
Smoker	Yes	No
Left ventricular hypertrophy	Yes	No
Family history of infarction	Yes	Yes
Absolute 10-year CHD risk	60%	< 2%
Relative risk reduction	40%	40%
Absolute benefit	24%	0.8%
Number needed to treat (for 5 years)	4	125

HDL, high-density lipoprotein; CHD, coronary heart disease.

correspondingly very different, namely 4 patients with the absolute risk of patient A and 125 patients with the absolute risk of patient B. Therefore, before recommending long-term and costly treatment which may have adverse effects, the decision to treat a hypertensive patient should be based on their absolute risk and not simply on their blood pressure reading.

Risk prevention tables and charts

There are several tools for estimating coronary heart disease risk, and most of them are based on the Framingham data, from the only published epidemiological study in which both men and women were included.

Framingham risk equations

These were developed to predict the 10-year risk of coronary heart disease, heart failure or stroke and the average risk in age- and sex-matched controls. The subjects from Boston, Massachusetts, were mainly white middle-class people. This is important, because certain high-risk groups (e.g. South Indian Asians) were not included. A reasonable but (by current standards) incomplete range of risk factors was measured. For example, family history, inactivity and obesity were not included, and the protective influence of high HDL levels and the high risk of high LDL levels were not appreciated at the time. However, it is difficult to include all emerging or potential risk factors in a risk assessment table until they have been validated, so this criticism could be applied in retrospect to any risk estimation tool.

Dundee coronary risk disk

This provides an estimate of a person's relative risk of coronary mortality matched for age and sex. It was derived in men only, and has not been independently validated in women and may not be applicable to other populations. It does not correlate very well with Framingham estimates.

British Regional Heart Study risk function

This has not been independently validated. It cannot be used to predict risk in women, and it may underestimate risk.

The predictive accuracy of any risk factor assessment system depends on the inclusion of all relevant prognostic information. This should include data from a large study population, including people of different ethnicity, so that the information is representative of the population to whom the results will be applied. These tools also require updating to include newly established risk factors, and should take account of protective risk factors.

Comparison of different risk charts and tables

There are several such charts and tables, and that proposed by the Joint British Societies (British Cardiac Society, British Diabetic Society and British Hyperlipidaemia Society) is probably the most accurate. The Sheffield table, the New Zealand charts and the European charts are less accurate in coronary risk prevention. There is a computer program available from the British Heart Foundation.

The Joint British Societies risk chart incorporates gender, age, smoking status, systolic blood pressure and total:HDL cholesterol ratio. The chart is relatively easy to use and accurate. Its limitations include the omission of other important risk factors (*see* Table 4.1 and Box 4.3). The classification of 'Yes/No' for smoking does not differentiate between a person who stopped smoking 60 cigarettes a day the week before and a person who has never smoked. Diabetic patients are assessed using a separate chart, which is illogical as they are at high risk and should be treated. Young people may be under-treated because they do reach the risk treatment threshold of 30%. For example, the current guidelines would not recommend treating a 30-year-old diabetic hypertensive female smoker with a high cholesterol level. However, treatment for old men would be recommended in view of their age and gender.

The Joint British Societies risk computerised assessment differs from the chart in that it incorporates diastolic blood pressure, serum cholesterol, HDL cholesterol, diabetes ('Yes/No') and left ventricular hypertrophy on electrocardiogram ('Yes/No'), as well as age, gender and systolic blood pressure. It has similar limitations to the chart because variables such as smoking and blood sugar level, which confer an incremental risk, are scored categorically as either 'Yes' or 'No'.

Using risk prevention tables and charts in primary care is not easy at present, but may become so with user-friendly desktop computer programs and the availability of straight-forward, up-to-date, comprehensive systems that integrate with patients' clinical data. Importantly, the risk assessment program should be based on clinical data and therefore applicable to the patients treated in the practice where the program is to be used. Other information showing the differential weighting of risk factors and the potential incremental and total benefits of modifying each of them would be helpful. This type of program could provide risk assessment relevant to the patient in front of you, audit facilities and graphic illustrations. It would also provide an interactive capability to allow patients to understand, participate and take the principal role in their own self-administered and motivated cardiovascular risk management.

> Calculating cardiovascular risk in order to help to decide treatment strategies in individual patients is only of value if the patient takes the treatment and makes other synergistic long-term lifestyle changes.

General practitioners and practice nurses are able to evaluate the risk of coronary heart disease with only moderate accuracy because not all of the required risk factors (e.g. HDL-cholesterol levels) may be available in the patients' records.

Different experts, different views

The majority of patients will not need specialist referral, and will be managed in primary care using risk tables and charts to guide treatment strategies for individual patients. Some patients may have been admitted to hospital after having an unheralded myocardial infarction, stroke or other cardiovascular problem, and only then have been found to have hypertension, hyperlipidaemia or diabetes. Treatment may have been started in hospital, or recommendations made to monitor the patient, with the GP deciding whether treatment is necessary.

> The patient may have seen different specialists with different opinions, and the primary care team will have to consider all of the advice, which may differ or even conflict. The primary care team will have to plan a strategy which is safe, sensible, effective and practical, and explain this to the patient and their family. The tactics will need constant review and updating because of the rapid changes in treatment protocols resulting from the plethora of sometimes confusing and conflicting research results.

Difficulties associated with prevention strategies

Initiating and ensuring long-term patient compliance with cardiovascular prevention is practically difficult. Effective management of this important but time-consuming work depends on good practice organisation and the knowledge, enthusiasm, skill and commitment of staff who are aware of the difficulties of persuading patients to change their day-to-day lives by stopping lifelong pleasurable habits and taking tablets on a long-term basis. Patients make these sacrifices in return for the possibility of living longer with a lower risk of developing a stroke, heart attack, heart failure or renal failure.

With an ageing and diverse population, this task is not getting any easier because the potential benefits are not immediately apparent to either the patient or the clinician. It is not surprising that even with the best of intentions and skilled, dedicated staff, patients find it very difficult to maintain long-term lifestyle changes. This difficulty is compounded by various factors, including patient compliance, current thresholds for starting certain drugs, local prescribing practices and availability of rehabilitation and smoking cessation programmes. In addition, there are significant regional variations in the prevalence and prognosis of patients with atheromatous disease due to age, ethnicity and lifestyle.

The role of the primary care team

Risk factor reduction clinics are now usually run by nurses in primary care. Patients should be educated about absolute cardiovascular risk and take responsibility for improving their risk profile with ongoing encouragement and monitoring by primary care services. All risk factors should be discussed. Patients should understand their own crucial role in their long-term health, and what changes they may need to make to their lifestyle.

The primary care team is uniquely placed to assess cardiovascular risk and to initiate, monitor and review interventions to improve a patient's long-term risk profile with a view to lowering their risk of cardiovascular events. In patients with established atheromatous vascular disease and those referred for specialist care, this may be in conjunction with a variety of hospital staff, including cardiologists, diabetologists, hypertension specialists, cardiac nurse specialists, pharmacists and rehabilitation team members. However, the long-term responsibility and burden of management will fall on those working in primary care.

The role of nurses

Nurses are playing an increasingly important and therapeutic role in risk factor management, and are key members of the primary care team. They are also closely involved in hospital-based risk management, and initiate secondary risk factor management for patients admitted with acute coronary syndromes and other patients with cardiovascular disease. Nurses also provide continuing care in the community.

Nurse-managed programmes have been shown to be effective in the management of single risk factors, including smoking cessation, lipid lowering, diabetes and hypertension. They now run comprehensive clinics for risk factor modification and rehabilitation.

Management protocols and teaching and training courses on these subjects have provided nurses with the skills and experience necessary to identify patients who may benefit from drug interventions and need specialist referral. These include patients who are resistant to treatment, those at high risk and those who want a specialist opinion.

Variations in the incidence and outcomes of coronary heart disease

Guidelines and management protocols have increased the homogeneity of clinical management. Areas of doubt exist, and it is important for clinicians to keep an open mind, questioning and evaluating new research data and deciding which new proposed interventions would improve patient care and outcome. Audit can be used to facilitate this approach.

There is well-recognised variation in cardiovascular disease outcomes in the UK, with comparatively high mortality rates in Scotland and some parts of the north of England. The causes of this variation are unclear, but it may be due to cultural, socioeconomic, age and lifestyle differences.

Diet has an important influence on cholesterol levels, particularly LDL-cholesterol, and on coronary heart disease mortality. The low LDL-cholesterol levels in Japanese and Chinese people from rural areas probably explain their low myocardial infarction rates despite their high rates of smoking. People with a low LDL-cholesterol level have a very low risk of infarction, and this can be used to help exclude infarction in patients who are admitted to hospital with chest pain.

Variations in secondary care management of coronary heart disease

Local variation in coronary heart disease morbidity and mortality is more difficult to measure, but clinicians may be aware of organisational arrangements whereby patients with acute presentations of coronary heart disease may be seen by non-cardiologists and would be less likely to undergo invasive investigation and intervention. Management protocols can only be effective if they are applied, and this depends on the clinical team making the correct diagnosis. Local variations in practice between cardiologists may also affect outcomes. Cardiologists trained in interventional techniques are more likely than non-interventionists to recommend an invasive and interventional strategy to patients with coronary artery syndromes. Patients admitted to a hospital with comprehensive cardiology and cardiac surgical facilities are more likely to undergo coronary angiography and myocardial revascularisation than patients who are admitted to a hospital without these facilities.

Specialists may have a different view of the importance of risk factors, and may advocate investigations or treatments that are not recommended in the local guidelines. For example, some cardiologists test for and treat high homocysteine levels with folic acid. Cardiologists vary in their attitude and approach to weight loss, diet and exercise. Some of them, for a number of reasons, leave risk management to their colleagues in primary care.

Advice for patients

- Your risk of developing heart disease depends on a number of risk factors. These are not the same as causes, but increase the chances of you developing furring up of the heart and other arteries.
- People who have risk factors may or may not need tablets. The decision is made by estimating your risk based on your age and other factors – for example, your blood pressure and cholesterol level. This means that even though you may have a friend who is not taking tablets, you need them because you are at greater risk of developing heart disease because you have risk factors that they do not have.

Further reading

Legal implications of guidelines

- Anderson KM, Odell PM, Wilson PWF *et al.* (1990) Cardiovascular disease risk profiles. *Am Heart J.* **121**: 293–8.
- Armstrong PW (2003) Do guidelines influence practice? *Heart.* **89**: 349–52.
- British Cardiac Society, British Hyperlipidaemia Association, British Hypertension Society and British Diabetic Association (2000) Joint British recommendations on prevention of coronary heart disease in clinical practice: summary. *BMJ.* **320**: 705–8.
- Cook RJ and Sackett DL (1995) The number needed to treat: a clinically useful measure of treatment effect. *BMJ.* **310**: 452–4.

- Department of Health (2000) *National Service Framework for Coronary Heart Disease*. Department of Health, London.
- Durrington PN, Prais H, Bhatnagar D *et al.* (1999) Indications for cholesterol-lowering medication: comparison of risk-assessment methods. *Lancet*. **353**: 278–81.
- Grimshaw JM and Russell IT (1993) Effect of clinical guidelines on medical practice: a systematic review of rigorous evaluations. *Lancet*. **342**: 1317–22.
- Hampton JR (2003) Guidelines – for the obedience of fools and the guidance of wise men? *Clin Med*. **3**: 279–84.
- Jones AF, Walker J, Jewkes C *et al.* (2001) Comparative accuracy of cardiovascular risk prediction methods in primary care patients. *Heart*. **85**: 37–43.
- McManus RJ, Mant J, Meulendijks CF *et al.* (2002) Comparison of estimates and calculations of risk of coronary heart disease by doctors and nurses using different calculation tools in general practice: cross-sectional study. *BMJ*. **324**: 459–64.
- Nash IS (2001) Practice guidelines in cardiovascular care. In: V Fuster, RW Alexander and RA O'Rourke (eds) *Hurst's 'The Heart'* (10e). McGraw Hill, New York.
- National Cholesterol Education Program (2001) Executive summary of the third report of the National Cholesterol Education Program (NCEP) expert panel on detection, evaluation and treatment of high blood cholesterol in adults (adult treatment panel III). *JAMA*. **285**: 2486–97.
- Poulter N (2003) Global risk of cardiovascular disease. *Heart*. **89** (**Suppl. 2**): ii2–5.
- Schwartz PJ, Breithard G, Howard AJ *et al.* (1999) The legal implications of medical guidelines – a Task Force of the European Society of Cardiology. *Eur Heart J*. **20**: 1152–7.
- Shaper AG, Pocock SJ, Phillips AN *et al.* (1986) Identifying men at high risk of heart attacks: strategy for use in general practice. *BMJ*. **293**: 474–9.
- Tunstall-Pedoe H (1991) The Dundee coronary risk-disk for management of change in risk factors. *BMJ*. **303**: 744–7.
- Wilson PW, D'Agostino R, Levy D *et al.* (1998) Prediction of coronary heart disease using risk factor categories. *Circulation*. **97**: 1837–47.
- Wolf PA, D'Agostino RB, Belanger AJ *et al.* (1991) Probability of stroke: a risk profile from the Framingham study. *Stroke*. **22**: 312–18.
- Wolf PA, D'Agostino RB, Silbershatz H *et al.* (1999) Profile for estimating risk of heart failure. *Arch Intern Med*. **159**: 1197–204.
- Wood D, De Backer G, Faergeman O *et al.* with members of the Task Force (1998) Prevention of coronary heart disease in clinical practice: recommendations of the second joint task force of European and other societies on coronary prevention. *Atherosclerosis*. **140**: 199–270.
- Wood D, Durrington PN, Poulter N *et al.* (1998) Joint British recommendations on prevention of coronary heart disease in clinical practice. *Heart*. **80** (**Suppl. 2**): S1–29.

CHAPTER 5

Lipid disorders and emerging risk factors for cardiovascular disease

Case studies

1 A 63-year-old man attends your surgery 2 weeks after leaving hospital following a heart attack. He is slim, a non-smoker, normotensive, and in addition to aspirin and atenolol has been prescribed a statin which he would like to stop because he has a 'good diet'. What advice would you give him?

2 A 28-year-old woman comes to see you, distressed after the sudden death of her 73-year-old father a few days previously, having had a 'high cholesterol'. She wants to know what she should do to avoid the same fate as her father.

3 An 83-year-old hypertensive woman with type 2 diabetes and frequent episodes of angina is brought to your surgery by her daughter, who lives with her. What would you do?

4 A 59-year-old man who has been on a statin for 6 months comes to see you 1 month after coronary angioplasty, complaining of aches in his thighs. What would you do?

5 A 60-year-old retired GP with well-controlled hypertension and diabetes, who is an occasional cigar smoker, asks for advice because his LDL is 4.0 mmol/l, his total cholesterol is 5.5 mmol/l and his triglycerides are 3.2 mmol/l. He was told by one of his ex-patients at the golf club that he should be on a statin and a fibrate. Do you agree with this?

Factors which determine successful management of lipid disorders

It is important to have a basic understanding of the physiology of lipids in order to appreciate their role as a risk factor in coronary artery disease. Management of hyperlipidaemia requires an understanding of the following:

- lipid physiology
- the patient's absolute coronary risk
- the importance of lipid lowering in primary and secondary prevention
- the patient's lifestyle and other coexisting clinical conditions

- the impact and limitations of lifestyle changes and drugs on lipid levels and other risk factors in long-term risk reduction
- lipid-lowering drugs
- the practical difficulties of patient compliance with advice and prescribed treatments.

The need for good advice given well

Perhaps most importantly, successful management ultimately depends on how the advice is given and the patient's ability to understand it and make the necessary long-term changes. This highlights the importance of the relationship that the patient has with the primary care team, and the complex art of giving a patient personal lifestyle advice which has often not been requested.

The treatment of hyperlipidaemia and hypertension requires similar professional skills for both conditions, and a comprehensive appreciation of cardiovascular risk in different patient groups. Lifestyle changes in these conditions are effective to some degree, and should be started before and continuously underpin drug interventions.

Patient variation in compliance with treatment

Patients vary in their willingness to take medication and follow medical advice. Some are very keen to take medication (e.g. non-prescribed aspirin to reduce their cardiovascular risk), even though they may be at low risk. Some older patients may consider suggested lifestyle changes or medication to be irrelevant or unacceptable. Young patients may take a similar view and feel immune from the distant possibility of a stroke or myocardial infarct. This understandable attitude may also explain the failure of smoking cessation and weight loss programmes for young people. Survivors of infarction are usually more compliant, at least initially after the event.

Effective primary and secondary prevention requires the patient to take responsibility for their health, but even with enthusiastic education and encouragement, it is unrealistic to expect all patients to maintain compliance in the long term. Reassurance and explanation should be given to patients who are anxious about the safety of long-term medication.

Improving compliance

A high proportion of patients take more than one tablet because they may, in addition to hyperlipidaemia, have hypertension, diabetes and coronary artery disease. Combination tablets and simplified once-daily doses timed to coincide with regular events in their daily schedule improve compliance. Patients, particularly the elderly, may also benefit from a visit by a community pharmacist.

It is important to review regularly all of the prescribed medication and their doses and to ask patients, or those who look after them, whether they take their tablets and if they think these have any resulting side-effects. Unless they are asked, patients may not wish to upset the doctor by 'confessing' that they do not take their tablets.

What do patients want to know about cholesterol?

They want to know if they have a high cholesterol level, if they need to worry about it, what food they should avoid, what food or supplements might help, and whether they need tablets.

Patients who are slim, exercise frequently and have a low-fat diet may not understand why they have a high cholesterol level. They may know someone who had a heart attack or heart operation who had a 'normal' cholesterol level and may want an explanation as to how this could happen and whether it could happen to them. They may want to know what high- and low-density cholesterol and triglycerides are, and what they can do to improve them. What are the 'good' foods to eat and which ones should they avoid? Is alcohol good or bad? Is red wine really 'good for the heart' and how much should they drink? What foods and drinks lower cholesterol levels? They increasingly ask and expect those who check their blood cholesterol level and manage it in primary care to answer these and other questions.

Explaining risk and who needs tablets

Most patients know that a high cholesterol level is undesirable and may lead to blocked arteries and heart attacks. The higher the cholesterol level, the greater the risk of cardiac events. Those who are tested and shown to have a 'normal' cholesterol level will be pleased and relieved to learn that they have 'passed' the test and can therefore carry on with their usual lifestyle. Those with hyperlipidaemia may be at low risk of cardio-vascular events, and may not need medication. In contrast, some patients with a 'normal' cholesterol level may be at high absolute risk of coronary heart disease. This may be confusing, and such patients will need a clear explanation about this and why the cholesterol level is not the sole determinant of medical treatment.

What are lipoproteins?

Lipoproteins are large molecules that transport cholesterol and triglycerides in the blood. They have a lipid core consisting of triglycerides and cholesterol esters, which is surrounded by phospholipids and apolipoproteins. They are classified according to their density, and there are five components:

- chylomicrons – these are the largest, and they contain the highest concentration of lipid
- very-low-density lipoproteins (VLDL) – made in the liver
- intermediate-density lipoproteins (IDL)
- low-density lipoproteins (LDL) – made in the plasma
- high-density lipoproteins (HDL) – these are the smallest, and they contain the lowest concentration of lipid.

About 70% of the plasma total cholesterol is carried in the LDL fraction, and 25% in the HDL fraction. Atherogenesis is mainly produced by LDL-cholesterol, whereas HDL-cholesterol is protective against atherosclerosis.

Cholesterol metabolism

The average person consumes 300 mg of cholesterol and 100 mg of triglyceride a day. It mixes in the bowel lumen with about 900 mg of biliary cholesterol, and this is then digested to form free cholesterol, fatty acids and mono- and diglycerides, which through the detergent effects of bile acids become part of micelles which are then transported to absorption sites in the gut lumen.

All of the triglyceride content is absorbed through the gut wall. Only 50% of the cholesterol is absorbed, and the remainder is excreted. Cholesterol esters are reconstructed to cholesterol in the gut luminal cells through the action of the enzyme acyl coenzyme A cholesterol acyltransferase (ACAT) and incorporated with triglyceride with 1% protein to become chylomicrons. Chylomicrons are formed after consumption of a fatty meal, and are then transported to the thoracic duct and to the bloodstream via the left subclavian vein. As they pass through the circulation, triglyceride 'fuel' is deposited in striated and cardiac muscle and adipose tissue. The cholesterol-ester-containing remnant is highly atherogenic, and under normal circumstances is rapidly assimilated by the liver.

Transport of lipids is mainly by the VLDL that is manufactured and secreted by the liver. Lipoprotein lipase extracts the triglyceride, leaving behind the atherogenic LDL. The LDL is extracted from the plasma by LDL-receptors on the liver cells. When intracellular cholesterol levels fall, the LDL-receptors are activated and cholesterol is drawn into the liver cells from the circulation for the production of more VLDL and bile acids.

Thus cholesterol homeostasis depends on absorption of cholesterol from the gut through the intestinal mucosal cells, and on hepatocyte cells, which control the rate of cholesterol extraction from the plasma into the liver.

New cholesterol drugs have been developed that reduce dietary and biliary cholesterol absorption across the intestinal wall without affecting the absorption of triglycerides and fat-soluble vitamins. An example of this type of drug is ezetimibe (see below).

Cholesterol, atheroma plaque formation and rupture

Cholesterol is an essential component of cell membranes, steroid-based hormones (e.g. sex hormones) and the bile acids that are produced by the liver. It is the main constituent of atheroma, which is deposited inside arterial walls and forms plaques. Under certain circumstances, the cap or top covering of these plaques may rupture, exposing the arterial wall. This leads to platelet aggregation and thrombus formation as part of the healing mechanism. In a heart artery, this may (unless the clot is broken down or dissolved by the body's own thrombolytic processes) result in a heart attack. The deposition of cholesterol in arterial walls causes similar problems in the cerebral arteries and leads to impaired blood and oxygen supply to the legs (claudication).

Risks of hypercholesterolaemia

There is a strong graded relationship between a total cholesterol level of > 4.6 mmol/l and coronary heart disease. The protective effect of HDL-cholesterol is probably as potent as the atherogenic effect of LDL-cholesterol, particularly in women.

Benefits of cholesterol reduction

Several trials have shown that reducing cholesterol levels decreases fatal and non-fatal myocardial infarction without increasing death from other causes. An 11% reduction in total cholesterol is associated with a 23% decrease in cardiovascular events. However, even a strict low-fat diet may result in only a 5% reduction in total cholesterol levels.

Lowering cholesterol levels slows the natural progression of coronary artery disease and may also 'clear' affected heart arteries, resulting in regression of atheroma. Cardiac event rates have also been reduced out of proportion to the usually small improvements in appearance on angiography.

LDL-cholesterol

The LDL-cholesterol level almost entirely accounts for the positive correlation between cholesterol levels and coronary heart disease. It is atherogenic, and a decrease in the level of LDL-cholesterol reduces the risk of coronary heart disease.

The minimum concentration of LDL-cholesterol required for atherogenesis in humans appears to be 2 mmol/l. The relative risk of coronary heart disease is < 2 with an LDL-cholesterol level of < 4 mmol/l, and 35 in patients with familial hypercholesterolaemia and an LDL-cholesterol level of > 6 mmol/l.

Triglycerides

Triglycerides are synthesised in the liver and transported with cholesterol as VLDL. Together with cholesterol as part of absorbed dietary fat, they constitute chylomicrons.

The most important clinical consequences of high triglyceride levels are coronary artery disease, cerebrovascular disease and peripheral vascular disease. Acute pancreatitis is a rare consequence of extremely high levels of triglycerides. No trials have been conducted to determine whether decreasing triglycerides in isolation from other lipids reduces cardiovascular risk. Measurement of triglyceride levels alone for estimation of cardiovascular risk has no advantage over measurement of total cholesterol levels. Most laboratories include triglyceride levels in the lipid profile.

Aggressive lipid lowering with statins may have effects other than cholesterol lowering. These include the following:

- stabilising atheromatous plaques by depleting them of the soft 'explosive' lipid core, thus making them less liable to rupture
- stabilising the endothelium
- inhibiting platelet aggregation
- modifying the behaviour of vascular smooth muscle cells.

These effects support the increasing use of statins in patients with vascular disease in any arterial territory, and in those with high LDL levels with or without a high total cholesterol level.

Similar beneficial effects have also been found with statin treatment in patients with carotid artery disease. Carotid artery intimal thickening (an early stage of atheroma) and cerebrovascular events are both reduced.

Risk factors for vascular disease

At least 80% of major coronary heart disease events in middle-aged men can be attributed to the three strongest risk factors, namely smoking, hypertension and serum total cholesterol levels.

Cardiovascular risk factors may be classified as follows:

- major independent risk factors
- lifestyle risk factors
- emerging risk factors.

Major independent risk factors
These include the following:

- age
- cigarette smoking
- diabetes
- hypertension > 140/90 mm Hg
- HDL < 1 mmol/l
- raised LDL levels
- family history of premature coronary artery disease
    (first-degree male relative < 55 years or first-degree female relative < 65 years)
- renal impairment.

Lifestyle risk factors
These include the following:

- obesity
- physical inactivity
- atherogenic diet.

Emerging risk factors
These include the following:

- homocysteine levels
- lipoprotein(a) levels
- prothrombotic factors and fibrinogen levels
- pro-inflammatory factors
- impaired fasting glucose

- subclinical atherosclerosis
- stress
- social class.

Measuring lipid levels: random or fasting?

Although total and HDL-cholesterol levels are not significantly influenced by consumption of a fatty meal, it is sensible to advise patients to have a fasting blood sample. The laboratory may not measure the HDL directly but estimate it from the LDL level, which would be affected by a recent fat-containing meal.

Risk assessment

Count the major risk factors. If there are two or more, perform a 10-year risk absolute coronary risk assessment. Patients with no more than one risk factor are at low risk and would probably have a 10-year coronary risk of < 10% and would not benefit significantly from drug interventions.

Principles of interventions in primary and secondary prevention

Patients with known vascular disease (i.e. previous infarct, revascularisation and peripheral vascular disease, cerebrovascular disease) are at high risk (the 10-year risk of a cardiovascular event is > 20%), so the threshold for initiating lifestyle changes and drug treatment is lower. LDL target levels should be lower (< 2.5 mmol/l), and these patients should be treated with a statin. Fibrates and nicotinic acid are used in addition for patients with raised triglyceride levels.

In contrast, patients at low risk (10-year risk < 10%) should be encouraged to take primary preventive measures, and would not usually need drug intervention unless their LDL level was > 4.8 mmol/l.

The principle of 'more to gain – more to lose'

The benefit of any intervention is greatest in those individuals who are at greatest risk from the condition treated, although the potential for side-effects or an operative complication may be correspondingly greater.

For example, thrombolysis for acute myocardial infarction may confer a greater morbidity and mortality benefit in an elderly patient with a large area of threatened heart muscle than in a young and otherwise fit patient with little jeopardised myocardium (heart muscle at risk of death due to lack of blood and oxygen).

Patients with coronary artery and other atheromatous disease have more to gain from aggressive lipid lowering and control of other risk factors (secondary prevention) than do low-risk individuals without vascular disease (primary prevention).

Health economics: influence of resources on guidelines

If statins cost the same as aspirin, a primary prevention case could be made for treating even 'low'-risk individuals (10-year risk < 10%). Patients with a 10-year risk as low as 6% would derive prognostic benefit from statins, with a reduction in coronary events and deaths from all causes. It has been estimated that this would involve treating nearly 60% of the UK population. Lowering the threshold for using statins has enormous cost implications in the UK because of the way in which most drugs are licensed and dispensed. Generic statins are available 'over the counter' (OTC) in some countries.

Variations in guideline recommendations

National guidelines formulated by the Joint British Societies make useful evidence-based recommendations for starting treatment for primary and secondary cardiovascular disease prevention.

Financial considerations influence treatment thresholds, which vary considerably between different countries and largely depend on medication and implementation costs. The scientific evidence shows that statins improve the prognosis in people with a 10-year cardiovascular risk of 10%. The Joint British Societies recommend statins only when the risk exceeds 15%, the Joint European Task Force on Coronary Heart Disease when the risk exceeds 20%, and the NHS framework on cardiovascular disease prevention at a risk of 30%. The US National Cholesterol Education Program (NCEP) recommendations use lower thresholds.

Most GPs use the Joint British Societies recommendations, which will be updated. The thresholds for using statins are partially set by NHS financial restraints. The current thresholds for initiating statins may well be lowered in the future, and possibly brought into line with the US guidelines published by the National Heart Lung and Blood Institute (NHLBI).

Summary of the Joint British Societies recommendations

The current guidelines make the following recommendations.

- A total cholesterol level of < 5 mmol/l and LDL level of < 3.0 mmol/l for both primary and secondary prevention. Around 60% of the population have a higher level than this. If despite lifestyle and dietary changes the absolute coronary risk remains above 15% and the total cholesterol level is > 5.0 mmol/l, a statin should be started, or if the triglyceride levels are raised in addition, a fibrate should be started.
- Calculate the 10-year coronary heart disease risk using the Joint British Societies assessment chart prior to initiating lifestyle changes or treatment. All cardiovascular risk factors should be addressed.
- Secondary causes of hyperlipidaemia should be corrected.

- Diabetics should be given a statin if their 10-year coronary heart disease risk exceeds 15%.
- Fibrates should be used if triglyceride levels are > 2.3 mmol/l despite a lipid-lowering diet.
- Lipoprotein analysis should include fasting total cholesterol, total triglycerides and HDL levels. The LDL can be calculated using the following formula:

LDL = TC – (TG/2.19 + HDL)

where TC = total cholesterol level and TG = triglyceride level.

Note: 'High' and 'low' cardiovascular risk are artificial and arbitrary terms. They will have different meanings for a patient, a doctor and a statistician. A middle-aged patient who is told that he has a 9% risk of dying from a heart attack within 10 years may feel that this is not a 'low' risk. However, an octogenarian given the same prognosis may feel quite reassured. Guidelines for cardiovascular risk reduction should be just that – guidelines – and interpreted and applied with an understanding of the patient's clinical condition, their overall risk profile and an appreciation of their wishes.

The following points are not detailed in the Joint British Societies recommendations.

- All patients (both primary and secondary prevention) should be given 'lifestyle advice'.
- Diabetics are at high risk, and the target blood pressure is lower in these patients.
- Patients with cardiovascular risk equivalents are not specified in the current Joint British recommendations.
- 'Targeting progressively more patients' highlights the uncertainty of treating patients who are at intermediate risk.

Priorities for cardiovascular risk management

First priority

These are patients with established coronary artery disease or other atherosclerotic disease (secondary prevention). Management includes the following:

- relevant lifestyle changes – stopping smoking, increasing exercise, eating healthier food
- blood pressure controlled to below 140/85 mmHg
- diabetes – optimal control of blood glucose level; blood pressure reduced to < 140/80 mmHg; total cholesterol reduced to < 5.0 mmol/l and LDL-cholesterol reduced to < 3.0 mmol/l
- cardioprotective drugs for 'selected' patients – aspirin, ACE inhibitors, β-blockers, statins.

Second priority

These are patients without known coronary heart disease or other atherosclerotic disease (primary prevention).

There are three groups to be identified and managed in a staged approach – the group with the highest risk first. All patients should be given relevant lifestyle advice.

1   Absolute 10-year CHD risk of > 30%:
   - blood pressure controlled to < 140/85 mmHg
   - total cholesterol reduced to < 5.0 mmol/l and LDL to < 3.0 mmol/l

- diabetes – optimal control of blood glucose, blood pressure controlled to 140/80 mmHg
- aspirin for patients aged > 50 years if male and/or hypertensive.

2   Absolute 10-year CHD risk of > 15%:
- 'target progressively more patients' and intervene as described above.

3   Absolute 10-year CHD risk < 15%:
- drug treatment is not required unless there is hypertension (> 160/100 mmHg) with associated target organ damage or familial hyperlipidaemia.

Cardiovascular risk equivalents

Patients with the following conditions are at equivalent cardiovascular risk to those who have coronary artery disease, and should be screened:

- known vascular disease (coronary, cerebrovascular, peripheral)
- hypertension
- abdominal aortic aneurysm
- diabetes
- transient ischaemic attacks
- previous stroke.

These patients should be considered for statins irrespective of their lipid levels.

Hypertensive patients, particularly men over 60 years of age, should be examined for an abdominal aortic aneurysm, and an ultrasound scan should be performed if necessary. Feel the foot pulses in all patients with claudication, hypertension and diabetes. Duplex ultrasound scanning should be performed if the patient has symptoms.

HDL target levels

A high HDL level is protective and lowers cardiovascular risk. HDL-cholesterol may act as a scavenger, collecting free cholesterol from peripheral tissues and transporting it to the liver. Ideally most of the total cholesterol should be HDL. A level of < 1 mmol/l is considered to be 'low', and a level above 1.5 is regarded as 'high'. There is currently no evidence from trials that increasing HDL levels decreases cardiovascular risk.

Vigorous sustained exercise (e.g. long-distance running) and moderate alcohol consumption are associated with high HDL levels.

Low HDL levels are associated with obesity, physical inactivity, severe renal failure, type 2 diabetes and cigarette smoking. Thiazides and β-blockers reduce HDL levels. There are no guidelines for managing patients with a low HDL level, which is an independent risk factor for coronary heart disease.

Causes of secondary hyperlipidaemia

Most patients with hyperlipidaemia have a 'primary' or genetic cause. The 'secondary' causes (see Table 5.1) should be considered and, where necessary, treated. This may result

Table 5.1:   Causes of secondary hyperlipidaemia and their effect on lipids

Disorder	Cholesterol	Triglycerides	HDL
Hypothyroidism	++	−	−
Type 2 diabetes	+	++	−
Renal disease	++	++	−
Obstructive liver disease	++	−	−
Alcohol	++	++	+
Thiazide	+	+	−
β-blockers	+	+	−
Anorexia nervosa	+++	−	−

− no increase; + mild increase; ++ moderate increase; +++ major increase.

in a substantial improvement in the lipid profile and render drug treatment for the hyperlipidaemia unnecessary. Tight control of diabetes and correction of hypothyroidism improve the lipid profile. Both β-blockers and thiazides have an unfavourable effect on lipids, and this should be considered in patients with hypertension and hyperlipidaemia.

Family history

A family history of death from coronary heart disease in either parent before the age of 55 years doubles an individual's risk of fatal and non-fatal myocardial infarction. The effect of family history as a risk factor is largely independent of other risk factors, implying that a separate mechanism is involved.

Hypertension

There is a strong and graded relationship between blood pressure and cardiovascular disease, but no clear threshold value which separates hypertensive patients who will experience future cardiovascular events from those who will not.

Diabetes

This is an important, common and modifiable cardiovascular risk factor. Diabetics should undergo comprehensive risk factor assessment. The treatment goal is to achieve normal blood sugar levels and correction of other modifiable risk factors. Diabetics have a high mortality rate both during and after acute myocardial infarction. The short- and long-term results of myocardial revascularisation with both angioplasty and coronary artery bypass are worse than those for non-diabetic patients.

Statins should be prescribed in diabetic patients with a coronary heart disease risk of > 15%.

Smoking

The risk of cardiovascular disease is proportional to the number of cigarettes smoked and how deeply the smoker inhales. The risks of pipe and cigar smokers are intermediate between those of non-smokers and cigarette smokers.

Renal impairment

Minor renal impairment is as powerful a cardiovascular risk factor as diabetes. Patients with cardiovascular disease and impaired renal function constitute a high-risk subgroup.

A minor elevation in serum creatinine levels is associated with an increased cardiovascular risk, including cardiovascular death, myocardial infarction and stroke. Impaired renal function independently increases the risk of death in hypertensive patients. Even minor renal impairment adversely affects both the outcome of patients with acute coronary syndromes or myocardial infarction, and the results of angioplasty and coronary artery surgery.

Pharmacological blockade of the renin–angiotensin system reduces cardiovascular risk in patients with renal impairment. Angiotensin-converting-enzyme (ACE) inhibitors should not be withheld from patients with cardiovascular disease because they have mild renal impairment. ACE inhibitors may increase the serum creatinine concentration, but should be continued with monitoring of renal function, and the dose should only be reduced if there are major increases in serum creatinine levels. The beneficial effects of these drugs against heart failure in patients with acute myocardial infarction are greater in patients with more severe renal impairment, and their efficacy is enhanced by β-blockers.

Exercise and diet

These lifestyle interventions are important and effective components of the primary and secondary prevention of coronary artery disease and atheromatous vascular disease in general. Regular aerobic (cardiovascular) exercise has a significant and graded effect in reducing cardiovascular mortality. Sedentary individuals have a 1.6-fold higher relative risk compared with highly active individuals. Exercise exerts a beneficial effect on blood pressure and serum lipids by reducing triglyceride levels, and it has a modest effect in reducing LDL levels and increasing HDL levels. Conversely, lack of exercise increases the risk of coronary heart disease and cardiovascular mortality.

Maintenance of a low-fat, low-calorie diet and regular exercise programme is very difficult, but it is both important and helpful, particularly in secondary prevention. Primary and secondary prevention clinics, particularly for high-risk individuals, should be offered to patients and are likely to be successful if they are run by enthusiastic, well-informed staff.

Obesity

Obesity is an independent risk factor for cardiovascular disease, and may have more prognostic importance in women than in men, and in young rather than in old people. Central obesity is measured using the waist:hip ratio, and this is a better predictor than overall adiposity (e.g. body-mass index). Obesity is positively correlated with fasting triglyceride and cholesterol levels.

Alcohol

Mild to moderate alcohol consumption reduces the risk of cardiovascular disease, and there is an inverse relationship between alcohol consumption and death from coronary heart disease. However, taking more than 2 units of alcohol per day may increase the risk of death from cancer and cirrhosis. There is no convincing evidence that red wine is superior to other types of alcohol in reducing the risk of cardiovascular disease.

There is no evidence from controlled trials that alcohol reduces total mortality, and there is insufficient evidence to encourage patients who do not drink alcohol to start.

Left ventricular hypertrophy

This is a common result of hypertension and a strong predictor of cardiovascular events, particularly when associated with a repolarisation change on the electrocardiogram.

Homocysteine

In 1959 it was first recognised that patients with homocysteinuria developed vascular abnormalities. High levels of homocysteine are a weak but independent risk factor for the development of vascular atherosclerotic disorders and thromboembolic disease. The concentration of homocysteine is inversely related to that of folate and vitamins B_{12} and B_6. High levels may also increase platelet aggregation and damage vascular endothelium. Increases of 5 µmol/l have been associated with significant increases in coronary heart disease, but after adjustment for confounding variables the association is not convincing.

The normal range of homocysteine levels in the blood is unclear. Levels are higher in males and in patients with renal impairment, and they increase with age and with deficiencies of folate and vitamin B_{12}. Homocysteine levels may be spuriously raised if blood is stored at room temperature. Their measurement is time consuming and expensive, and is currently not widely available or requested.

Folate is present in green leafy vegetables. Folate treatment at a dose of 0.8 mg per day can reduce the homocysteine level by 25%.

Although there is some laboratory and clinical evidence for considering homocysteine as a potential risk factor for coronary artery disease, as yet there is no evidence that reducing homocysteine levels with folate decreases vascular morbidity or mortality.

Screening for homocysteinuria for either primary or secondary prevention with a view to treatment with folic acid is not recommended.

Lipoprotein(a)

First discovered in 1963, lipoprotein(a) is synthesised in the liver, and it consists of an LDL particle linked to a molecule of apo(a) protein (a large protein similar to plasminogen). Lipoprotein(a) levels increase with LDL-cholesterol levels, are higher in black than in white populations, and are higher in all patients with renal disease, in diabetics and after myocardial infarction. High levels of lipoprotein(a) combined with high LDL levels have been associated with a high risk of coronary artery disease, but this finding is not consistent, and the mechanism is unknown. It is unclear whether it is an independent risk factor or whether reducing the levels of lipoprotein(a) decreases cardiovascular events. For this reason it is not routinely measured.

Fibrinogen

This is a key component of fibrin clots, platelet aggregation and blood viscosity. Fibrinogen levels are raised in patients after myocardial infarction. Fibrinogen is synthesised in the liver. Levels are higher in women than in men and in smokers than in non-smokers, and increase with age, alcohol consumption, renal impairment, glucose intolerance, obesity, and after the menopause.

Stress at work has been shown to be associated with raised levels of fibrinogen. Fibrinogen levels are decreased by weight loss, reduced alcohol consumption, exercise and bezafibrate and platelet inhibitors. A fibrinogen concentration of > 3.1 g/l is associated with relative risks of coronary heart disease of 1.6 in men and 2.9 in women.

Fibrinogen is not routinely measured, and at present there are no specific fibrinogen-lowering drugs.

Other prothrombotic factors have been investigated, but their prognostic importance is unclear. Concentrations of tissue plasminogen activator and factor VII are strongly correlated with triglyceride levels and hypercoagulability.

Chlamydia pneumonia

Although it was proposed that previous infection with *Chlamydia pneumoniae* increased the risk of coronary artery disease, subsequent studies have no convincing association.

Dietary recommendations for patients with hyperlipidaemia

The general principle is to eat as little fat (preferably none) as possible. Some individuals may appreciate referral to a dietitian, and this should be discussed with the patient. Not surprisingly, patients become very confused after being given often complicated advice, including the percentages of saturated fat (< 7%), polyunsaturated fat (< 10%), monounsaturated fat (< 20%) and total fat (30%) relative to their total calorie intake, together with less than 200 g of cholesterol per day.

How these amounts are measured is difficult for medical staff to understand and explain! The simpler the advice, the more likely the patient is to follow it. You may wish to give them a list of fatty foods which they should avoid completely.

Oat bran, 50–100 g per day, and soya protein, 25 g per day, each reduce total cholesterol levels by 2–3%.

One portion of oily fish per week is recommended because it contains omega-3 fatty acids, which are protective against coronary heart disease, susceptibility to cardiac arrhythmia, blood clotting and plasma triglycerides. Omega-3 fatty acids are thought to protect against fatal myocardial infarction and sudden death. This view is supported by the low risk of coronary heart disease-related death in Japan, where the national diet includes large amounts of raw oily fish.

Hormone replacement therapy in women: effect on lipids

Observational studies showed that hormone replacement therapy (HRT) might protect women against coronary heart disease, but randomised clinical trials have not confirmed this.

Hormone replacement therapy does not protect women against death, coronary heart disease or myocardial infarction. In diabetic women, it significantly increases the risk of death from all causes, and of coronary heart disease, although the reasons for this are unclear.

Oestrogens elevate triglyceride levels, particularly when given orally, and may occasionally precipitate acute pancreatitis, so should be avoided in women with very high triglyceride levels. These levels should be checked before starting treatment. Patch oestrogen may need to be given, as this has little effect on triglyceride levels. Oestrogen reduces LDL-cholesterol levels and increases HDL-cholesterol levels.

Stress

Job-related stress and effort–reward imbalance increase cardiovascular mortality. One possible mechanism for this may be that high stress levels (low salary, low level of job control, lack of social approval and few career opportunities) are associated with hypertension, raised LDL-cholesterol levels, raised fibrinogen levels and reduced fibrinolytic activity.

Although stress at work may be associated with a doubling of the risk of cardiovascular death among employees, as yet there is no evidence that stress reduction decreases this risk.

Social class

The mortality from coronary heart disease is lower, and is decreasing more quickly in social class I than in social class V. The reasons for this are unclear, but are probably multifactorial, including diet, exercise, smoking and obesity.

Treating the elderly

Although lipid trials have excluded patients over 75 years of age, it is accepted that patients above this age with established coronary artery disease should be managed in the same way as younger patients, and that statins should be used where appropriate in full consultation with the patient. An ageist approach is likely to be resented by fit octogen-arians with symptomatic vascular disease. The decision to start a statin in a symptom-free elderly patient with an isolated raised LDL level is more difficult, and their views about wanting to avoid their first and possibly final heart attack should be respected.

Ethnic risks

South Asians have a 50% higher risk of developing coronary heart than white people living in the UK, while Afro-Caribbeans have a lower risk. South Asians are at greater risk from cardiovascular disease, and show a tendency to have a low HDL level, high triglyceride levels, diabetes, obesity and hypertension (metabolic syndrome). Coronary artery disease tends to be more diffuse, and the arteries appear to be smaller, possibly because there is widespread vascular disease.

Drug therapy for lipid disorders

Treatment for lipid disorders is usually lifelong. It is important to warn the patient about the potential side-effects of all drugs before prescribing. Remember that not all symptoms are side-effects.

Statins

Statins specifically inhibit HMG CoA reductase (the rate-limiting step in cholesterol synthesis). They have made a major impact on the treatment of patients who have or are at risk of vascular disease. They reduce VLDL and LDL levels and induction of the LDL-receptors. Their main effect is the reduction of LDL-cholesterol levels, although atorvastatin decreases triglyceride levels as well.

Statins have several possible modes of action in addition to reducing LDL-cholesterol levels. These include a direct effect on endothelial function, reducing the inflammatory reactions (levels of C-reactive protein fall) and changes in arteries, plaque stabilisation, and reducing thrombus formation.

They are generally well tolerated, and are the most effective lipid-lowering drugs. They do not increase morbidity or mortality or the risk of cancer. Compared with placebo, statins do not cause changes in liver enzymes, and produce no significant increase in myalgia, myositis or myopathy, or a raised creatine kinase level.

A response is seen within 4 weeks. If the patient cannot tolerate them, try a different statin or one of the other groups of drugs described below which may be used together with a statin in patients with persistently high lipid levels, or in those with a high-risk profile. Doubling the dose of statin to the recommended maximum dose achieves a modest lowering of the LDL and total cholesterol levels. Although some physicians prescribe statins to be taken at night to slow down the endogenous cholesterol pathway, which may be more active at night (it may be suppressed during the day by fatty meals), the timing of the dose does not seem to be clinically important.

The two most commonly used and effective statins are simvastatin and atorvastatin, but new ones are available.

Statins:

- reduce major coronary events by 30%
- reduce cardiac mortality
- reduce coronary procedures (angioplasty and bypass surgery)
- reduce stroke
- reduce total mortality.

They are effective and should be prescribed to patients after myocardial revascularisation, even if cholesterol levels are normal.

Highest-dose statins for patients with resistant hyperlidaemia

Each doubling of a statin dose results in a 6% reduction in LDL-cholesterol levels, but it is not yet known whether this translates to a significant lowering of coronary heart disease risk.

Adverse effects of statins are dose dependent, with 2–3% increases in liver enzymes which only rarely result in jaundice. The risk of myopathy increases from 0.2% to 0.6% with statin doses of 80 mg compared with doses of 40 mg (using simvastatin, atorvastatin or pravastatin). These adverse event rates are low, but 80 mg doses have been used in trials for only 6 months on average, so there is little evidence for their long-term safety profile. It is recommended that patients who are on highest-dose statins, particularly the elderly or frail, those with multi-system disorders and those on drugs which may interact, are monitored more closely.

Effects of statins:

Statins reduce LDL-cholesterol levels by 30%, and reduce triglyceride levels by 20%.

Side-effects of statins

Compared with placebo, statins do not cause significant changes in liver enzymes, and produce no significant increase in myalgia or myositis.

Side-effects include the following:

- myopathy (rare, but increased risk if the patient is taking fibrates, too). There is pain, tenderness and weakness, and a tenfold increase in creatine phosphokinase activity. Stop the statin and monitor the patient both clinically and with regard to creatine phosphokinase activity
- joint pains
- increased liver enzymes (1% of patients). Check liver function tests after 2 months and then every 6 months. Moderate elevation of transaminases should be monitored, and the statin does not need to be stopped unless it continues to rise or reaches three times the upper limit of normal. It may normalise with continued treatment or reduced dosage. The alkaline phophatase and glutamyl transferase (gamma-GT) levels are not helpful and do not need to be monitored
- gastrointestinal problems.

Under-use of statins in primary care

GPs and nurse practitioners are becoming increasingly experienced in running lipid clinics, taking blood samples for lipid levels in the surgery, and treating patients for both primary and secondary prevention. However, for reasons that are unclear, only around half of the total number of patients at risk who should be on statins are being treated. Possible reasons include practitioners' inexperience, lack of awareness of the benefits, over-caution or a concern for thrift. Few clinicians prescribe statins to the recommended maximum dose.

Bile-acid sequestrants (e.g. cholestyramine, colestipol)

These have now been largely replaced by statins. Patients find them difficult to take because of their side-effects, namely gastrointestinal pain, wind and constipation. They also affect the absorption of other drugs. They reduce LDL-cholesterol levels by 15–30% and raise HDL-cholesterol levels by 3–55%.

Bile-acid sequestrants may increase triglyceride levels, and are contraindicated in hypertriglyceridaemia. They reduce the absorption of fat-soluble vitamins, and therefore supplementary vitamins A, D and K are required for patients on long-term treatment.

They also reduce major coronary events and decrease cardiac mortality. They are not absorbed, so are the drugs of choice in young women (who may become pregnant) and children. They are useful in combination with statins, and act synergistically to reduce LDL-cholesterol levels.

Nicotinic acid (niacin)

This is used only rarely. Nicotinic acid:

- lowers LDL-cholesterol levels by 5–25%
- lowers triglyceride levels by 20–50%
- raises HDL-cholesterol levels by 15–35%.

Its side-effects include flushing, hyperuricaemia, upper gastrointestinal side-effects and liver damage. It is contraindicated in liver disease, diabetes, severe goat, peptic ulcer and patients taking warfarin. It reduces major coronary events, but its effects on total mortality are unclear.

Nicotinic acid is available over the counter, and is cheap, safe and useful as combination therapy with statins in patients with high triglyceride levels or persistently raised LDL-cholesterol levels.

Fibrates (e.g. gemfibrozil, fenofibrate, clofibrate)

Fibrates lower triglyceride levels effectively, elevate HDL-cholesterol and reduce LDL-cholesterol levels by 18%. They are mainly used to reduce the risk of acute pancreatitis in patients with high triglyceride levels. Clofibrate is now rarely used as a trial showed that it was associated with an increase in gastrointestinal tumours and mortality.

Fibrates reduce the progression of coronary artery disease and reduce coronary heart disease events and non-fatal infarction. They are recommended for high-risk patients with high cholesterol and triglyceride levels.

Side-effects include muscle pain and raised creatine kinase levels, particularly in patients with renal impairment or hypothyroidism, and when statins are taken in addition.

Fish oils

Greenland Eskimos, who eat whale and seal meat, which contains omega–3 poly-unsaturated fatty acids (n3-PUFA), have lower levels of total cholesterol, triglycerides, LDL and VLDL, but increased HDL levels and, importantly, lower rates of coronary heart disease compared with Danish people. In addition, men who eat some fish every week have lower rates of heart disease than those who eat no fish. Other studies have not confirmed this, and the protective role of fish oils in preventing coronary heart disease remains unproven. Fish oil levels do not correlate with the incidence of myocardial infarction, and a large dose of n3-PUFA has no effect on re-stenosis after coronary angioplasty. However, in one study fish oils did decrease all-cause mortality after myocardial infarction, but not by reducing cholesterol levels. N-3 fatty acids have anti-arrhythmic properties, and may reduce the risk of sudden death after myocardial infarction.

Patients should be advised to eat fish twice a week.

Cholesterol absorption inhibitors

These are new drugs which may prove to be important as adjunctive treatment in resistant cases. They target the exogenous pathway.

Ezetimibe is a new drug which appears to be safe and acts synergistically with statins, resulting in a reduction in LDL-cholesterol levels of around 40%, compared with 30% with a statin alone. It acts by inhibiting the absorption of around 50% of dietary and biliary cholesterol. It acts synergistically with statins, resulting in an additional 20% lowering of cholesterol levels. Ezetimibe, 10 mg, every morning, reduces LDL-cholesterol levels by an additional 14%, and slightly more in patients with familial hypercholes-terolaemia. It does not interfere with the absorption of triglycerides or fat-soluble vitamins.

It is a useful additional drug to use if the LDL-cholesterol level remains high despite the maximum recommended or tolerated dose of statin.

Unusual lipid abnormalities

These may need specialist referral. Family members should be evaluated.

Patients with very high LDL levels (> 4.9 mmol/l) may need a statin plus bile acid sequestrants plus nicotinic acid, but warn the patient about the high risk of side-effects.

Very high triglyceride levels (> 4.0 mmol/l) are associated with the following:

- obesity
- physical inactivity
- cigarette smoking
- excess alcohol consumption
- type 2 diabetes
- chronic renal disease
- high carbohydrate intake
- steroids.

Secondary causes of hyperlipidaemia

These are listed above, and should be treated vigorously.

Uncommon genetic causes of hyperlipidaemia

Familial hypercholesterolaemia

The heterozygote form is inherited as an autosomal dominant and occurs in 1 in 500 people, so most GPs would have at least four patients with this condition.

Patients have very high LDL-cholesterol (> 5.0 mmol/l) and total cholesterol (> 8.0 mmol/l) levels, a family history of hypercholesterolaemia and/or premature coronary artery disease. Look for tendon xanthomata and an arcus (significant in patients under 50 years of age). Affected patients need aggressive treatment (often all three classes of lipid-lowering drugs) and specialist referral for diagnosis and monitoring of vascular disease.

Children of affected individuals should be screened at the age of 12 years. Screening of family members provides a 50% yield. They should be referred to a specialist.

The homozygous form is very rare, and affected individuals usually die at a very young age from accelerated atherosclerosis.

Patients with hyperlipidaemia who should be referred to a specialist

These include the following:

- those with resistant hyperlipidaemia
- those with cardiac symptoms
- those who experience side-effects to drugs
- those with other risk factors which are difficult to control
- non-compliant patients
- those with possible side-effects

- patients with mixed hyperlipidaemia who may need fibrates and statins
- patients who want to be referred.

Advice for patients with hyperlipidaemia

- You can and should do a lot for yourself, and we will help you.
- Try to change to a healthy low-fat diet.
- Losing weight, exercising regularly, avoiding fatty foods and stopping smoking will greatly reduce your risk of a heart attack and stroke.
- These measures will also improve your chances of a longer and healthier life after a heart attack, coronary artery bypass surgery or angioplasty. You should be taking a statin if you have had any of these conditions.
- These measures are very important if you have any cardiovascular risk factor, particularly diabetes, hypertension or if you are overweight.
- Make sure that your blood pressure is checked regularly, and if it is high take treatment for life.

Answers to case studies

1 Ask the patient if he understands what happened to him, whether he is taking the medication prescribed, and what kind of exercise he is doing and how frequently. Ask him about his diet and whether he wants to attend a rehabilitation programme. Explain that he would benefit from a statin, and suggest that he tries one.

2 Check the patient's lipids. Unless there are indications for drug intervention, reassure her and give her primary preventive advice. Offer to see her again at any time if she is anxious.

3 Perform a full cardiac evaluation, lipid profile, full blood count, electrolytes and thyroid function tests, and start the patient on anti-anginal treatment, including aspirin, a statin, a low dose of β-blocker and GTN spray if she is able to use it. Advise her not to over-exert herself for the next few days, and explain that if her symptoms do not improve within 48 hours or if she continues to experience chest discomfort at rest, she may need to be admitted to hospital.

4 Examine the patient, consider a statin-induced myopathy, check the creatine phosphokinase (CPK), C-reactive protein (CRP), erythrocyte sedimentation rate (ESR) and liver function tests, and if necessary stop the statin. Consider other causes of muscle pain.

5 Start the patient on a statin and check his lipids after 2 months.

Further reading

General

- Department of Health (2001) *National Service Framework for Coronary Heart Disease.* Department of Health, London.

- Wood D, Durrington P, Poulter N *et al.* (1998) Joint British recommendations on prevention of coronary heart disease in clinical practice. *Heart.* **80 (Suppl. 2)**: S1–29.

Cholesterol

- Expert Panel on Detection, Evaluation and Treatment of High Blood Cholesterol in Adults (2001) Executive summary of the third report of the National Cholesterol Education Program (NCEP) expert panel on detection, evaluation and treatment of high blood cholesterol in adults (adult treatment panel III). *JAMA.* **285**: 2486–97.
- Neaton J and Wentworth D (1992) Serum cholesterol, blood pressure, cigarette smoking and death from coronary heart disease. The Multiple Risk Factor Intervention Trial Research Group. *Arch Intern Med.* **152**: 56–64.

Smoking

- Irbarren C, Tekawa IS, Sidney D *et al.* (1999) Effect of cigar smoking on the risk of cardiovascular disease, chronic obstructive pulmonary disease and cancer in men. *NEJM.* **340**: 1773–80.

Renal function

- Culleton BF, Larson MG, Wilson PW *et al.* (1999) Cardiovascular disease and mortality in a community-based cohort with mild renal insufficiency. *Kidney Int.* **56**: 2214–19.

Exercise

- Sandvik L, Erikssen J, Thaulow E *et al.* (1993) Physical fitness as a predictor of mortality among healthy, middle-aged Norwegian men. *NEJM.* **328**: 533–7.

Obesity

- Hubert HB, Feinlib M, McNamara PM *et al.* (1983) Obesity is an independent risk factor for cardiovascular disease: a 26-year follow-up of participants in the Framingham Heart Study. *Circulation.* **67**: 968–77.

Alcohol

- Criqui MH and Ringel BL (1994) Does diet or alcohol explain the French paradox? *Lancet.* **344**: 1719–23.
- Mukamal KJ, Conigrave KM, Mittlemen MA *et al.* (2003) Roles of drinking pattern and type of alcohol consumed in coronary heart disease in men. *NEJM.* **348**: 109–18.
- Thun MJ, Peto R, Lopez AD *et al.* (1997) Alcohol consumption and mortality among middle-aged and elderly US adults. *NEJM.* **337**: 1705–14.

Left ventricular hypertrophy

- Dunn FG, McLenachan J, Isles CG *et al.* (1990) *J Hypertens.* **8**: 775–82.

Lipoprotein(a)

- Harjai KJ (1999) Potential new cardiovascular risk factors: left ventricular hypertrophy, homocysteine, lipoprotein(a), triglycerides, oxidative stress and fibrinogen. *Ann Intern Med.* **131**: 376–86.

Triglycerides

- Avins AL and Neuhaus JM (2000) Do triglycerides provide meaningful information about heart disease risk? *Arch Intern Med.* **160**: 1937–44.

Fish oils

- Kromhout D, Bosschieter EB and de Lezenne-Coulander C (1985) The inverse relationship between fish consumption and 20-year mortality from coronary heart disease. *NEJM.* **313**: 1205–9.
- Vollset SE, Heuch I and Bjelke E (1985) Fish consumption and mortality from coronary heart disease. *NEJM.* **313**: 820–21.

Hormone replacement treatment

- Grodstein F and Stampfer M (1995) The epidemiology of coronary heart disease and estrogen replacement in postmenopausal women. *Prog Cardiovasc Dis.* **38**: 199–210.
- Lokkegaard E, Pederse T, Heitmann BL *et al.* (2003) Relation between hormone replacement therapy and ischaemic heart disease in women: prospective observational study. *BMJ.* **326**: 426–8.
- Rossouw JE, Anderson JL, Prentice RL *et al.* (2002) Risks and benefits of estrogen plus progestin in healthy postmenopausal women: principal results from the Women's Health Initiative randomized controlled trial. *JAMA.* **288**: 321–33.

Homocysteine

- Boushey CJ, Beresford SA, Omen CS *et al.* (1995) A quantitative assessment of plasma homocysteine as a risk factor for vascular disease. Probable benefits for increasing folic acid intake. *JAMA.* **274**: 1049–57.
- Clarke R, Daly L, Robinson K *et al.* (1991) Hyperhomocysteinaemia: an independent risk factor for vascular disease. *NEJM.* **324**: 1149–55.
- Danesh J and Lewington S (1998) Plasma homocysteine and coronary heart disease: systematic review of published epidemiological studies. *J Cardiovasc Risk.* **5**: 229–32.
- Mayer EM, Jacobsen DW and Robinson K (1996) Homocysteine and atherosclerosis. *J Am Coll Cardiol.* **27**: 517–27.

Family history

- Myers RH, Kiely DK, Cupples A *et al.* (1990) Parental history is an independent risk factor for coronary artery disease: the Framingham study. *Am Heart J.* **120**: 963–9.

Stress

- Hemingway H and Marmot M (1999) Psychosocial factors in the aetiology and prognosis of coronary heart disease: systematic review of prospective cohort studies. *BMJ.* **318**: 1460–7.
- Kivimäki M, Leino-Arjas P, Luukkonen R *et al.* (2002) Work stress and risk of cardiovascular mortality: prospective cohort study of industrial employees. *BMJ.* **325**: 857–60.

CHAPTER 6

Atherosclerosis imaging and screening

Case study

1　A 40-year-old symptom-free but stressed business executive with no cardio-vascular risk factors is worried about the possibility of having heart disease because his father died at the age of 80 years, apparently from a heart attack. He asks you whether he should have an electron beam computed tomogram, which is claimed to provide diagnostic information about the presence of heart disease. What advice would you give him?

Aims of atherosclerosis imaging

Most coronary events (sudden cardiac death, unstable angina or myocardial infarction) occur in patients with coronary artery stenoses of < 50%. Patients with atherosclerosis affecting the carotid or peripheral arteries or aorta are at similar cardiovascular risk to patients with coronary heart disease.

The challenge for clinicians responsible for cardiovascular prevention is to detect coronary atherosclerosis and to predict which individuals are at risk of coronary events. Atherosclerosis imaging using various techniques has been used to detect atherosclerosis in arteries, with the aim of identifying patients at risk from cardiovascular events who would benefit from prevention measures. The techniques used include carotid artery ultrasound scanning, coronary calcium scanning, cardiovascular magnetic resonance imaging (MRI) scanning and the ankle–brachial index.

Cost–benefit analysis of atherosclerotic imaging in high- and low-risk individuals

The value and limitations of atherosclerotic imaging are illustrated by comparing the number needed to treat and the cost implications for patients at high and low cardio-vascular risk.

High-risk individuals

If a treatment reduces the relative risk of cardiovascular death by 25%, then if a high-risk individual has an absolute 10-year risk of 20%, 20 patients will need to be treated for 10 years to prevent one death.

Low-risk individuals

If a low-risk individual has a 10-year risk of cardiovascular death of 1%, then 400 individuals will need to be treated for 10 years to save one life.

Drawbacks of atherosclerotic imaging in low-risk individuals

Before these various techniques are recommended for clinical use, they must be shown to provide accurate, reliable, reproducible, cost-effective information which adds significantly to conventional cardiovascular risk scoring assessments. At present, there is doubt concerning the widespread use of these techniques in routine clinical practice.

- Atherosclerotic imaging, including electron beam computed tomography and nuclear perfusion imaging, is not recommended for asymptomatic individuals.
- The application of atherosclerotic imaging is theoretically best suited to intermediate-risk patients, but before clinicians apply it to these patients, a larger body of supporting evidence is needed to show the incremental benefit of obtaining the information that imaging provides.
- Because most of our knowledge of the characteristics of vulnerable plaque is derived from referred populations in pathology studies, the applicability of the data to clinical screening populations must be demonstrated.
- Data are needed on the incremental value of new imaging techniques for clinical risk assessment. The methodology used for cardiac imaging needs to be standardised and its reproducibility and variability defined, especially for emerging technologies.
- Selecting intermediate-risk patients for plaque burden assessment by imaging technology has potential advantages, but more studies are needed in low- and high-risk patients.
- There is a paucity of high-quality outcome and cost-effectiveness data for atherosclerosis imaging, and therefore long-term outcome data are needed to develop models of cost-effectiveness.

Imaging and other diagnostic tests used for cardiovascular diagnosis and prognosis are most appropriately employed in patients at 'intermediate' coronary risk. This can be defined as an annual risk of 0.6–2% (10-year risk of 6–20%), whereas 'low' risk can be defined as an annual coronary event risk of < 0.6% (10-year risk of < 6%) and 'high risk' as an annual risk of > 2% (10-year risk of 20%).

These tests will not provide further *diagnostic* information in patients with angina or proven coronary artery disease (e.g. angiographically documented coronary artery disease). In *low-risk* individuals, the tests are more likely to provide misleading information and complicate clinical decision making. At present, atherosclerotic imaging tests are most appropriately used in individuals at *intermediate* risk.

However, there is currently insufficient evidence to support the use of any form of atherosclerotic imaging in individuals in any risk group, and the use of these tests cannot be recommended. They do not provide additional diagnostic or prognostic information over conventional coronary risk scores combined (where appropriate) with non-invasive stress testing. In addition, there is no evidence that they are cost-effective.

Carotid artery ultrasound scanning

This can be used to image carotid artery intima-media thickness, which may be increased in hypertension, and to image atherosclerotic plaques. Doppler quantification of carotid artery disease may show obstruction to flow if there is a stenosis of < 50%. Intima-media thickness increases with age, and this complicates the interpretation of the results. Serial measurements performed by the same person on the same machine may in the same individual provide useful information about the change in the condition or the response to treatment. The technique cannot be recommended as a screening test.

Electron beam computed tomography (EBCT) scanning

It has been known for many years that the presence of calcium in the walls of coronary arteries seen on X-ray fluoroscopy increases the probability of coronary artery disease, although its prognostic significance is unknown. It does not have incremental predictive value over clinic cardiovascular risk assessment. Electron beam computerised axial tomography is a new and expensive technique, not available in NHS hospitals, that is used for coronary calcium scanning. It exposes the patient to a considerable dosage of ionising radiation, equivalent to approximately 15 chest X-rays. The test provides a 'calcium score'. For men, the probability of having any detectable coronary calcium is roughly equivalent to their age. For women, the probability is 10 to 15 points below their age. EBCT scanning is marketed as a component of a risk factor evaluation, but its prognostic value is unclear, and in the only published study that directly assessed the additive value of coronary calcium scores with regard to the predictive value of measurements of conventional risk factors, the CT results provided little incremental predictive information. EBCT scanning has equivalent predictive value to exercise testing.

Comparison of EBCT scanning with coronary angiography

In contrast to angiography, EBCT scanning does not provide reliable information on intraluminal disease (inside the artery), but the derived 'score' provides a guide as to whether the individual may have vascular disease.

Compared with coronary angiography, EBCT scanning has a sensitivity of 80% and a very low specificity of 40% (less useful than flipping a coin in excluding coronary artery disease, and therefore of particular concern in low-risk individuals). The published literature shows that it has an extremely high false-positive rate, and the clinical and economic implications are considerable.

Around 50% of scans detect unexpected cardiac findings which, when investigated, are almost always of negligible clinical importance. The high false positive rate engenders considerable and unnecessary anxiety in many asymptomatic, low risk patients.

The proposed rationale for the use of EBCT scanning is that it can 'quantify' atheromatous plaque. Patients with unstable angina may have a high score, but this test would add little to either the diagnosis or the prognosis in this high-risk group. The score is usually low in patients at low risk (e.g. in young people who do not have arterial wall calcification).

Young patients with acute coronary syndromes usually do not have hard calcific coronary artery stenoses, but rather inflamed ulcerated plaques and thrombus. An EBCT scan can be misleading in this young or middle-aged group (false-negative results). Similarly, elderly people in whom coronary artery calcification is expected may have no intraluminal disease, and this results in a high false-positive rate.

The inter-observer variability of around 24% and the major variability (50%) in the calcium score reported by the same observer in the same patient scanned on two consecutive days raise important issues about the applicability of this new imaging modality, particularly in those patients in whom it is advocated as a method of monitoring response to lipid-lowering treatment.

The test provides little useful additional clinical information for monitoring vascular disease or for guiding and monitoring treatment in either high- or low-risk patients. It cannot yet be recommended in asymptomatic patients or as a screening test for selecting asymptomatic patients for invasive investigations. Recommending asymptomatic patients to adopt a healthy lifestyle, and the indications for treating hyperlipidaemia, hypertension or diabetes, or to stop smoking, would not be affected by the results of a calcium score.

Much more information is required in individuals with intermediate cardiovascular risk before EBCT scanning is recommended. At present, exercise testing remains the test of first choice in patients at intermediate risk. EBCT scanning may be indicated in the rare case of a patient at intermediate coronary risk (10–20% 10-year risk) in whom other non-invasive tests are contraindicated or the results cannot be interpreted. Otherwise it is a costly waste of resources.

A thorough clinical assessment incorporating a risk assessment analysis with simple blood tests and judicious use of exercise testing will suffice for virtually all patients.

Cardiac magnetic resonance imaging (CMRI)

This has potential for imaging and characterising atherosclerotic plaque, and can differentiate between different plaque components (fibrous cap, calcium and lipid core). This may provide prognostic information, as patients with lipid-rich, unstable, inflamed plaques may be at particularly high risk of coronary events. Carotid arteries are easier to image than the aorta or coronary arteries. Cardiac magnetic resonance imaging is not widely available, and there are no data on its prognostic value. It is comparatively reproducible and accurate, but it has no place at present in routine cardiovascular risk assessment.

Ankle–brachial index (ABI)

This is the ratio of the systolic blood pressure at the ankle divided by the systolic blood pressure in the arm. When a stenosis in a peripheral artery reaches a critical level, a decrease in effective perfusion pressure occurs distal to the stenosis, and this is roughly equal to the severity of the occlusive disease.

The test is painless, simple to perform and is used in vascular clinics. It detects advanced peripheral artery disease but does not detect early plaque formation. An abnormal ABI is a value of ≤ 0.9, and this has a sensitivity of around 90% and a specificity of about 98%. It can detect subclinical disease, and 40% of patients with abnormal ABI results are symptom free.

The test is fairly reproducible, but not sufficiently so to recommend its use for serial testing, although it may be used for population screening. It provides incremental predictive information over clinical risk assessment. Its clinical impact is limited by the low prevalence of abnormal test results in individuals under 60 years of age.

Screening for coronary heart disease in symptom-free individuals

The chapters dealing with risk assessment and Bayesian analysis provide the necessary background information for this section.

Exercise testing

Exercise testing in symptom-free patients with a low pre-test probability of coronary heart disease is of limited diagnostic value. In common with other non-invasive tests of

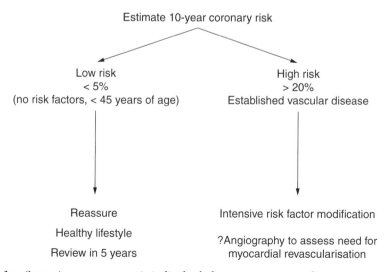

Figure 6.1:   Screening asymptomatic individuals for coronary artery disease.

ischaemia, it should only be performed after a careful consideration of the pre-test likelihood of coronary artery disease in the individual. A 'positive' test result in an individual at low risk is likely to be a 'false-positive' result, and must be interpreted with caution, with a knowledge of the patient's clinical state. A 'negative' test result in a high-risk patient is likely to be a 'false-negative' result, and should not affect the need to withhold long-term preventive treatment. The main indication for exercise testing is the assessment of reversible ischaemia in individuals at intermediate risk.

Answers to case study

1   At present there is insufficient evidence to recommend atherosclerotic imaging, particularly electron beam computed tomography. It does not provide incremental diagnostic or prognostic information over a clinical assessment of cardiovascular risk or exercise testing.

Further reading

- Burke AP, Virmani R, Galis Z et al. (2003) Task Force # 2. What is the pathologic basis for new atherosclerosis imaging techniques? *J Am Coll Cardiol.* **41**: 1874–86.
- Daly C, Saravanan P and Fox K (2002) Is calcium the clue? *Eur Heart J.* **23**: 1562–6.
- Detrano RC, Wong ND, Doherty TM et al. (1999) Coronary calcium does not accurately predict near-term future coronary events in high-risk adults. *Circulation.* **99**: 2633–8. [Errata (2000) *Circulation.* **101**: 697, 1355].
- Greenland P and Gaziano JM et al. (2003) Selecting asymptomatic patients for coronary computed tomography or electrocardiographic exercise testing. *NEJM.* **349**: 465–73.
- Mark DB, Shaw LJ, Lauer MS et al. (2003) Task Force # 5. Is atherosclerosis imaging cost-effective? *J Am Coll Cardiol.* **41**: 1906–17.
- Pasternak RC, Abrams J, Greenland P et al. (2003). Task Force # 1. Identification of coronary heart disease risk: is there a detection gap? *J Am Coll Cardiol.* **41**: 1863–74.
- Redberg RF, Vogel RA, Criqui MH et al. (2003) Task Force # 3. What is the spectrum of current and emerging techniques for the non-invasive measurement of atherosclerosis? *J Am Coll Cardiol.* **41**: 1886–98.
- Taylor AJ, Merz CNB and Udelson JE (2003) Executive summary. Can atherosclerosis imaging techniques improve the detection of patients at risk for ischaemic heart disease? *J Am Coll Cardiol.* **41**: 1860–2.
- Wilson PWF, Smith SC, Blumenthal RS et al. (2003) Task Force # 4. How do we select patients for atherosclerosis imaging? *J Am Coll Cardiol.* **41**: 1898–906.

CHAPTER 7

Obesity and diet

Case studies

1 A 48-year-old woman who is moderately overweight and who finds it difficult to maintain an optimum weight asks you whether she should go on the Atkins diet. What would you advise her?
2 A 60-year-old man who is overweight, inactive and drinks one bottle of red wine a day comes to see you 2 weeks after leaving hospital for management of unstable angina. He believes that red wine prevented him from having a heart attack, and wants you to confirm this. What would you tell him?
3 A 36-year-old diabetic man with a family history of premature coronary heart disease has succeeded in giving up smoking, but is now overweight and wants help. How would you help him?

Role of the primary care team in the management of obesity

Primary care is a focal point for the management of obesity and its complications. Many primary care units have dedicated staff who run obesity and diet clinics. Effective treatment of this increasingly common medical condition requires skill, enthusiasm and perseverance. Patients should be helped to understand the importance of maintaining an optimum weight, and how this will reduce their risk of cardiovascular disease and make them feel better.

Diagnosing obesity

Definitions of excess body weight in relation to body mass index are as follows:

- normal: 18.5–24.9 kg/m^2
- overweight: 25–29.9 kg/m^2
- obese: > 30 kg/m^2.

Obesity affects over half the UK population, and a larger proportion of the population is overweight. Most of us know if we are overweight, and obese patients understand that they have a problem.

A good set of weighing scales and a height ruler are used to record weight and body mass index (BMI) calculated as weight (in kg) divided by height (in m^2). Special scales are necessary for obese patients. Body mass index is the preferred index for measuring obesity, and it minimises the effect of height on body weight. An increased BMI increases the risk of death from a cardiac cause.

> Obesity is a disease which causes morbidity and mortality, and for which the patient has responsibility and the ability to control it.

Pathology and risks of obesity

The prevalence of obesity has increased worldwide. The condition is common in all age groups in the UK, and is becoming even more common, particularly in children. This is due both to the popularity of 'fast food' (which has a high fat, salt and sugar content) and to children leading a more sedentary life, doing less sport in and out of school. Adults in the UK are also working long hours. The UK population is aware that exercise is an important part of a healthy lifestyle, but in general remains inactive and has an unhealthy diet.

Obesity, cardiovascular disease and heart failure

Obese people are predisposed to diabetes, hypertension, left ventricular hypertrophy, stroke, heart failure and heart attack. Overweight children may become overweight adults because dietary and lifestyle habits established in childhood are difficult to change. It is perhaps interesting to observe that proportionately few elderly people are obese. In fact most elderly people are slim.

Obesity and cardiac death

Obesity increases the risk of cardiac death. The mechanism may be due to premature coronary artery disease, heart failure or sudden death due to arrhythmia related to left ventricular dilatation and hypertrophy. Ventricular ectopic beats, possibly leading to more serious ventricular arrhythmias, are more common in hypertrophic hearts. The hypertrophy is not concentric as in hypertension, but eccentric, so the cardiac enlargement in obesity may not simply reflect associated hypertensive heart disease. Obesity results in an increase in blood volume and cardiac output. There are also abnormalities in haemodynamics, with increased cardiac work during exercise.

Genetics of obesity

The reasons why some people like to eat more in one meal than others remain unclear. Appetite is dependent on hormonal signals from adipose tissue providing feedback to the hypothalamus. A genetic link to childhood obesity has been reported. Melanocyte-stimulating hormone produced in the hypothalamus stimulates the melanocortin-4-receptor (MC4R), which may account for 6% of cases of obesity by influencing the appetite and eating behaviour in affected people.

Obesity as a cardiovascular risk factor

> Obesity is now considered to be as important an independent risk factor for cardiovascular disease and heart failure as diabetes, hypertension and smoking.

Therefore obesity as an isolated condition (although it would be unusual for an obese patient to have no other risk factor) increases the risk of stroke and myocardial infarction. However, it is commonly associated with type 2 diabetes mellitus, hypercholesterol-aemia, and hypertension. These conditions are more resistant to treatment in obese patients. They act synergistically as cardiovascular risk factors, so patients with two or more of these conditions are at particularly high risk for cardiac events.

Obese survivors of myocardial infarction have a higher subsequent cardiac risk (i.e. are more likely to have another possibly fatal infarct or to develop angina or heart failure) compared with thin patients.

The metabolic syndrome

The metabolic syndrome may affect around 25% of the population, and consists of the following:

- visceral obesity
- atherogenic dyslipidaemias (low levels of HDL-cholesterol and elevated levels of total cholesterol, LDL-cholesterol and triglycerides)
- elevated levels of C-reactive protein
- hypertension
- glucose intolerance that contributes to insulin resistance (the core of the problem) and a heightened risk of diabetes, thrombosis and cardiovascular disease.

This syndrome is a major risk factor for cardiovascular disease. Overweight patients should be evaluated for this increasingly common condition, and treated vigorously to reduce their cardiovascular risk.

Obesity and heart failure

The higher the body mass index, the greater the risk of heart failure. The risk of heart failure in obese people is twice as high as that in individuals with a normal body mass index. This risk appears to be independent of other risk factors associated with obesity.

The symptoms of obesity are similar to those of heart failure (breathlessness, orthopnoea and oedema), and this makes it difficult to diagnose heart failure in obese people.

Obesity and sleep apnoea syndrome

Obese people often have sleep apnoea and hypoventilation. Sleep apnoea is an important trigger of pulmonary hypertension, and has been implicated in the development of coronary heart disease. Affected patients are characteristically obese, fall asleep in the middle of the day and snore loudly because of upper airways obstruction. They have prolonged episodes of apnoea, which frighten their family or other observers. Sleep apnoea responds to weight loss, and continuous positive airways pressure treatment, but surgery to the upper airways may occasionally be necessary.

Benefits of weight loss

Overweight patients with heart conditions, particularly hypertension, type 2 diabetes and hypercholesterolaemia, should be encouraged to lose weight and exercise regularly.

- *Hypertension* may resolve after significant weight loss, so patients with suspected hypertension may not need to start medication, or may be able to stop their tablets.
- *Type 2 diabetes* may be controlled by diet and weight loss alone.
- A low-fat diet and exercise may render statin treatment unnecessary in patients with *mild hyperlipidaemia*.
- Patients should also be told that *weight loss improves survival after heart attacks and lowers the risk of stroke.*
- Usually, *a weight loss of 4 kg allows antihypertensive medication to be reduced,* possibly by reducing the sensitivity of blood pressure to sodium levels.

Most overweight patients with angina or heart failure improve symptomatically after they lose weight. Because there have not been any randomised controlled trials of weight reduction in obese patients with coronary artery disease, it is unclear whether weight loss alone reduces the risk of cardiac events in secondary prevention. Such a trial may never be undertaken, so this is an example of a situation where common-sense medical practice and advice override evidence-based medicine. Even in the absence of 'evidence', over-weight coronary patients should be helped and encouraged to lose weight, because weight loss reduces cardiovascular risk.

Benefits of a low-fat diet

Reducing fat intake results in a lower blood cholesterol level and a lower risk of death and cardiovascular events. In patients with coronary artery disease, this benefit occurs even in patients with a normal cholesterol level. This has formed part of secondary cardiovascular prevention, involving the prescribing of statins to virtually all patients with coronary artery disease (survivors of an infarct or those who have had angioplasty or bypass surgery) and other forms of vascular disease.

A low-fat diet reduces the frequency and severity of angina, and this may be explained by a change in the behaviour or vasomotion of coronary arteries through an action on nitric oxide.

The US National Cholesterol Education Program Population Panel has estimated that adherence to their recommendations would reduce the cholesterol level in the population by 10%, with an associated reduction in the development of atherosclerosis and its effects on the heart and brain arteries. This 10% reduction in the cholesterol level in the population would prevent 30% of all coronary heart disease events. Treating the patients in the top 10% category of cholesterol levels with lipid-lowering drugs would reduce 20% of coronary events.

Attitudes to and perceptions about diets

Some patients may be very sensitive about their weight, and may not want to discuss what they regard as a very personal issue. Before giving dietary advice, it is worth asking the patient if they want to lose weight. It should not be assumed that all overweight or obese patients want to lose weight. Most do, but do not wish to change their diet. Others are prepared to diet so long as they can eat and drink what they want. This is the common perception of a 'good' diet.

Some patients may feel that diets and changes in eating habits are for fat people who simply want to improve their appearance. Giving well-intentioned dietary advice to patients who find it offensive or insulting is both dispiriting and a waste of valuable time. However, most patients with cardiac conditions are pleased to receive advice, and expect it when they visit the surgery. Indeed, patients with cardiac conditions may be disappointed if dietary advice is not given.

Most patients are interested to know how their diet affects their heart and their health, and would expect to be asked about their fat, sugar and carbohydrate intake in the same way as they would expect to be asked about smoking and alcohol consumption. They may have read or heard about certain additives, minerals or vitamin supplements, and may ask their GP or practice nurse about these and whether they should take them.

The public is now better informed about diet and 'lifestyle', and knows that certain foods with a high fat and sugar content are 'bad' and increase the risk of coronary heart disease. Although patients may find it very difficult to follow the dietary advice offered, they usually like to know how their diet compares with what is recommended. Most of us underestimate the amount of fat and alcohol that we consume.

Patients want a quick painless 'fix' with significant weight loss that will be noticed by others. Dieting is popular, and it is a perpetual feature in lifestyle magazines for both men and women. This explains the popularity of the very large number of diet books proposing fashionable and fad diets. There are many 'wonder' diets, but in general they are tried by the desperate and result in frustration and disappointment rather than weight loss.

Patients need to understand that if they eat less food, particularly fat and carbo-hydrate, and drink less alcohol, they will lose weight, feel better, live longer and probably need fewer tablets. These benefits will be lost if they revert to their 'old habits' of eating and drinking, which will inevitably lead to their regaining the weight they worked so hard to lose. The difficulty in losing weight is not the theory, but its practice and maintenance!

Fats

Fats are essential in small amounts to transport vitamins A, D, E and K in the blood, and to manufacture prostaglandins and cell membranes. They add flavour, texture and aroma to food, and promote a feeling of fullness.

Saturated fats and cardiovascular disease

These are lauric, myristic, palmitic and stearic acids. They are hard at room temperature. Foods rich in saturated fat include meat and dairy products, and vegetable oils (e.g. coconut and palm oil). It has been known for over 20 years from the landmark Seven Countries Study that there is a direct relationship between the quantity of saturated fat intake and coronary heart disease event rates. Finland, with high levels of saturated fat intake, had the highest coronary heart disease mortality, and Japan, with the lowest saturated fat intake, had the lowest mortality. Japanese people who migrated to the USA developed higher cholesterol levels and a correspondingly higher rate of coronary heart disease events. The UK, particularly Scotland, has a high incidence of coronary heart disease compared with Mediterranean countries, and the population has a high intake of saturated fat. An explanation for the lower coronary mortality rate in obese Italians compared with obese Americans lies in their saturated fat intake. Italians eat more olive oil and pasta and less animal fat and drink more red wine than Americans, who consume a diet high in saturated fat, including hamburgers and hot dogs.

Trans-Fatty acids

These are found in vegetable oils, margarines, shortening agents in cakes and biscuits, and in milk, butter and cheese, and they increase cholesterol levels.

Unsaturated fatty acids

These lower LDL-cholesterol levels when substituted for saturated fat. They are liquid at room temperature.

- *Polyunsaturated fatty acids* include corn, sunflower, sesame and soybean oils. They increase weight because of their high calorie content. Polyunsaturates were recommended when saturated fat intake was higher, but now it is recommended that although they are less dangerous than saturated fat, their intake should be restricted and not used to lower cholesterol levels.

- *Monounsaturated fatty acids* reduce LDL-cholesterol levels, and common sources include rapeseed, olive and peanut oils, avocados and almonds.

Giving dietary advice

Dietary advice, like all medical advice, should be given with a background knowledge of the patient's medical condition, sympathetically, simply and with enthusiasm and interest. Patients need frequent monitoring and continuing support and encouragement, as dietary 'relapse' is common.

It is very important for patients to prove to themselves that they are able to lose weight if they change their eating habits, and that they will feel better and fitter and sleep better after they have lost weight.

Overweight or obese patients should be asked to record what they eat during a normal day, from the time they get up until they go to bed.

Diet clinics in primary care

These are effective, and patients generally like them because there is a medical atmosphere and they are taken seriously. They are usually run by a nurse, and may be organised on a one-to-one level or as a group. They may be part of a cardiovascular prevention clinic.

Aims of low-fat diet

These include the following:

- reducing total fat intake
- reducing saturated fat intake
- reducing dietary cholesterol
- reducing salt intake
- reducing weight.

A decrease in carbohydrate intake in conjunction with reduced fat intake is the initial step in treating type 2 (non-insulin-dependent) diabetes.

How to persuade patients to change their eating habits

To many people, the word 'diet' implies deprivation, hardship and suffering. People who tell others that they are on a diet may feel virtuous, brave and proud – all justifiable emotions. Others may feel embarrassed and consider their eating habits to be private information.

Some patients may find it preferable and less stressful or insulting if dietary recommendations for lowering their cardiovascular risk – for treatment of hypertension or hypercholesterolaemia – are not prescribed as a 'diet' but as suggestions for a long-term modification of their way of eating and living. They may find this concept less threatening and depressing. Exercise without dieting does not result in adequate weight loss.

Prescribed diets

These are difficult to understand because they recommend limits on dietary components. The National Cholesterol Education Programme (NCEP) diet for the population for primary prevention suggests restrictions of total fat to < 30% of total energy intake, saturated fat to < 10% of total energy intake, and dietary cholesterol to < 200 mg per day. The NCEP diet for patients with vascular disease recommends restricting saturated fat to < 7% of total energy intake.

The problem with recommendations of this type is that patients may not understand the terms used and what the percentages mean in practice. They need simple advice, and this explains the success and popularity of the 'Weight Watchers' and 'Slimmers World' diets, which are essentially fat and calorie reducing. The weekly weigh-ins and encouragement, the feeling of guilt of those who know why they have been unsuccessful, and the pride and sense of achievement of those who have succeeded, all provide a major incentive for the dieter.

Comparison between low-carbohydrate and low-fat diets

The amount of weight loss and its duration depend on the amount and duration of calorie reduction. Patients who are willing to try to lose weight must understand that dieting is a lifelong commitment, although not necessarily a continual daily burden. The occasional desire to feast is understandable, not life-threatening and, if planned, may be an incentive for the patient both before and after the dietary lapse.

Effect of low-fat diets on lipid levels

Total cholesterol levels fall by approximately 10%, depending on the pre-diet cholesterol intake.

The Mediterranean diet

The benefits of a 'Mediterranean diet' have been recognised since the 1950s. It is based on a diet low in saturated fat but rich in fruit, vegetables, whole-grain cereals, couscous, polenta, bulgar, beans, legumes and nuts, moderate amounts of fish, poultry and wine and occasional red meat. Olive oil is the main source of fat.

The traditional Mediterranean diet is associated with a lower total mortality, coronary mortality and mortality from cancer. The cause of this benefit is unknown, but it may be related to a combination of dietary components, olive oil and moderate amounts of wine.

The low-fat, high-carbohydrate diet

This is typified by the Asian diet, with a very low intake of saturated fat and cholesterol. It results in low total and LDL-cholesterol levels.

The low-fat, low-carbohydrate diet

This is a short-term 'no'-fat, very-low-carbohydrate diet designed for obese patients who may have diabetes, hypertension, hyperlipidaemia or vascular disease. It is particularly useful to help patients 'kick start' weight loss prior to cardiac surgery or before starting on antihypertensive or diabetic treatment. It is not dangerous, and is a slightly more explicit and rigid form of the diet recommended by the British Heart Foundation.

It is difficult but effective. Patients must be willing and able to stick to a major change in eating habits for at least 1 month. The diet should be combined with daily exercise.

Most patients will lose at least 5 kg in the first month and 3 kg in the second month, and a steady weight loss should continue until the patient achieves their goal weight. Patients should be seen regularly and weighed. When the patient has achieved their desired weight, they will need advice about future eating habits. Further supervision reduces the likelihood of relapse.

The principles of the diet may be continued long term, and patients can use a strict form of the diet for short periods to reduce their weight when they wish. Patients can stay on the diet for several months, although they tend to complain that it is boring (which it is – unless imagination and creativity are used).

Low-fat, low-carbohydrate diets result in significant weight loss and a reduction in total cholesterol, LDL-cholesterol and triglycerides.

What is allowed?
There is no restriction on the amount of fish, chicken, salad, fruit and vegetables (except potatoes and corn). The only cheese allowed is very-low-fat cottage cheese. Skimmed milk and olive oil may be used for cooking and in salads. Patients should drink as much water as they want.

What is forbidden?
- Fat: butter, cream, saturated fat oils, spreads, mayonnaise, confectionary, chocolate, cheese.
- Carbohydrate: cereals, sweets, alcohol, crisps, nuts, bread, crackers, biscuits, cakes, potatoes and pasta. Red meat is allowed once a week. Eggs should be avoided. Prepared supermarket foods, even the 'low-fat' kind, may contain high levels of fat and salt, which is relevant in patients with hypertension and heart failure.

Low-fat diets rich in fish, fruit, vegetables and whole grains, combined with exercise maintained over a long time, have been shown to reduce the rate of death from cardiovascular causes. Fat intake should represent less than 30% of the total calorie intake.

Patients should be encouraged to cook and prepare their food imaginatively. They are very happy and proud when they lose weight. Constipation is rare, due to the high fibre content, and diarrhoea is very unusual. Patients should be monitored and encouraged to continue with the diet until they have achieved their optimum weight or body mass index, and when they do, they can very gradually introduce a small amount of carbohydrate.

After they have achieved their target weight, they may then relax the diet but adhere to the main principles, and revert to the diet for a few days at a time if their weight starts to creep up.

High-protein, high-fat, low-carbohydrate diet

This is currently fashionable, and is the basis of the popular Dr Atkins diet. Like most diets, it is effective in some patients who like the freedom and encouragement to eat protein and fat while reducing their total calorie intake. The diet allows unlimited fat and protein intake, but prohibits carbohydrate and fruit and vegetables. Not surprisingly, it increases the cholesterol and triglyceride levels, and this is very undesirable in patients with coronary artery disease or who are at risk of developing coronary artery disease. Patients often complain of unpleasant constipation and wind. Weight loss with these diets is due to the duration of the diet and the restriction of calories, but not to the reduction in carbohydrate intake alone.

Two recent studies have shown that, compared with a traditional low-fat diet (< 30% of the total calorie intake), a low-carbohydrate diet followed for 90 days resulted in a greater weight loss. After 1 year, there was no significant difference in weight between the patients in the two groups, probably because of non-compliance, and this highlights the well-known difficulty, particularly among those who are obese and who have a fondness for food, of maintaining a healthy eating habit. The potential problems of a long-term low-carbohydrate, high-fat, high-protein diet are listed in Table 7.1. Nevertheless, the dangers of severe obesity probably outweigh those of a high fat diet in an otherwise healthy person.

Table 7.1: Comparison of low-carbohydrate and low-fat diets

Variable	Low-carbohydrate, high-fat diet	Low-fat diet
LDL-cholesterol	No change	Decrease
HDL-cholesterol	Moderate increase	Slight increase
Triglycerides	Moderate decrease	Slight decrease
Caloric restriction	Not necessary Induced ketosis reduces calorie intake	Necessary
Food choices	Very restricted	Moderately restricted
Rate of weight loss	Rapid initially with diuresis	Gradual with some diuresis
Potential long-term concerns	Calciuria (decreased bone mass and renal stones) Caution about high protein in patients with renal or liver disease Atherogenicity (high fat and low fruit and vegetable grain intake) Fibre and vitamin deficiency	None

It is important to ask all patients if they are on a particular diet or are taking any dietary supplements (conventional or homeopathic). Supplements may have 'an effect' in lowering cholesterol levels, but this may not translate into a reduction in coronary heart disease.

Fish oils

Oils found in oily fish (e.g. salmon, mackerel, swordfish) contain n-3 fatty acids which may provide protection against cardiovascular disease, possibly by reducing ventricular arrhythmias and sudden death. There may be other beneficial effects of oily fish on triglycerides levels, blood pressure and clotting mechanisms. It is recommended that oily fish is eaten twice a week.

Dietary fibre

This is an important part of a balanced diet. Insoluble fibre is roughage and reduces constipation. Sources that have a high content of insoluble fibre include blackberries, beans, parsnips, pears, whole-grain bread and wheat bran. Soluble fibre is found in oatbran, dried beans, grains, green vegetables and fruit. It reduces total and LDL-cholesterol by altering bile acid metabolism.

Soya protein

This lowers cholesterol levels, but the mechanism is unclear. It contains isoflavanoids and antioxidants, and may affect platelets and thrombin.

Coffee

Boiled coffee increases total and LDL-cholesterol levels due to the alcohols in the oil droplets (cafestrol and kahweol). Although drinking more than five cups of coffee a day has been shown to increase the risk of coronary artery disease, drinking one or two cups per day probably has no effect on either lipid levels or coronary heart disease rates.

Garlic

One half to one whole clove of garlic a day decreases total cholesterol by 9%, but there is no good evidence that garlic has any beneficial effect on coronary heart disease.

Alcohol

Alcohol is calorific, fattening, and increases triglyceride levels, blood pressure and, importantly, HDL-cholesterol levels. In excess it leads to hypertension, cardiomyopathy and arrhythmia (ectopics and atrial fibrillation).

Moderate alcohol consumption (1 to 2 units per day) decreases cardiovascular mortality, and this could be explained by the increase in HDL-cholesterol. It has been suggested that red wine consumption might explain the low cardiac mortality rate in France (the 'French paradox'). The French eat quite a lot of fat, including cheese, but the population has high HDL-cholesterol levels. Alcohol also increases endogenous tissue plasminogen activator and lowers fibrinogen levels. However, a study comparing red and white wine showed no difference in LDL-cholesterol oxidation.

Consumption of alcohol in moderation appears to exert a more striking beneficial effect in women, who have a lower threshold for developing cardiomyopathy.

Drug treatment

Sibutramine

This drug has been licensed for the treatment of obese patients with a body mass index of $> 30 \, \text{kg/m}^2$, and for patients with a body mass index of $> 27 \, \text{kg/m}^2$ if they have diabetes or dyslipidaemias. It inhibits the reuptake of noradrenaline and serotonin in the brain, and so reduces appetite. Most patients take 10 mg every morning. It should be used as part of a weight-reducing programme combined with exercise and a low-calorie diet.

It can be expected to result in a 5–10% weight loss, with associated benefits in the lipid profile.

It may result in an increase in blood pressure, so blood pressure monitoring is advised during treatment. It should be used with caution in patients with arrhythmias and coronary heart disease, and is contraindicated in patients with recent myocardial infarction (within the previous 6 weeks).

Advice for patients

- A healthy diet and maintenance of an optimum weight are important. Eating a healthy diet, not smoking and taking regular exercise will reduce your risk of heart disease and diabetes and increase your chances of survival after a heart attack. It will also make you feel better and more energetic.
- The less you eat, the more weight you will lose.
- The quickest way to lose weight is a no-fat, very-low-carbohydrate diet that includes plenty of natural food – salad, fruit and vegetables, fish and moderate amounts of meat.
- A key part of a healthy diet is reducing the amount of fat you eat. Try to avoid saturated fat (butter, cream, cheese, fast food), food cooked in fat (crisps, chips, deep-fried food), chocolate, eggs, liver and fatty meat.
- Avoid salt and salty food.
- Moderate alcohol consumption (2 units per day) is acceptable. There is no convincing evidence that red wine is better than white. However, alcohol is fattening, and ideally should be avoided completely while you are trying to lose weight.

Answers to clinical cases

1 This patient should not go on the Atkins diet. Instead she should be advised to follow a conventional low-fat, high-fibre diet containing plenty of fruit, vegetables and fish and a moderate amount of alcohol, as advised by the British Heart Foundation.

2 Tell this patient that moderate wine consumption is acceptable and might be good for him, but that one bottle a day is too much. He should have a cardiovascular risk assessment, have his cardiac medication checked and be advised about diet, weight and exercise. He may already have had or be

scheduled for coronary angiography, and this will provide the information that he wants about the reasons for his recent heart problem.

3   This patient appears keen to reduce his cardiovascular risk. Anyone who succeeds in stopping smoking should be able, with help and support, to change their eating habits. Discuss various dietary approaches, point out specifically the potential benefits, and either enrol him in a cardiovascular prevention clinic at your surgery or, if possible, see him yourself until he is on the right path. He will need continual supervision. All other cardiovascular prevention measures, including exercise, are important.

Further reading

- Albert CM, Campos H, Stampfer MJ *et al.* (2002) Blood levels of long-chain n-3 fatty acids and the risk of sudden death. *NEJM.* **346**: 1113–28.
- Barsch GS, Farooqi IS and O'Rahilly S (2000) Genetics of body-weight regulation. *Nature.* **404**: 644–51.
- Bravata DM, Sanders L, Huang J *et al.* (2003) Efficacy and safety of low-carbohydrate diets: a systematic review. *JAMA.* **289**: 1837–50.
- Foster GD, Wyatt HR, Hill JO *et al.* (2003) A randomised trial of a low-carbohydrate diet for obesity. *NEJM.* **348**: 2082–90.
- James WPT, Astrup A, Finer N *et al.* for the STORM Study Group (2000) Effect of sibutramine on weight maintenance after weight loss: a randomised trial. *Lancet.* **356**: 2119–25.
- Kenchaiah S, Evans JC, Levy D *et al.* (2002) Obesity and the risk of heart failure. *NEJM.* **347**: 305–13.
- Keys A (1980) *Seven Countries: a multivariate analysis of death and coronary heart disease.* Harvard University Press, Cambridge, MA.
- LaCroix AZ, Mead LA, Liang KY *et al.* (1986) Coffee consumption and the incidence of coronary heart disease. *NEJM.* **315**: 377–82.
- Must A, Spadano J, Coakley EH *et al.* (1999) The disease burden associated with overweight and obesity. *JAMA.* **282**: 1523–9.
- National Cholesterol Education Program (1990) *Report of the Expert Panel on Population Strategies for Blood Cholesterol Reduction.* US Department of Health and Human Services, Washington DC.
- Royal College of Physicians (1998) *Clinical Management of Overweight and Obese Patients with Particular Reference to the Use of Drugs.* Royal College of Physicians, London.
- Samaha FF, Iqbal N, Sesadri P *et al.* (2003) A low-carbohydrate as compared with a low-fat diet in severe obesity. *NEJM.* **348**: 2074–81.
- Trichopoulou A, Costacou T, Bamia C *et al.* (2003) Adherence to a Mediterranean diet and survival in a Greek population. *NEJM.* **348**: 2599–608.
- Wirth A and Krause J (2001) Long-term weight loss with sibutramine: a randomised controlled trial. *JAMA.* **286**: 1331–9.

CHAPTER 8

Smoking

Case studies

1 An 81-year-old man who has smoked 40 cigarettes a day for at least 60 years and who is hypertensive with a history of previous transient ischaemic attack comes to your surgery complaining of chest pain. Apart from reviewing his treatment for hypertension, checking his blood pressure, checking his diabetic status and advising him to stop smoking, what else would you do?

2 A 43-year-old man attends your surgery 2 weeks after a heart attack. He is symptom free and has not been able to stop smoking, and would like your help. What would you do?

3 A 64-year-old woman who smokes 20 cigarettes per day, with cor pulmonale and chronic obstructive airways disease comes to see you with a chest infection. What would you do?

4 An 18-year-old girl who smokes 10 cigarettes a day wants to start on the oral contraceptive pill. What would you do?

5 A 52-year-old woman with a long history of depression, alcoholism and previous oesophageal pain, and who smokes 30 cigarettes a day, comes to see you complaining of chest pain. What would you do?

Prevalence and risks

An estimated 13 million people smoke in the UK, with an equal proportion of males and females. Smoking is more prevalent in those of lower socioeconomic class and lower educational status. It is becoming more common in young girls and boys, so school education and prevention programmes are important. It can become an addiction shortly after starting the habit.

Smoking is the single largest cause of death, disability, preventable illness and unnecessary health expense in the UK. It is a direct cause of cancer of the lung, larynx, mouth, oesophagus and bladder, and it contributes to the development of cancer of the kidney, bladder, pancreas and cervix. It is the main cause of chronic obstructive pulmonary disease, which may result in right heart failure. It has been estimated to cause 17–30% of all cardiovascular deaths. Smoking shortens the lifespan by an estimated 10 years. About 50% of smokers die of a smoking-related illness.

Smoking and cardiovascular disease

Cardiovascular disease is the commonest smoking-related cause of death, with 25% of deaths in the 35–69 years age group being due to tobacco. Mortality after myocardial infarction is lower in patients who stop smoking compared with those who continue. Furthermore, the risk of a coronary event declines rapidly after stopping smoking. After 2–3 years of abstinence the risk of such an event is similar to that for individuals who have never smoked.

Passive smoking

With passive smoking the cardiovascular risk increases by 25%, and the lung cancer risk increases by 30%.

Smoking and cardiovascular risk

Middle-aged men who smoke more than 20 cigarettes a day have a two to three times higher risk of a major cardiac event compared to non-smokers of the same age. The risk of developing coronary heart disease is dose related. The cardiovascular morbidity and mortality risks for women are similar to those for men, but the risk of fatal myocardial infarction is 13 times higher if they use the oral contraceptive pill.

Effects of nicotine on the cardiovascular system

1 Atherosclerosis:
   - direct damage to arterial endothelium
   - increased smooth muscle proliferation
   - reduced endothelial-dependent vasodilatation
   - reduced HDL-cholesterol levels.

2 Thrombosis:
   - increased platelet stickiness
   - increased fibrinogen levels
   - increased plasma viscosity
   - increased arterial wall stiffness and tendency for plaque rupture.

3 Coronary artery spasm:
   - coronary vasoconstriction.

4 Arrhythmias:
   - cathecholamines may decrease the threshold for arrhythmias
   - increased oxygen demand
   - reduced oxygen-carrying capacity.

Benefits of smoking cessation

The risk of coronary heart disease falls by 50% 1 year after cessation, and after 4 years it is similar to that for a person who has never smoked. This benefit also applies to smokers aged over 60 years.

Smoking cessation reduces restenosis after coronary angioplasty, and reduces graft stenosis after coronary artery surgery and peripheral vascular surgery.

After smoking cessation, the risks of cancer and chronic obstructive pulmonary disease both fall progressively to near the levels in non-smokers.

Cigars

Cigar smokers are at similar risk to cigarette smokers. Because cigars vary in length and tobacco content, and whether the smoker inhales and how quickly the cigar is smoked, it is difficult to predict the risk according to the cigar size.

Pipe smokers

There is no evidence that pipe smokers are at lower risk of cardiovascular disease than cigarette smokers. Pipe smokers may in fact be at greater risk because of the amount of nicotine smoked in each pipe and the length of time for which the smoker keeps sucking and inhaling on the pipe.

Benefits of smoking cessation

Smoking cessation should be the main focus of risk reduction for patients with vascular disease, and should be managed like heroin and cocaine addiction. Stopping smoking reduces the 10-year risk of death by over half (from 54% to 18%). It is the single most important intervention conferring the greatest symptomatic and prognostic benefit. Patients who continue to smoke are at three times greater risk of death than those who quit.

Problems with smoking cessation

Addiction

Nicotine is highly addictive. In approximately 50% of people, withdrawal results in depression, insomnia, irritability, anxiety, difficulty in concentration, restlessness, increased appetite and weight gain. The symptoms appear within a few hours, peak at 1 to 2 days and last for several weeks at least, and in some people for many months.

Weight gain

Most people gain at least 3 kg in weight and some gain much more. Fear of weight gain is a potent deterrent for people (particularly women) who would otherwise want to stop smoking, so this needs to be addressed in smoking cessation programmes which should, where appropriate, address all of the risk factors.

Role of primary care physicians in smoking cessation

A smoking cessation programme is an important primary care service with major primary and secondary cardiac prevention and general health benefits. Ideally it should be combined with other cardiac risk factor interventions.

Partners, spouses, relatives, work colleagues and schoolfriends

The influence of other smokers on the smoking habits of the patient are difficult to quantify, but should not be underestimated. There are few data on this. Smokers find it understandably exceptionally difficult to stop smoking, even with motivation, if they are in close contact at home or at work with other smokers who may feel resentful if told that they should stop smoking. Peer pressure among schoolchildren is a well-recognised and powerful influence that induces children to smoke.

Smoking cessation programmes

Unfortunately, smoking cessation programmes and treatments have a very low success rate, and success ultimately depends on the smoker wanting to stop smoking, making a serious and sustained effort and being prepared to suffer the withdrawal symptoms, which can last for a long time. Some quitters claim that the desire to smoke is always there.

It is not enough simply to advise patients to stop smoking. A two-minute 'lecture' or admonishment by a doctor has little long-term effect. The success of a consultation advising a patient to stop smoking will depend on how the message is conveyed to the patient and, most importantly, on the patient's willingness and motivation to stop. Patients are more likely to stop smoking after a heart attack, or after coronary angiography has shown important coronary artery disease necessitating myocardial revascularisation.

Smoking cessation advice given by more than one primary care health professional is more effective than such advice given by only one clinician. Success rates improve when additional advice is given by a specialist, and when intense, frequent and prolonged sessions are provided. The resource implications are substantial, and need to be supported.

Smokers usually need to make major changes to their lifestyle because of the situations in which they smoke. For example, people often smoke in pubs and restaurants, under stressful circumstances, and when they are around other smokers.

No-smoking areas in public places, places of work and public transport facilities should help to reduce the incidence of smoking.

The 4 A's primary care approach to help patients to stop smoking

- Ask: identify smokers in the practice.
- Advise: strongly advise all smokers to stop, and explain the risks of continuing and the benefits of stopping.
- Assist: set a 'stop date', and offer nicotine replacement, a smoking cessation clinic, written supplementary materials and motivational advice, and encourage relatives and friends to offer support and encouragement.
- Arrange: follow-up advice and clinics.

Patients know that smoking is dangerous, but even after a heart attack they find it difficult to stop smoking completely and permanently. Patients who do not quit are often embarrassed about what they might perceive as a character defect, and do not want to tell the doctor or nurse that they have not stopped.

Success of smoking cessation clinics

Patients should be helped with a smoking cessation programme that combines group, drug and behavioural therapy, and this combined approach results in 40% of participants stopping smoking for at least 1 year. This programme can be led by suitably trained, enthusiastic staff who may themselves have quit smoking successfully. A joint collaborative programme could be established between neighbouring practices.

Nicotine replacement treatment

This improves the smoking cessation rate. Patient preferences for gum, skin patches or spray vary. Prescribe the form of nicotine replacement that the patient finds most acceptable.

The long-term success rate of nicotine patches in helping smokers to stop the habit is low. Only 5% of people remain abstinent from smoking 8 years after using a nicotine patch for a single 12-week treatment period.

Bupropion

This is a non-nicotine-based treatment for use in smoking cessation. It is effective and well tolerated. It is as effective as nicotine replacement and significantly more effective than placebo as an aid to stopping smoking at 1 year of follow-up after an 8-week treatment period. It has been recommended as an aid to smoking cessation by the National Institute for Clinical Excellence, and is available on NHS prescription. It is an antidepressant with noradrenergic and dopaminergic activity. Despite its mode of action, it does not appear to affect blood pressure.

It is recommended for smokers who are particularly refractory to other treatment. The recommended dose is 150 mg twice a day, usually for 7 weeks. It should be started a day or two before the intended start of smoking cessation and continued for 2 to 3 months. It is contraindicated in epileptics and those with a tendency to seizures. It has no significant cardiovascular side-effects, and can be used in patients with coronary artery disease.

When used in conjunction with group and individual counselling techniques, bupropion is twice as effective as placebo in helping patients to quit smoking. Side-effects include a dry mouth and insomnia, and it is contraindicated in patients with epilepsy, psychosis or severe panic disorders.

The indications for buproprion include the following:

- motivated addicted smokers who are keen to quit
- nicotine dependence
- patients involved in a support programme.

Clonidine

This is an α-blocker that is used to treat hypertension. It has been used to dampen nicotine withdrawal in doses of 0.1 mg to 0.4 mg daily for 2 to 6 weeks. It is indicated for patients who prefer not to receive nicotine replacement. It can be used in both oral and patch forms. The side-effects include sedation, dry mouth and postural hypotension.

Other forms of therapy

The Cochrane group found that hypnotherapy, acupuncture and aversion therapy had no significant effect in helping patients to quit smoking.

The future

Although prevention is better than cure, it is unlikely that the sale of tobacco will be made illegal. A programme of education in schools and the banning of advertising would probably be the most effective interventions.

Advice for patients

- The nicotine, tar and carbon monoxide in cigarettes are very dangerous and cause irreparable damage to your heart, your arteries and your lungs.
- Stopping smoking is more important than anything else you can do yourself to improve your health and reduce your risks of having a heart attack, a stroke or lung cancer. Your health will improve from the day you stop.

- We understand how difficult it is to stop, and we will help you.
- Even though we are willing to help you, this is something that you have to want to do, and to do for yourself and your family.
- If you smoke after a heart bypass operation, balloon angioplasty or a heart attack, it is likely that the arteries will block off and you will put yourself at risk of a heart attack or developing angina.
- Your angina will almost certainly improve if you stop smoking.
- Smoking is the most important cause of 'furring up' of the arteries of the legs. If you continue to smoke, the blood supply to your legs and feet may stop and this may be very serious.
- Women on the oral contraceptive pill who also smoke are at high risk of developing heart disease, and if they cannot stop smoking they should stop the pill.
- Come to our smoking cessation clinic. Your friends, partner or spouse should try to help you to stop. Cutting down is not stopping.
- You have to set yourself a 'stop date', understand and be prepared for the effects of withdrawal from a very addictive habit, change your daily routine and get away from the habits associated with smoking. This may be the pub, so you will have to be prepared to sacrifice parts of your lifestyle that you enjoy. Take one day at a time. It takes several months to 'kick the habit', but it will be worth it.
- Don't worry about putting on weight. You will not put on weight if you do not alter your eating habits. When you stop smoking your appetite may increase because you will rediscover your sense of smell and taste. Just be careful, but enjoy!
- There are a number of smoking cessation aids which can help, but you have to do the main part.
- Nicotine replacement and bupropion may help if you are having difficulty on your own.
- Nicotine replacements (patches, gum, lozenges, etc.) contain nicotine, but are safer than cigarettes.
- Bupropion (Zyban) may help, but may not completely take away the urge to smoke. The course lasts for 8 weeks, and we can give it to you on the NHS. It may cause side-effects.
- Some people have found hypnotherapy and acupuncture helpful. Do whatever works for you.

Answers to case studies

1   There is only a small chance that this patient will be motivated to stop smoking, but he should be offered advice and a smoking cessation clinic. The risks of continuing smoking and the benefits of smoking cessation should be discussed with him. All of his risk factors should be evaluated carefully and treated. He should be on aspirin if he can tolerate this.

2   Find out whether this patient wants to stop smoking, and give him advice and outline to him the importance of stopping. Early after an infarct is a good opportunity to help him stop smoking using all available techniques. His risk of further cardiac events should be evaluated, and if he has not seen a cardiologist, he should be referred to one.

3   Treat the chest infection, exclude lung cancer and optimise the patient's cardiac treatment. Even though it is unlikely that she will either want or be able to stop smoking, she should be given advice and help in a realistic and sympathetic way.

4   Discuss the vascular and thrombotic risks of the combination of smoking and the oral contraceptive pill, and discuss other forms of contraception if the patient insists on continuing to smoke.

5   This patient may have coronary artery disease and angina. The history is important, but it may be difficult to obtain. She should be referred for cardiac evaluation, and if the cardiac tests show a low probability of coronary artery disease, she should be investigated for oesophageal reflux and other gastrointestinal problems. It is unlikely that she will respond to advice to stop smoking or a smoking cessation programme, but if you have the resources and she is willing to consider this, she should be offered the opportunity. She may need further specialist input for her other problems.

Further reading

- Chambers R, Wakley G and Iqbal Z (2001) *Cardiovascular Disease Matters in Primary Care.* Radcliffe Medical Press, Oxford.
- Iqbal Z, Chambers R and Woodmansey P (2001) *Implementing the National Service Frameworks for Coronary Heart Disease in Primary Care.* Radcliffe Medical Press, Oxford.

These two books published by Radcliffe Medical Press contain sensible practical advice for primary care professionals about setting up smoking cessation clinics.

- Critchley J and Capewell S (2004) *Smoking cessation for the secondary prevention of coronary heart disease.* Cochrane Database Systematic Review (1) CD003041.
- Hirsch AT, Treat-Jacobson D, Landon HA *et al.* (1997) The role of tobacco cessation, anti-platelet and lipid-lowering therapies in the treatment of peripheral arterial disease. *Vasc Med.* **2**: 243–52.
- National Institute for Clinical Excellence (2002) *Guidance on the Use of Nicotine Replacement Therapy (NRT) and Bupropion for Smoking Cessation.* Technology Appraisal Guidance. No. 39. National Institute for Clinical Excellence, London.
- Tonstad S, Farsang C, Klaene G *et al.* (2003) Bupropion SR for smoking cessation in smokers with cardiovascular disease: a multicentre, randomised study. *Eur Heart J.* **24**: 946–55.
- Yudkin P, Hey K, Roberts S *et al.* (2003) Abstinence from smoking eight years after participation in a randomised controlled trial of nicotine patch. *BMJ.* **327**: 28–9.

CHAPTER 9

Benefits and risks of exercise and rehabilitation

Case studies

1 A 57-year-old previously fit man comes to see you 1 week after an un-complicated myocardial infarction. He wants to know when he can go back to the gym to do some cycling, treadmill work and weight-lifting. What advice would you give him?

2 A 38-year-old man joins your practice and tells you that he has familial hypertrophic cardiomyopathy. He would like to join the local gym, but he needs a doctor's letter confirming that he is fit. What would you do?

3 A 64-year-old man has mild hypertension, a slightly raised cholesterol level and borderline diabetes. He is very reluctant to take any tablets, and feels fine. What would you do?

4 A 55-year-old woman who is the carer for her elderly and immobile mother asks you if there is anything that can be done to improve the quality of both their lives. What would you suggest?

Introduction

Most people in the UK do not take enough physical exercise to benefit their health. Physical inactivity is a strong, graded risk factor for coronary heart disease. Physical inactivity doubles the risk of developing cardiovascular disease.

Regular exercise is inexpensive and has many health and cardiovascular benefits. It should constitute part of daily activities for people of all ages for primary and secondary cardiovascular prevention and for treating established cardiac disease. Even a single exercise session has beneficial effects on triglyceride levels, systolic blood pressure and insulin sensitivity. There is a linear decline in the risk of coronary artery disease with increasing levels of physical activity. Walking fast for one hour every day has been shown to reduce cardiovascular events by 28%.

Primary care health professionals have a pivotal role and a responsibility to educate patients and encourage them to exercise.

Regular exercise:

- prevents atherosclerotic coronary artery disease
- reduces mortality after myocardial infarction

- improves the cardiovascular risk profile
- improves exercise capacity in patients with stable angina, heart failure and claudication
- lowers blood pressure
- prevents the development of non-insulin-dependent diabetes by lowering blood glucose levels
- helps in the treatment of obesity
- lowers plasma fibrinogen levels and improves haemostatic parameters
- improves the lipid profile, with increases in HDL-cholesterol levels
- improves the psychological state.

Effects of regular exercise on cardiovascular risk factors

Lipid profile

> Regular exercise reduces lipid levels slightly, but when combined with a low-fat diet it may render drug treatment for hyperlipidaemia unnecessary.

Total cholesterol is reduced by at least 6%, LDL-cholesterol is reduced by 10% and HDL-cholesterol increases by 14%. The effects are enhanced by a low-fat diet and weight loss. The beneficial effects of exercise on the lipid profile are most pronounced in overweight patients with high triglyceride levels and low HDL-cholesterol levels. It is difficult to separate the independent effects of exercise, because people who are motivated to exercise regularly usually change their diet, too.

Obesity

Exercise alone has a modest effect on weight loss (approximately 3 kg) over a period of several months. When combined with diet, most people can lose 8 kg.

Hypertension

Regular physical activity prevents the development of hypertension and lowers blood pressure. Sedentary people have a 35% higher risk of developing hypertension compared with active people. Gentle cardiovascular exercise (e.g. running, cycling) reduces diastolic blood pressure, whereas heavy isometric exercise (e.g. weight-training) may increase systolic blood pressure and left ventricular wall thickness.

> Regular exercise, particularly when combined with weight reduction, may reduce blood pressure sufficiently to render antihypertensive treatment unnecessary in patients with mild hypertension.

Diabetes

Exercise has a beneficial effect on blood glucose levels and insulin sensitivity. Glucose production by the liver is decreased. Exercise and weight loss prevent the onset of non-insulin-dependent diabetes, but it is less clear whether they prevent insulin-dependent diabetes. Glycosylated haemoglobin is reduced by 1%.

Smoking

Regular exercise increases the likelihood of successful smoking cessation.

Thrombosis

Individuals who are physically active are at lower risk of cardiovascular events. In older people (aged over 60 years), fibrinogen levels are reduced by 13% and active tissue plasminogen activator is decreased by 140%. These changes have also been seen in younger people and in patients after myocardial infarction. In addition, platelet aggregation is reduced after regular exercise. Endothelial function is improved, and this may also account for the reduced thrombotic tendency after regular exercise.

Autonomic effects

Regular exercise increases parasympathetic tone and decreases sympathetic tone, and these combined effects may contribute to the reduction in cardiovascular risk. Regular exercise in young people results in a resting bradycardia. Neurally mediated syncope or near syncope in trained individuals is due to a high vagal tone.

Psychological effects

People exercise because they will feel and look better and fitter, and this can help depression and anxiety. People who exercise regularly are also more likely to be concerned about their health and make other lifestyle changes. It may be possible to harness their enthusiasm to help other patients.

Haemodynamic effects of exercise

These depend on the following:

- the type of exercise performed – isotonic (e.g. jogging, swimming or cycling) or isometric (e.g. weight-lifting)
- the muscles used (upper vs. lower body)
- body position.

Exercise results in increases in heart rate, systolic blood pressure, cardiac output and VO_2 (a measure of energy expenditure and oxygen utilisation). Diastolic blood pressure falls during exercise, due to peripheral vasodilatation. These factors lead to an increase in myocardial oxygen demand, and this is the basis of exercise stress testing in the evaluation of patients with known or suspected coronary artery disease. The stress test evaluates whether the myocardial blood and oxygen supply can meet the imposed demands.

Normal coronary arteries dilate with exercise, but this response is impaired in patients with atheroma. Chest tightness and breathlessness may develop in patients with an impaired myocardial oxygen supply, and muscle fatigue and breathlessness may develop in those with impaired heart muscle function.

Training effects

Regular endurance training results in muscular, cardiovascular and neurohumoral changes which improve functional capacity and strength, allowing the individual to exercise more efficiently – that is, to higher workloads with a lower heart rate.

Muscular changes

There are increases in skeletal muscle mitochondria, myoglobin, capillary density and metabolic enzymes. This promotes aerobic metabolism and increased exercise capacity with lower lactate levels through the use of fatty acids rather than glycogen for energy production. Isometric resistance exercise results in muscle-cell hypertrophy.

Cardiovascular changes

Increases in left ventricular wall thickness result from increases in afterload due to a rise in total peripheral resistance and systolic blood pressure. Exercise training results in less myocardial ischaemia in patients with coronary artery disease, and this is manifested as an increased exercise time to the onset of angina and an increased exercise time before the onset of ST depression, probably because of the mechanisms listed above.

Neurohumoral changes

The resting heart rate is increased due to an increase in parasympathetic tone, a decrease in sympathetic tone and a reduction in circulating catecholamines.

Detraining

The benefits of training are lost quickly, within 3 weeks or less, and this is apparent to all who stop regular exercise for any reason.

Cardiovascular benefits of exercise

There is a progressive decrease in cardiovascular events with increasing intensity of cardiovascular exercise. Walking at 3 mph for 1 hour each day has been shown to reduce the risk of cardiovascular events in healthy women by at least 30%, and overall in men and women by as much as 50%. These beneficial effects are probably due to a combination of the effects that exercise has on cardiovascular risk factors.

Exercise programmes in primary care

How much?

All people who are able to do so should exercise to at least moderate levels in order to break into a sweat and become breathless, for 30 minutes every day, with an average weekly calorie expenditure of 1400 calories. The American Heart Association recommends a weekly calorie expenditure of 700–2000 calories. Cycling for 20 minutes against a moderate resistance to 70% of age-predicted maximum heart rate expends approximately 240 calories.

Cardiovascular mortality decreases with increasing daily calorie expenditure and increasing exercise duration.

Cardiovascular risk decreases with increasing intensity and duration of exercise. Therefore the more exercise the better, in nearly everyone.

What is moderate exercise?

Moderate exercise is achieved by walking briskly at 3 to 4 mph for long enough to become breathless. Slower but sustained walking may be adequate for elderly people, because they have a lower peak heart rate and less exercise is required to achieve a training effect. Carrying weights increases the work performed and the exercise intensity. Any exercise is better than none, so walking the dog or playing nine holes of golf is better than sitting, although a round of golf would constitute at most only very mild cardiovascular exercise. In general, irrespective of the fitness of the individual in question, exercise should result in a doubling of the resting heart rate for at least 30 minutes a day.

What exercise should be recommended?

It does not matter whether exercise is taken inside or outside the home. Treadmills are useful because they allow increases in speed and inclination and result in less impact trauma to the leg and foot joints. Cycling and stair climbing should also be encouraged, and these are useful forms of exercise.

All muscle groups should be exercised and stretched. Isometric exercise should be performed carefully and after guidance, and is not recommended for patients with certain cardiac conditions (see below). The level and duration of exercise should be tailored to the individual. For example, after myocardial infarction a patient may have had a pre-discharge exercise test which would provide prognostic information, form the basis of an exercise prescription and reassure the patient and their family that exercise is safe and should form part of their daily activities and secondary prevention programme.

Both walking and vigorous exercise are associated with a substantial reduction in the incidence of cardiovascular events in postmenopausal women, irrespective of race, ethnic group, age or body mass index.

> Exercise should be considered as important as aspirin by patients with coronary artery disease, and as beneficial as diuretics by those with heart failure.

Exercise for the elderly and physically less able

Although it may be impossible for elderly, bed-bound or chair-bound patients to perform conventional cardiovascular exercise, they may nevertheless be able, with help and encouragement, to do passive exercise and breathing exercises. Elderly people can remain active and independent for longer if they are encouraged to remain physically and mentally active.

Home- or health-centre-based programmes may be possible with enthusiastic helpers and some guidance from experienced professionals. These may be physiotherapists or nurses who have gained experience in a neurological or cardiac rehabilitation unit. Cardiac rehabilitation will be discussed later.

In whom is exercise potentially dangerous?

Sudden cardiac death due to ventricular tachycardia and ventricular fibrillation may occur in young fit athletes with inherited or congenital cardiovascular abnormalities. It may also occur in patients with coronary artery disease or structural heart disease (e.g. severe hypertrophic cardiomyopathy or aortic valve stenosis).

Sudden cardiac death in young athletes

The risk is low, probably less than 1 in 200 000. Death typically occurs either during or immediately after exercise.

It is not standard practice in the UK to screen all athletes for cardiovascular disease, because of the high prevalence of false-positive results and the cost implications. High-risk individuals should be evaluated on the basis of the nature and severity of the cardio-vascular condition and the classification of the sport involved.

The current recommendations for participation in competitive sports are summarised in Table 9.1.

Screening young athletes at high risk

Individuals at high risk include those with symptoms, the abnormalities listed in Table 9.1 or a family history of premature cardiac disease or sudden death. Screening should include history and examination, resting ECG and two-dimensional echocardiogram to look for structural and functional abnormalities. Stress testing is required to evaluate those with suspected coronary artery disease, and ambulatory ECG recordings are needed for those with palpitation.

Seeding an exercise philosophy for life in the young

People in the UK are exercising more than their parents and grandparents did, and this encouraging trend should continue if schoolchildren are encouraged to view exercise as a 'life skill'. This would necessitate political will and support. Competitive school sports

Table 9.1: Current recommendations for participation in competitive sports

Diagnosis	Recommendations
Hypertrophic cardiomyopathy	Should not participate in competitive sports
Congenital coronary artery anomalies	Should not participate in competitive sports unless they have been revascularised and have no residual ischaemia
Wolff-Parkinson-White syndrome	Can participate if there is no structural heart disease, palpitation or tachycardia
	Can participate after successful accessory pathway ablation
Dilated cardiomyopathy	Cannot participate in competitive sports
Coronary artery disease	Can participate in the absence of symptoms, ischaemia or induced arrhythmia, and if there is normal left ventricular function
Marfan's syndrome	Should not participate in competitive sport if there is a family history of sudden death or if there is aortic root dilation
	May participate in competitive sport if there is no aortic root dilation or a family history of sudden death
Myocarditis	Should not participate in competitive sport until cardiac function is normal
Aortic stenosis	Mild stenosis (< 20 mmHg) – can participate
	Moderate stenosis (< 40 mmHg) – low-intensity sport only
	Severe stenosis (> 40 mmHg) – cannot participate in any competitive sport

should be seen as part of a step towards this long-term lifestyle and engagement in the fun and enjoyment of sport, comradeship and teamwork, rather than being deprecated. Getting children and young people into the 'exercise habit' is a key part of helping them to adopt a healthy lifestyle in their adult years.

Cardiac rehabilitation

Approximately 300 000 people have a heart attack each year in the UK, with 140 000 deaths. Cardiac rehabilitation involves patient education, comprehensive secondary prevention, psychological measures to reassure patients, and exercise training. It has proven benefits after myocardial infarction, resulting in a 34% reduction in cardiac mortality and a 29% reduction in recurrent infarction. Ideally, cardiac rehabilitation after infarction should start at the time of hospital admission. It also has benefits in patients after coronary artery surgery, and in heart failure. It is most useful in patients who have lost confidence after a heart attack, or who find their cardiac condition difficult to accept or understand.

Cardiac rehabilitation can be performed safely, effectively and cheaply in primary care, but the quality of the programme depends on the enthusiasm and skills of the multi-disciplinary staff and, most importantly, of the patients and their families.

What is involved?

The patient

The patient should be willing, motivated and interested in prevention and the measures needed to improve the prognosis, and they must be prepared to use the 6- to 8-week programme of two attendances a week as a springboard for continuing self-help health-care and a lifelong commitment to regular exercise. They must take long-term, full-time control of their life and be committed to a healthy lifestyle.

The staff

Staff should receive training in a good unit, have appropriate life support skills and knowledge of defibrillation, and be given updated literature and teaching aids. Patients at high risk may need a hospital-based programme and access to staff with advanced life support training. The general thrust of each component of the programme, as outlined above, can be modified depending on the type of patient attending. Each member of the team should be encouraged to inject their own personality and, when appropriate, humour and warmth into the sessions. Without this, the sessions can become lifeless and 'sterile', and may have little impact and consequently little long-term effect.

Pre-enrolment evaluation

The patient's history can be obtained from pro formas and practice records. The blood pressure and resting heart rate should be recorded. Signs of heart failure should be sought. Patients with angina at rest, important arrhythmias, uncontrolled hypertension, or pulmonary oedema at rest should be assessed by a doctor and treated before they start the rehabilitation programme.

Facilities

A suitable space, resuscitation facilities, exercise cycles and/or treadmills or other exercise equipment, including stairs and rowing or ski machines, can be used for cardiovascular exercise. Gentle weights or medicine balls are useful for some patients. The sessions are usually run by a nurse and/or physiotherapist. Medical input adds an extra dimension. This team may be complemented by interested, trained and educated lay helpers who can provide useful reassurance, particularly if they have recovered from a heart attack or coronary artery surgery and have been through a rehabilitation programme.

The programme

Patients should be taught the principles and practice of cardiovascular prevention, and should be allowed to ask questions about their health, medical history, life stresses and anxieties. They may need specialist help for depression or psychological problems, including personal, marital or sexual problems.

The programme offers the opportunity for the primary care team to review the patient's medical history, risk factor status, diet, medication and drug compliance.

The long-term benefits of a rehabilitation programme depend on the ability of the patient to accept and follow the advice given, but this is difficult for most people, and the short-term benefits often disappear within a year. New information from clinical trials will result in new recommendations, and these need to be passed on to patients. Primary care is probably the most effective arena in which primary and secondary prevention can be offered and updated on a continuing basis, but this has major resource implications. Effective long-term risk reduction requires lifelong commitment from patients and primary care input.

Risk of death during cardiac rehabilitation

This is approximately 1 per 170 000 patient hours of participation.

Exercise training for patients with coronary heart disease

Until the advent and widespread use of aspirin, β-blockers, angiotensin-converting-enzyme (ACE) inhibitors, thrombolytics and acute coronary angioplasty, regular exercise and other risk factor interventions were the only effective secondary preventive therapies available after myocardial infarction. Exercise training for 2 to 6 months following myocardial infarction, combined with smoking cessation and dietary changes, reduced total mortality by 20%, cardiovascular mortality by 22%, fatal reinfarctions by 25% and sudden death at 1 year by 37%. Current drug treatments have greatly reduced mortality and morbidity after infarction, so the benefits of exercise training may not be as great, but it is still worthwhile when combined with other interventions.

In patients with mild to moderate angina, exercise training improves exercise capacity by the haemodynamic mechanisms mentioned above.

Exercise training for patients with congestive heart failure

Exercise training improves exercise capacity but not survival.

Exercise training for patients with peripheral vascular disease

Regular exercise increases claudication distance by 180% or approximately 225 m to the onset of pain, and should be strongly recommended to all suitable patients with claudication. The greatest improvement is seen when patients are exercised to maximal levels (maximum tolerated pain). The mechanism responsible for this is unclear, but may relate to opening of collaterals. These results are as good as those for surgical and pharmacological therapies.

Athlete's heart and cardiovascular responses

Patients may ask about the potential cardiac dangers of regular training and sport. This would include elite athletes and those who participate in high-level competitive sports. It is important for primary care physicians to be aware of the effects of exercise on the heart – including which clinical and investigative findings are abnormal and require further evaluation, and which are normal and do not.

It is important to distinguish athlete's heart from hypertrophic cardiomyopathy. A diagnosis of hypertrophic cardiomyopathy excludes an athlete from competition, with adverse financial, psychological and physical consequences. Patients with hypertrophic cardiomyopathy typically have severe left ventricular hypertrophy on echocardiography, but some have only slight hypertrophy, making it difficult to distinguish the two conditions, which may also coexist.

ECG changes

Approximately one-third of athletes have an abnormal ECG, and most of them have no underlying cardiac disease and are at low risk.

The enhanced parasympathetic and reduced sympathetic tone resulting from training may cause any of the following:

- resting bradycardia
- increased sinus arrhythmia (increased heart rate variability with breathing)
- prolonged PR interval (first-degree heart block)
- steep take-off of the ST segment
- voltage criteria of left ventricular hypertrophy are particularly likely in slim endurance athletes (e.g. long-distance runners)
- atrioventricular conduction delay
- Mobitz type I second-degree atrioventricular block, which may be apparent on the ECG
- Mobitz type II second-degree atrioventricular block, which is rare in athletes and is more likely to be due to conduction tissue disease.

The commonest ECG changes seen in athletes are ST-segment abnormalities (increased voltages, early take-off) and widespread T-wave changes. These may pose a diagnostic and management problem, and require a specialist opinion because they may also signify other cardiac disease. When combined with echocardiographic evidence of *symmetric* left ventricular hypertrophy, these ECG changes of athlete's heart must be distinguished from the steep T-wave inversion and classic *asymmetric* hypertrophy of hypertrophic obstructive cardiomyopathy (HOCM), which may coexist in approximately 1% of athletes and is the commonest cause of sudden death in young people. The situation is complicated when HOCM results in *symmetric* left ventricular hypertrophy (as may be seen in hypertension). Therefore it is important to detail the patient's athletic activities, blood pressure and ECG findings if an echocardiogram is requested. If there is diagnostic doubt, the patient should be referred.

Vasovagal syndrome

Compared with strength-trained athletes, endurance-trained athletes have an increased tendency to faint due to postural hypotension. The mechanisms include enhanced vagal tone, reduced sympathetic tone and increased lower limb venous capacity. Tilt-table responses may be abnormal. Individuals who experience troublesome symptoms should be referred for a specialist opinion, and may require dual-chamber pacing to protect them from fainting due to an impaired heart rate response in the presence of a low blood pressure.

Left ventricular hypertrophy

Significant left ventricular hypertrophy (> 12 mm; upper limit of normal is 11 mm) is rare, occurring in 2% of athletes (principally in rowers, canoeists, cyclists and distance runners who perform regular isometric and isotonic large-muscle-bulk exercise). It is an adaptation to exercise, and is reversible after a few months. Severe wall thickening (> 16 mm) is unusual in athletes, and is more likely to be due to hypertrophic cardiomyopathy. Causes other than endurance exercise should be considered in athletes with more than mild left ventricular hypertrophy. Approximately 15% of individuals may develop increased left ventricular cavity size suggestive of dilated cardiomyopathy.

Cardiac murmurs

Athletes may have a larger stroke volume and increased blood velocity due to vigorous cardiac function. The commonly heard systolic murmur in young slim people may be normal and due to increased flow across both the right and left ventricular outflow tract, or in athletes it may be due to vigorous cardiac function. Systolic murmurs are usually benign. Diastolic murmurs are always pathological. Echocardiography is helpful when investigating the possibility of structural heart and valve disease.

Table 9.2: Comparison of athlete's heart and hypertrophic obstructive cardiomyopathy (HOCM)

	Athlete's heart	HOCM
Echocardiography		
Maximal left ventricular wall thickness	Mild (< 13 mm)	≥ 16 mm
Left ventricular hypertrophy type	Concentric	Asymmetric Variable
Left ventricular cavity size	Large	Small
Diastolic function	Normal	Impaired
Left atrial size	Normal	Dilated
Regression of hypertrophy with detraining	Regression	No regression
Family history	Nil of hypertrophy	More likely
ECG	See above	Septal Q-waves, deep T-wave inversion, left axis

Risk and causes of sudden cardiac death in athletes

Sudden cardiac death in athletes is extremely rare, averaging approximately 1 per year among 500 000 young people, and is more common in males. This is lower than the prevalence of hypertrophic cardiomyopathy in young people (0.2%).

The commonest causes of sudden death in *young* individuals during exercise are hypertrophic cardiomyopathy (over 50% of cases) and coronary artery anomalies (13%), and less commonly congenital aortic stenosis (6%) and myocarditis (7%).

Atherosclerotic plaque rupture, acute myocardial infarction and ventricular fibrillation are the most frequent causes of sudden death in adult athletes. The annual risk of death for symptom-free healthy joggers had been estimated to be 1 in 18 000, but this may be similar to or less than the risk for a similar age-matched symptom-free non-jogging population.

The risk of death is increased in usually sedentary individuals who take up vigorous exercise, and is higher if they have cardiovascular risk factors. The risk is lower in individuals who have exercised regularly over a long period of time.

Identifying high-risk individuals before they start exercise training

Exercise testing to detect reversible ischaemia is recommended in individuals with a history of coronary artery disease (angina or infarction revascularisation). It is not recommended in low-risk, symptom-free individuals because of the low prevalence of obstructive coronary artery disease.

A significant proportion of athletes who had experienced exercise-related cardiac events had prodromal symptoms which were ignored. Therefore a full cardiac evaluation, including stress testing, is recommended for athletes who develop cardiac symptoms, and for those with a family history of an inherited cardiac disorder or a family history of 'unexplained' premature death below the age of 40 years (*see* Table 9.1). Therefore athletes with palpitation, syncope, chest pain or surprising shortness of breath require specialist referral and full evaluation.

Advice to give patients

- Regular exercise halves the risk of developing heart disease and stroke, and should be part of a healthy lifestyle that includes modification of all cardio-vascular risk factors.
- The more exercise the better. Aim to get hot, sweaty and breathless for 30 minutes a day. Any form of exercise that is convenient, comfortable and can be performed regularly is appropriate. Get into the habit and make it a fixed part of your daily routine.
- Elderly people should walk, swim or cycle to comfortable levels every day. This keeps them fitter, more alert and independent for longer. Any exercise is better than nothing.

- Exercise and achieving optimum body weight reduces the risk of diabetes and makes you feel better, more energetic and less depressed.
- Exercise reduces the risk of developing high blood pressure, and is an important part of its treatment.
- Exercise is part of the treatment for heart failure and for patients recovering after heart attacks, but should be undertaken carefully after an exercise test.
- Exercise lowers the risk of developing osteoporosis.

Answers to case studies

1   If the patient is symptom-free and has no signs of heart failure on examination, arrange a symptom-limited exercise test if he has not already had one. If he has a satisfactory exercise test with no ischaemia and a normal blood pressure he is at low risk for subsequent cardiac events and could go back to the gym, but should be advised to take it easy. He should avoid heavy weight-lifting for 4 weeks. Check his medication and fasting lipids (if this has not already been done), and ask him if he would like to join a rehabilitation course. If he develops symptoms or ischaemia, he should be referred back to the cardiologist for further investigation and coronary angiography.

2   Confirm with the patient's previous GP or specialist that the diagnosis is correct. Patients with hypertrophic obstructive cardiomyopathy are advised not to participate in competitive sports. This patient should be advised that moderate exercise is safe and he should be instructed by an experienced sports trainer. He should be told that he can jog or cycle gently but must not overexert himself by exceeding 70% of his age-predicted maximal heart rate. He can swim, walk, and play golf and leisurely tennis. It is difficult to restrict young active men. We need to educate patients that sudden vigorous exertion resulting in rapid increases in heart rate and systolic blood pressure is potentially dangerous, but that this depends on the nature and severity of the underlying heart disease.

3   It is possible that regular daily exercise combined with a careful diet might delay the time when he will require tablets. The only way to find out is to try it. He may need some guidance on an exercise prescription, and will require monitoring.

4   This is a difficult and common problem, and it may require a multi-disciplinary approach. It might be possible to make the patient's mother more mobile and independent and to improve the fitness and morale of the daughter if they both did some exercise. The mother will need careful evaluation of her musculoskeletal (arthritis) and neurological (Parkinson's disease, cerebrovascular disease) systems, a general medical evaluation (haematological, biochemical and thyroid status) and home assessment. Passive exercise, activities to increase her muscle tone and power, and standing, sitting and general mobility exercises should be practised under the supervision of a physiotherapist experienced in working with this age group.

Further reading

- Atterhog JH, Jonsson B and Samuelson R (1979) Exercise testing: a prospective study of complication rates. *Am Heart J.* **98**: 572–9.
- Billman GE, Schwartz PJ and Stone HL (1984) The effects of daily exercise on susceptibility to sudden cardiac death. *Circulation.* **69**: 1182–9.
- Coats AJ (2000) Exercise training in heart failure. *Curr Control Trials Cardiovasc Med.* **1**: 155–60.
- Huston TP, Puffer JC and Rodney WM (1985) The athletic heart syndrome. *NEJM.* **313**: 24–32.
- Manson JE, Greenland P, LaCroix AZ *et al.* (2002) Walking compared with vigorous exercise for the prevention of cardiovascular events in women. *NEJM.* **347**: 716–25.
- Maron BJ (1998) Athlete's heart and sudden cardiac death. In: EJ Topol (ed.) *Comprehensive Cardiovascular Medicine.* Lippincott-Raven Publishers, Philadelphia, PA.
- Maron BJ (2002) Hypertrophic cardiomyopathy: a systematic review. *JAMA.* **287**: 1308–20.
- Mittleman MA, Maclure M, Tofler GH *et al.* (1993) Triggering of acute myocardial infarction by heavy physical exercise. Protection against triggering by regular exertion. *NEJM.* **329**: 1677–83.
- Noakes TD (1987) Heart disease in marathon runners: a review. *Med Sci Sports Exerc.* **19**: 187–94.
- O'Connor GT, Buring JE, Yusuf S *et al.* (1989) An overview of randomised trials of rehabilitation with exercise after myocardial infarction. *Circulation.* **80**: 234–44.
- Powell KE, Thompson PD, Caspersen CJ *et al.* (1987) Physical activity and the incidence of coronary heart disease. *Annu Rev Public Health.* **8**: 253–87.
- Siscovick DS, Weiss NS, Fletcher RH *et al.* (1984) The incidence of primary cardiac arrest during vigorous exercise. *NEJM.* **311**: 875–7.
- Thompson PD, Klocke FJ, Levine BD *et al.* Task Force 5: Coronary Artery Disease (1994) Recommendations for determining eligibility for competition in athletes with cardiovascular abnormalities. Twenty-Sixth Bethesda Conference, 6–7 January 1994. *J Am Coll Cardiol.* **24**: 880–5.
- Thompson PD (ed.) (2001) *Exercise and Sports Cardiology.* McGraw-Hill, New York.
- Thompson PD and Moyna NM (2001) The therapeutic role of exercise in contemporary cardiology. *Cardiovasc Rev Rep.* **22**: 279–84.
- Vongvanich P, Paul-Labrador MJ and Merz CN (1996) Safety of medically supervised exercise in cardiac rehabilitation center. *Am J Cardiol.* **77**: 1383–5.

CHAPTER 10

Diabetes and the heart

Case studies

1 A 76-year-old overweight diabetic woman with a long history of hypertension comes to see you complaining of leg aches and cold feet. What would you do?
2 A 38-year-old Asian man with type 1 diabetes complains of chest pain which does not sound like angina. He is worried about his heart because his father died of a heart attack at the age of 65 years. What would you do?
3 An 88-year-old man with hypertension and diabetes presents with angina. What would you do?

Diagnostic criteria for diabetes

Diabetes can be diagnosed if the fasting glucose concentration is > 7.1 mmol/l or the glucose concentration 2 hours after a glucose load is > 11.1 mmol/l. An intermediate state of impaired glucose tolerance or subclinical glucose intolerance is a fasting glucose of > 6.1 mmol/l and < 7.0 mmol/l.

Cardiovascular risk associated with diabetes

Diabetes is becoming increasingly common in the UK due to the lifestyle that tends to involve taking too little exercise, an unhealthy diet and consequent obesity. Of the 1.4 million people in the UK who have diabetes, 85% have type 2 diabetes. It is estimated that by 2010, 3 million people will have diabetes (most of them with type 2 diabetes), many of whom will be children and young adults. Children who do little exercise and who eat a lot of carbohydrate and sugar are a high-risk group and require special attention.

The Framingham Study showed that, after controlling for the effects of major cardiovascular risk factors, diabetes increased the relative risk of developing coronary heart disease to 66% in men and 203% in women who were followed up for 20 years. Female diabetics appear to be more vulnerable to cardiovascular risk than male diabetics. The risk of cardiovascular disease and mortality due to myocardial infarction is increased further in diabetics with microalbuminuria and proteinuria or any other risk factor (*see* Chapter 15).

Coronary heart disease is the major cause of death in diabetics. Over 75% of diabetics aged over 40 years will die from a cardiovascular cause, and diabetics are more likely than non-diabetics to die from their first cardiovascular event. The mortality of adult diabetics without coronary heart disease is similar to that of non-diabetics with coronary heart disease, which suggests that type 2 diabetes confers a similar risk to established coronary heart disease. After a first coronary event, 50% of patients with diabetes may die within 1 year, and half of those die before they reach hospital. One-third of young, insulin-dependent (type 1) diabetics die of coronary heart disease by the age of 50 years. Subclinical glucose intolerance also increases cardiovascular risk, so all patients with one or more cardiovascular risk factors should be screened for diabetes and monitored.

> Diabetics constitute a particularly high-risk group who require early diagnosis, energetic and effective cardiovascular risk factor identification, and lower thresholds for intervention.

Compared to non-diabetics, diabetics are at greater risk of the following:

- obstructive coronary artery disease
- peripheral vascular disease
- renal artery stenosis
- angina
- myocardial infarction and its complications
- heart failure
- cerebrovascular disease.

They are also more likely to require the following:

- coronary artery surgery
- coronary angioplasty
- peripheral vascular intervention
- long-term medical treatment and monitoring of risk factors.

In addition, they have a poorer short- and long-term success rate after the following:

- coronary angioplasty (although this may be improved with new adjunctive medications and stents)
- coronary artery surgery, which has been the preferred approach to revascularisation
- myocardial infarction.

Pathology

Vascular problems

Diabetes increases atherogenesis via several mechanisms, including glycosylation of proteins and lipoproteins and oxidative damage, prothrombosis, impaired fibrinolysis and high levels of atherogenic LDL particles. Compared with non-diabetics, diabetic patients are more susceptible to accelerated atherogenesis and obstructive and unstable vascular disease, with a greater tendency to plaque rupture, platelet activation and thrombosis. These processes underlie the clinical consequences listed below.

Renal problems

These increase cardiovascular risk and mortality and the incidence of hypertension, which compounds the risks. They are determined mainly by genetic influences and only partially by glycaemic control.

Diabetes results in a *pre-nephropathy* phase characterised by subclinical albuminuria (microalbuminuria detected by radioimmunoassay and not dipstix) and subsequently *nephropathy* with proteinuria, decreasing glomerular filtration rate and increasing blood pressure. The cardiovascular mortality rate is 37 times higher in patients with nephropathy, and nearly all of them have significant coronary artery disease. It is four times higher in patients without proteinuria. This underpins the use of angiotensin-converting-enzyme (ACE) inhibitors in diabetics.

Microalbuminuria is associated with a prothrombotic profile with raised LDL-cholesterol, decreased HDL-cholesterol, raised lipoprotein(a) levels and raised activity of plasminogen activator inhibitor, factor VII and plasma fibrinogen.

Diabetic management in primary care

Shared care between hospital diabetic clinics and primary care with active patient education by diabetic trained nurses is now well established.

The importance of global risk assessment and a lowered threshold for intervention

Obesity, hyperlipidaemia and hypertension often coexist. A vigorous, global approach to risk factor improvement in diabetics reduces cardiovascular risk and improves prognosis. Estimation of absolute cardiovascular risk using the Joint British Societies risk chart or Cardiac Risk assessor computer program is helpful when rationalising treatment decisions.

Multi-factorial risk factor assessment and intervention combined with long-term monitoring for the recognition and management of diabetic complications therefore constitute a major, ongoing burden of work in primary care.

The results of recent trials have provided evidence for vigorous lipid lowering and tight control of blood pressure and blood sugar levels in reducing cardiovascular morbidity, retinopathy and proteinuria. Thus diabetic patients will often be taking more than one form of medication, and attract and deserve considerable healthcare resources because they are likely to derive considerable benefit from risk factor treatment.

The benefits of risk factor intervention are commensurately greater in diabetics, and this is the rationale for the lower thresholds for risk factor interventions in diabetics.

The metabolic syndrome

The well-recognised association of a raised blood sugar level, dyslipidaemias and hypertension in obese people has been recognised for several years, and the term 'metabolic syndrome' arose from the National Cholesterol Education Program (NCEP) Third Adult Panel (ATP-III). The syndrome is due to insulin resistance, and the current diagnostic criteria include the presence of at least three of the following:

- serum triglyceride level > 3.8 mmol/l
- serum HDL-cholesterol level < 1.0 mmol/l
- blood pressure > 130/85 mmHg
- waist girth > 102 cm
- fasting blood glucose level > 7 mmol/l.

This relatively recently characterised syndrome is common, affecting around 25% of men and women, and is due to insulin resistance. The prevalence increases from 7% in people aged 20–30 years to 40% in those aged 60 years or over.

It appears that obese patients have insulin resistance which then tends to progress, with resulting dyslipidaemias, hypertension and/or type 2 diabetes. The syndrome and its complications may be missed in individuals with low or borderline levels, but it is advisable to keep them under surveillance. The metabolic syndrome may explain the presence of coronary artery disease in young patients who might otherwise be thought to have a genetic cause. A large proportion of patients with metabolic syndrome progress to diabetes, and conversely a large proportion of diabetics would have fulfilled the criteria for a diagnosis of metabolic syndrome several years earlier. It is possible that patient education may have prevented or delayed the onset of the syndrome.

The metabolic syndrome is associated with vascular inflammation, with raised C-reactive protein levels.

The management goal is to prevent morbidity and mortality due to type 2 diabetes and cardiovascular disease. Relatively modest lifestyle changes can substantially reduce the risk of type 2 diabetes in mildly hyperglycaemic individuals. The management of patients with vascular disease and the metabolic syndrome centres on vigorous risk factor correction.

> Lifestyle changes, particularly diet and weight loss combined with daily exercise, are recommended for patients with the metabolic syndrome. It is important that patients understand that vascular disease may be present at the time when diabetes is diagnosed.

Statins and a fibrate may be needed to raise the HDL-cholesterol level and lower the triglyceride and LDL-cholesterol levels. Metformin and thiazolidinediones (e.g. rosiglitazone) are insulin sensitisers that may play a role in patients without diabetes, but at present there are few data to support this approach. The management of hypertension is discussed in Chapter 12.

An integrated approach to risk factor modification for diabetics

In primary care, specialised clinics should aim to provide continuing, long-term education and training for patients and their families to help them to manage their diabetes and all other risk factors. Patients are more likely to take control of their condition and their compliance with medication and lifestyle interventions will be improved if they understand what diabetes is, how it can affect them, and how a disciplined and healthy lifestyle can improve their chances of a longer and healthier life.

Patient self-help groups guided by interested, dedicated and inspiring clinicians may be a useful facility in primary care, and this together with other aspects of diabetic management may provide an instructive audit and evaluation topic.

Principles of diabetes management

These have changed over the last few years against the background of major trials, including the United Kingdom Prospective Diabetes Study Group (UKPDS) and the Heart Outcomes Prevention Evaluation (HOPE) Study Investigators. Furthermore, our understanding of the pathophysiology and natural history of diabetes and its complications has resulted in increasingly aggressive risk factor intervention, and this is likely to continue.

Epidemiological extrapolation of data from the UKPDS study showed that a 1% reduction in HbA_{1c} would be associated with a 21% decrease in the risk of any diabetic complication, a 21% decrease in death due to diabetes, a 31% decrease in microvascular complications and a 14% reduction in the risk of macrovascular events.

Modern management of diabetes should target the following high-risk patients:

- those with established vascular disease (previous myocardial infarction, myocardial revascularisation, cerebrovascular and/or peripheral vascular disease)
- patients, particularly females, who have one or more major cardiovascular risk factors, particularly hypertension, hyperlipidaemia and obesity
- diabetics with microalbuminuria
- diabetics with nephropathy (macroalbuminuria)
- diabetics with retinopathy
- Asians
- patients with poor glycaemic control.

Management should focus on reducing the absolute risk by using lower thresholds for intervention, including the following:

- the early identification of glucose intolerance in patients at risk of cardiovascular disease (those with a family history or one or more risk factors)
- sympathetic, clear, tailored and reinforced dietary advice
- tight control of blood sugar levels (diabetics with myocardial infarction should be treated with insulin and glucose)
- achievement of optimal body weight
- tight blood pressure control

- smoking cessation
- encouraging regular exercise
- aggressive lipid lowering
- ACE inhibition with or without an angiotensin II antagonist for hypertension, heart failure, post-myocardial infarction, vascular disease, microalbuminuria or multiple risk factors
- aspirin treatment both for those with cardiovascular disease and for those without it.

Non-insulin-dependent diabetes

Patients with non-insulin-dependent diabetes have a two- to fourfold higher risk of cardiovascular disease, and women appear to be at particularly high risk, although the reasons for this are unclear. Hypertension is common. The degree and duration of hyperglycaemia largely determine microvascular complications, but these influences do not extend to macrovascular complications.

Smoking

Smoking cessation is very important in diabetics, and may reduce the risk of myocardial infarction by 50% within 1 year of quitting. Diabetics are likely to derive greater benefit from smoking cessation than non-diabetics.

Hypertension

Diabetic patients should be checked and monitored carefully for hypertension. The latter affects 40% of patients with type 2 diabetes by the age of 50 years, and 60% of patients by the age of 75 years. The UKPDS trial showed that tight blood pressure control reduced diabetes-related deaths and microvascular events, stroke and heart failure, but not myocardial infarction.

Current treatment guidelines for diabetic patients

- All patients, whether diabetic or not, should be treated if their blood pressure is > 160/100 mmHg.
- The target blood pressure is 140/80 mmHg unless the patient has microalbuminuria or macroalbuminuria, when the target is lowered to < 130/80 mmHg.
- Diabetic patients with hypertension and one or more other risk factors and organ damage require aggressive and effective blood pressure control.
- Patients with diabetes and a blood pressure of > 140/80 mmHg with organ damage and a 10-year coronary heart disease risk of > 15% should be treated.
- Patients with microalbuminuria and/or macroalbuminuria and a blood pressure of > 130/80 mmHg should be treated.

Choice of drug for diabetic patients with hypertension

The main aim is to choose a drug, or usually a combination of drugs, that is effective and which the patient can tolerate. The UKPDS trial showed that atenolol and captopril were similarly effective in reducing the incidence of diabetic complications. However, ACE inhibitors and angiotensin-II-receptor blockers have advantages over other drugs, and are the pharmacological treatment of first choice in patients with microalbuminuria and in the following situations.

- Patients with heart failure – diuretics may also be necessary.
- Patients should be switched to an angiotensin-II-receptor blocker if they cannot tolerate an ACE inhibitor, usually because of a cough.
- Blood pressure control may be improved by the addition of an angiotensin-II-receptor blocker to an ACE inhibitor, although there will be no further improvement in microalbuminuria.
- Afro-Caribbean patients respond poorly to β-blockers and angiotensin-II-receptor blockers, and usually respond better to the calcium-channel blockers and diuretics.
- β-blockers, combined when necessary with calcium antagonists, are useful in patients with angina, post myocardial infarction, or in patients who cannot tolerate other drugs.

Hyperlipidaemia

Type 2 diabetes typically results in a raised triglyceride level and a reduced HDL-cholesterol level.

> The vascular event rates in adult diabetics of all ages (both male and female), with and without vascular disease, are reduced by high-dose statins, which should therefore be considered in all diabetics. Fibrates should be used in addition for hypertriglyceridaemia.

Primary prevention targets for cholesterol and lipid fractions for diabetics are the same as for secondary prevention targets in patients without diabetes:

- total cholesterol < 5.0 mmol/l
- fasting triglyceride < 2.0 mmol/l
- LDL-cholesterol < 3.0 mmol/l
- HDL-cholesterol > 1.1 mmol/l
- total cholesterol:HDL cholesterol < 3.0 mmol/l.

Angina and coronary artery disease

Diabetes results in accelerated atherosclerosis, and diabetics without coronary artery disease are likely to have a similar rate of myocardial infarction, cardiovascular death and other events to that in non-diabetics who have had an infarct. Diabetics have a blunted or diminished awareness of angina but, compared with non-diabetics, are more likely to have coronary artery disease. Silent ischaemia and infarction are therefore more common in diabetics.

Medical treatment

The principles of medical treatment of angina in diabetics are similar to those for non-diabetics, but coexisting risk factors should be treated aggressively and at lower thresholds in accordance with absolute risk estimation.

Note: Smoking cessation, weight loss, dietary control and exercise are crucial.

Prophylactic short-acting and long-acting nitrates, calcium antagonists, β-blockers and, in resistant cases, potassium-channel openers are used.

> Aspirin is recommended for all diabetics with vascular disease and also for those without vascular disease, although this is not based on randomised clinical trial evidence.

ACE inhibitors improve endothelial function in patients with coronary artery disease. The HOPE study showed that ramipril produced significant reductions in the risk of the combined outcome of death, myocardial infarction and stroke and nephropathy.

> ACE inhibitors should be prescribed for diabetic patients with vascular disease, more than one risk factor or microalbuminuria.

Renal function

Renal function should be evaluated before procedures using radiographic contrast media, which can precipitate renal failure in patients with renal impairment. Pre-procedure or pre-operative fasting may also induce renal failure in susceptible patients. The use of non-cardiac drugs with potential renal side-effects (e.g. non-steroidal anti-inflammatory drugs) should be initiated very cautiously and renal function must be monitored.

Diabetic control

The UKPDS trial showed that tight glycaemic control (glycosylated haemoglobin concentration of < 7%) reduced microvascular complications. Insulin and dextrose infusions may need to be given to patients who are not allowed to eat peri-operatively.

Five main steps have been proposed in treating type 2 diabetes.

1 Lifestyle change

Assess the patient's psychological state and lifestyle, and discuss and educate them about lifestyle modifications. If the target HbA_{1c} is not achieved, go to step 2.

2 Monotherapy

Introduce metformin in patients with a BMI of > 25 kg/m^2 unless:

- there are contraindications or the drug is poorly tolerated
- there is renal impairment (creatinine concentration > 130 μmol/l)
- there is a risk of renal impairment because of a history of cardiac or hepatic failure.

If this is the case, and in patients with a BMI of < 25 kg/m^2, introduce an insulin secretagogue (e.g. sulphonylurea).

If the target HbA$_{1c}$ is not achieved, go to step 3.

3 Combination therapy

Consider metformin plus an insulin secretagogue (standard sulphonylurea or prandial glucose regulator) combination therapy if there are no renal problems or tolerability issues.

Consider metformin plus glitazone if:

- metformin plus an insulin secretagogue is contraindicated or not tolerated
- the patient has a BMI > 25 kg/m^2.

Consider an insulin secretagogue plus glitazone if:

- there is renal impairment (serum creatinine concentration > 130 μmol/l)
- there is a risk of sudden deterioration in renal function because of a history of cardiac or hepatic failure.

If the target HbA$_{1c}$ is not achieved, go to step 4.

4 Insulin therapy

Reassess psychological issues and any lifestyle changes, and give or obtain appropriate support.

Discuss and agree change of treatment to insulin.

Initiate 10 IU of basal insulin (NPH insulin at bedtime; insulin glargine at any time, but always at the same time of day).

- Titrate the dose to achieve target fasting blood glucose concentration (4.0–7.0 mmol/l) slowly over a period of weeks.
- Continue treatment with metformin.
- Discontinue other anti-diabetic agents.
- Review other medications/interventions as appropriate.

If the HbA$_{1c}$ target is not achieved, introduce short- or rapid-acting insulins prior to meals, and review other medications.

Myocardial revascularisation

Revascularisation strategies in diabetics with angina are more complicated because the underlying coronary artery disease is more likely to be diffuse, affecting the entire length of the artery. This makes angioplasty and coronary artery surgery technically difficult and an unattractive option because of the higher short-term and long-term risks. The infection risks are higher. Tight glycaemic control during the peri-operative and long-term post-operative phases is important and influences the outcome.

Coronary artery bypass surgery

Diabetes is an independent predictor of short-term morbidity and long-term survival after coronary artery surgery. This probably relates to the higher risk of widespread and progressive vascular disease and associated renal disease. Technical problems, including the manipulation of an atheromatous and calcified aorta (resulting in emboli), and graft insertion into a diffusely diseased and narrowed distal coronary artery, contribute to peri-operative and long-term morbidity and mortality from infection, graft occlusion and myocardial infarction.

Renal failure may develop in patients with pre-existing diabetic renal disease. It may also occur when coronary artery surgery is performed shortly after the use of large volumes of contrast medium for angiography or angioplasty.

Infection and slow healing of the leg vein harvest sites may present difficult problems for the primary care team.

Coronary angioplasty

Before the advent and wider use of coated coronary artery stents and glycoprotein IIb/IIIa inhibitors in diabetics, coronary artery bypass surgery was shown to offer diabetic patients a better 5-year survival, mainly because of the high restenosis rates after angioplasty in diabetics.

Associated renal disease and renal artery stenosis pose an increased risk of renal failure with the use of radiographic contrast media during angiography.

Diabetics are more likely to have diffuse multi-vessel coronary artery disease, rather than focal lesions.

Peripheral vascular disease increases the technical difficulties of vascular access and post-procedure complications. Patients with carotid and cerebrovascular disease are at risk of cerebrovascular events. Patients should be screened for associated vascular disease before revascularisation is performed, so that the risks of the chosen approach are minimised.

Combined angioplasty and coronary angioplasty

Hybrid approaches using both angioplasty and minimally invasive direct coronary artery bypass grafting with internal mammary arterial conduits are a relatively new development which may offer improved short- and long-term outcomes, although there are no data to support this at present.

Myocardial infarction

The risk of myocardial infarction increased to 50% in men and 150% in women, and 30% of diabetics die as a result of infarction.

Silent ischaemia and autonomic neuropathy may explain the absence, blunting or atypical symptoms of myocardial infarction in diabetics. The complications of infarction, including sudden death, are more common in diabetics because of the nature of their coronary artery disease, their atherogenic and prothrombotic predisposition, and late or non-presentation to emergency medical care, resuscitation, thrombolysis and intervention. Patients who survive the acute ischaemic event are more likely to have larger infarcts and associated heart failure and cardiogenic shock.

Tight blood sugar control by means of insulin has been shown to improve survival after infarction, but the UKPDS trial showed only a borderline reduction in the risk of infarction. Other current secondary preventive treatments in the management of acute myocardial infarction apply to and should be used in diabetics. These include primary coronary angioplasty, medical thrombolysis, and other medical interventions such as aspirin, β-blockers and statins. ACE inhibitors should be used to prevent left ventricular remodelling, heart failure and microvascular complications.

Diabetic cardiomyopathy

Occasionally, diabetics may develop heart failure due to a diabetic cardiomyopathy, and this is distinct from the much more common situation of muscle damage resulting from myocardial infarction.

Screening diabetic patients for coronary heart disease

At present this is only recommended for patients prior to major non-cardiac surgery and renal transplantation, where the presence of significant coronary artery disease and ischaemia may adversely affect the operative success, and where myocardial revascularisation would improve the outcome.

The most accurate and direct approach for assessing coronary anatomy is to perform coronary angiography rather than non-invasive imaging. Stress testing may be helpful in certain patients, but nuclear perfusion imaging has a low sensitivity (5–10%) in asymptomatic patients.

Advice for patients

- Your diabetes puts you at greater risk of furring up of all your arteries, so we must work together to make sure that your diabetes is very tightly controlled. You will have a lower risk of heart trouble, stroke or circulation problems in your legs if your diabetes is well controlled. This involves a lot of work and self-discipline, but it will be worth it. It is important that you understand how you can control your future by modifying your lifestyle.
- All of the factors which contribute to furring up of the arteries need continuous vigorous attention, and this includes smoking, blood pressure, cholesterol, your weight and your diet.
- There are a number of tablets which will help you, and we need to make sure that they are suitable for you.

Answers to case studies

1   This patient needs to be assessed for vascular disease affecting her legs, and also for coronary heart disease and carotid artery disease. She should have her glucose state checked, together with her blood count, lipid status and renal function. She should be referred to the peripheral vascular team, and if she has not seen the diabetologists recently, she should be reviewed. An ECG might show signs of ischaemia or hypertension. She will need help with and advice about her diet, glucose control and exercise. Her blood pressure will have to be tightly controlled. She should be on an ACE inhibitor if possible, plus aspirin and other appropriate medication.

2   Examine the patient's heart and blood pressure, feel his peripheral pulses, check his glucose and lipid status and arrange an exercise test. If he has a good exercise performance and no signs of reversible ischaemia, then he can be reassured. Estimate his absolute coronary risk and initiate preventive treatment as necessary.

3   This patient needs a comprehensive assessment, and hopefully his symptoms will be adequately controlled on medical treatment. If this is not possible, angioplasty is an option to be considered.

Further reading

Reviews

• McGuire DK and Granger CB (1999) Diabetes and ischaemic heart disease. *Am Heart J.* **138**: S336–75.
• Timmis AD (2001) Diabetic heart disease: clinical considerations. *Heart.* **85**: 463–9.

Epidemiology

• Fuller JH, Shipley MJ, Rose G *et al.* (1983) Mortality from coronary heart disease and stroke in relation to degree of glycaemia: the Whitehall study. *BMJ.* **287**: 867–70.
• Kannel WB and McGee DL (1979) Diabetes and cardiovascular risk factors: the Framingham study. *Circulation.* **59**: 8–13.
• Stamler J, Vaccaro O, Neaton JD *et al.* (1993) Diabetes, other risk factors, and 12-year cardio-vascular mortality for men screened in the multiple risk factor intervention trial. *Diabetes Care.* **16**: 434–44.

Myocardial revascularisation

• Marso SP, Lincoff AM, Ellis SG *et al.* (1999) Optimizing the percutaneous interventional outcomes for patients with diabetes mellitus: results of the EPISTENT (Evaluation of Platelet IIb/IIIa Inhibitor for Stenting Trial) diabetic substudy. *Circulation.* **100**: 2477–84.
• The Bypass Angioplasty Revascularisation Investigation (BARI) Investigators (1996) Compari-sons of coronary bypass surgery with angioplasty in patients with multivessel disease. *NEJM.* **335**: 217–25.

Risk factor intervention

- Executive Summary of The Third Report of the National Cholesterol Education Program (NCEP) (2001) Expert panel on detection, evaluation and treatment of high blood cholesterol in adults (Adult Treatment Panel III). *JAMA.* **285**: 2486–97.
- United Kingdom Prospective Diabetes Study (UKPDS) Group (1998) Tight blood pressure control and risk of macrovascular and microvascular complications in type 2 diabetes (UKPDS 38). *BMJ.* **317**: 703–13.
- United Kingdom Prospective Diabetes Study (UKPDS) Group (1998) Efficacy of atenolol and captopril in reducing risk of macrovascular and microvascular complications in type 2 diabetes (UKPDS 39). *BMJ.* **317**: 713–20.
- United Kingdom Prospective Diabetes Study (UKPDS) Group (1998) Intensive blood-glucose control with sulphonylureas or insulin compared with conventional treatment and risk of complications in patients with type 2 diabetes (UKPDS 33). *Lancet.* **352**: 837–53.
- Yusuf S, Sleight P, Pogue J *et al.* for the Heart Outcomes Prevention Evaluation (HOPE) Study (2000) Effects of ramipril on cardiovascular and microvascular outcomes in people with diabetes mellitus: results of HOPE study and MICRO-HOPE substudy. *Lancet.* **355**: 253–9.

Treating type 2 diabetes

- Barnett AH, Capaldi B, Farooqi A *et al.* (2003) Treating to target in Type 2 diabetes: from lifestyle changes to insulin therapy. *Mod Diabetes Manag.* **4**: 2–5.

CHAPTER 11

Peripheral arterial disease

Case studies

1 A 78-year-old hypertensive man who smokes 20 cigarettes a day comes to see you with pain in the buttock and down the leg when he walks, stands or bends. The symptoms are not affected by walking. What would you do?

2 An 85-year-old diabetic woman with a previous myocardial infarction and a long history of angina and claudication asks you whether chelation therapy would be helpful? What advice would you give her?

3 A 47-year-old previously fit man presents with an acutely ischaemic foot. It is white, pulseless and painful. What would you do?

4 A 76-year-old man with a long history of both coronary artery disease and peripheral vascular disease, and who had a femoro-popliteal bypass 10 years ago, presents with recurrent claudication in the same leg, and absent foot pulses, but the foot is not threatened. You refer him back to the vascular surgeon, who does not consider that either angioplasty or bypass is possible. What advice would you give the patient?

Primary care approach to patients with peripheral arterial disease

Peripheral vascular disease is part of a widespread atheromatous process that affects all arterial territories. Patients with angina and coronary heart disease often have peripheral arterial disease which may only become apparent after myocardial revascularisation enables them to walk faster and for longer distances. Patients with non-cardiac vascular disease should be screened for coronary heart disease. The management of patients with peripheral arterial disease involves cardiovascular risk factor screening and aggressive management, and should be undertaken in primary care.

The role of primary care in managing peripheral arterial disease includes the following:

- increased awareness of peripheral arterial disease and its consequences
- improving the identification of patients with symptomatic peripheral arterial disease
- initiating a screening programme for patients at high risk
- improving risk factor management for patients with symptomatic peripheral arterial disease
- increasing rates of detection of individuals with asymptomatic disease

- arranging an exercise test
- referring the patient either to an exercise training clinic or to a vascular surgeon.

Symptoms and risk

The pathology, risk factors and principles of management of peripheral arterial disease are similar to those for coronary heart disease. At least 50% of patients with peripheral arterial disease do not have claudication and may therefore go undiagnosed. Those with claudication may be misdiagnosed as having arthritis or other musculoskeletal disease. With or without symptoms, patients have a sixfold increase in mortality within 10 years compared with patients without peripheral arterial disease. A comprehensive evaluation for atheromatous disease should be performed before revascularisation for any arterial territory. This is particularly important prior to myocardial revascularisation, because coexisting vascular disease increases the peri-operative risk, particularly of renal failure. Similarly, coronary artery disease increases the risk of peripheral artery surgery.

Management of peripheral vascular disease necessitates the following:

- an anatomical and functional assessment
- exclusion of non-atheromatous causes of claudication
- a comprehensive survey and prompt and aggressive treatment of risk factors
- effective lifestyle, medical and, where necessary, revascularisation interventions.

Prevalence

In common with vascular disease in other arterial territories, peripheral vascular disease is becoming more common because people are living longer and risk factor management may simply delay the timing of onset of the disease. Around 20% of people aged 65–75 years have reduced leg pulses on clinical examination, but only 25% of them have symptoms. Symptoms of arterial disease depend on the patient's level of activity.

Claudication

Symptoms

These occur when the artery is narrowed by at least 50%. A long but less severe stenosis may also result in poor flow and claudication. Claudication is defined as pain in the calf, buttock or foot or tightness or cramp on walking, that is relieved by rest. It is not relieved by continued walking. It is present in 15–40% of patients with peripheral vascular disease. Patients may experience cold feet and calf cramp at night, which can be relieved by hanging the leg out of the bed.

Patients may be unable to perform their normal activities and become deconditioned and dependent on others.

It is important to assess the severity of symptoms by recording the claudication distance and asking whether the patient experiences rest pain.

Signs

These include reduced foot pulses, arterial bruits and ischaemic skin changes with ulcers in severe disease.

Diagnosis

The ankle–brachial index is the most effective method of diagnosis. This involves wrapping a blood pressure cuff around the leg just above the ankle, inflating the cuff to above the systolic pressure, and listening with a hand-held Doppler device for the return of blood flow as the cuff is deflated. Systolic pressures are measured in both the posterior tibial and dorsalis pedis arteries, and the higher of the two systolic readings is compared with the Doppler-detected systolic pressure in the brachial artery. An ankle to brachial pressure ratio of < 0.9 is diagnostic of peripheral arterial disease.

An ankle–brachial index of < 0.5 is associated with a 5-year survival of 63%. An ankle–brachial index of 0.7–0.9 is associated with a 5-year survival of 91%. It is not yet used as a screening tool in primary care.

Risk factor checklist

- Smoking is the commonest and most important risk factor, and patients must be advised of the risks of smoking and the potential benefits of stopping.
- Blood pressure.
- Diabetes.
- Lipid profile.
- Renal function – because peripheral vascular disease is commonly associated with renal artery stenosis and renal impairment.
- β-blockers may aggravate claudication symptoms and either they may need to be stopped or the dose may need to be reduced.

The differential diagnosis of leg pain includes the following.

- Venous claudication – this results in a bursting sensation that affects the whole leg and is relieved by elevating the leg.
- Nerve root pain – this results in a poorly localised, shock-like pain that affects both legs and is relieved by sitting down.
- Inflammatory vasculitis (Buerger's disease) – this affects the small and medium-sized arteries and veins of the arms and legs in young people, predominantly male smokers. There may be thrombosis of peripheral vessels leading to ulceration and gangrene. More than one limb is affected, and proximal vessels are usually normal. Referral to an expert vascular unit is required, and revascularisation strategies are usually of little value. Management is based on smoking cessation, local treatment of ulcers, anti-thrombotics and occasionally sympathectomy. Amputation may be necessary, particularly if the patient continues to smoke.

Natural history (*see* **Figure 11.1**)

The leg

This has improved since the introduction of aggressive and effective medical treatment and exercise prescriptions. For most patients the symptoms and prognosis improve, and they should be told this. Around 25% of patients deteriorate. Major limb amputation is rarely necessary.

Overall vascular prognosis

Because peripheral vascular disease is usually a manifestation of generalised atheromatous disease, and is more common in the elderly, the overall vascular prognosis is poor. Around 30% of patients will die, and a further 10% will have a non-fatal infarct. Around 60% of patients survive for 5 years with no vascular complications (*see* Figure 11.1).

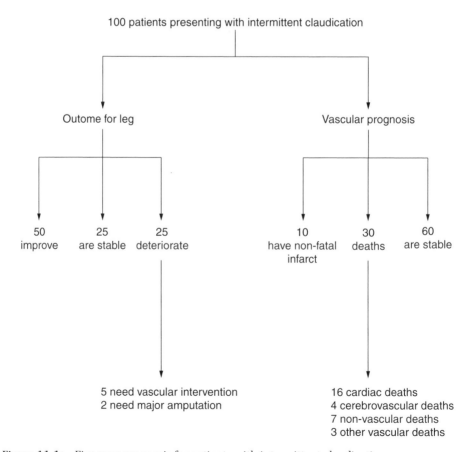

Figure 11.1:   Five-year prognosis for patients with intermittent claudication.

Atheroembolism

Embolisation of atheromatous material from plaques may result in ischaemic infarction. This may affect the kidneys with acute renal failure, and one or both legs depending on the source of the embolism. Patients present with acute severe pain and an ischaemic foot and/or leg that is cold, pale and is either pulseless or has reduced pulses. If atheroembolism is suspected, patients should be referred to an experienced vascular unit for prompt investigation and treatment.

Management of peripheral artery disease

All risk factors must be addressed vigorously (*see* Chapters 5, 7, 8, 9, 10 and 12) and conjointly together with a lifelong exercise programme.

Antiplatelet medication

Aspirin
This acts by blocking the cyclo-oxygenase pathway and reducing thromboxane-induced platelet aggregation. It decreases the risk of non-fatal and fatal vascular events and cardiovascular mortality by an average of 20%. It should be used in both primary and secondary prevention. It improves patency rates after revascularisation that has been performed using bypass grafting or angioplasty. All patients should be given aspirin 75 mg. Compared with placebo, aspirin prevents 19 fatal and non-fatal cardiovascular events per year for every 1000 patients treated.

Clopidogrel
This should be tried in the 10% of patients who cannot tolerate aspirin. Clopidogrel is a thienopyridine, and it blocks the activation of platelets by adenosine diphosphate. It has a similar side-effect profile to aspirin, and is used in patients with vascular disease for both primary and secondary prevention. Clopidogrel may be more effective than aspirin in reducing ischaemic events in patients with atheromatous disease in other arterial territories. It may be used in addition to aspirin in high-risk patients, and for long-term treatment after angioplasty and stent implantation. Clopidogrel prevents 24 fatal and non-fatal cardiovascular events per year for every 1000 patients treated.

Smoking cessation

Cigarette smoking increases the risk of peripheral vascular disease by fourfold, and continued smoking increases the rate of progression of disease and the likelihood of leg amputation. Smoking cessation reduces the progression of disease and cardiovascular events, including death, and is probably the single most important (but possibly also the most difficult) intervention.

Diabetes

Diabetics have a fourfold higher risk of developing peripheral vascular disease compared with non-diabetics.

The HbA_{1c} should be reduced to below 7.0%, and tight glycaemic control, combined with correction of hypertension and other risk factors, has been shown to reduce the risk of peripheral vascular disease by 34%. Tight glycaemic control alone has little or no proven benefit in reducing the risk of amputation.

Lipids

Although reducing total cholesterol and LDL-cholesterol levels has not, in isolation from other risk factor modification, been shown to improve claudication symptoms or prognosis (possibly because of the small sample sizes involved), aggressive lipid lowering using dietary interventions, exercise, statins and cholesterol-absorption blockers should be used to achieve a target LDL-cholesterol concentration of < 2.5 mmol/l and a total cholesterol concentration of < 5.0 mmol/l.

Hypertension

Hypertension increases the risk of peripheral vascular disease by threefold. All anti-hypertensive drugs may be used in patients with peripheral vascular disease. In the absence of bilateral renal artery stenosis, and using careful biochemical monitoring, angiotensin-converting-enzyme (ACE) inhibitors, particularly in diabetics, are the drug of first choice and may be used for patients with peripheral vascular disease without diabetes or hypertension.

Patient education

The prognosis as shown above should be explained, as should the potential benefits of risk factor improvement and the consequences of inadequate risk factor control.

Exercise training

Daily vigorous walking or cycling combined with aggressive risk factor modification will improve exercise performance and quality of life. Regular exercise, walking for 30 minutes at a time, improves pain-free walking time by 180%. Exercise training appears to be more effective than medication, and the benefits are noticeable within a few weeks.

Patients should be told to walk until they claudicate, and then to stop and to start again. Potential mechanisms responsible for the benefits of exercise training include increased muscle strength, improved vascular function and dilatation, and improved muscle metabolism.

Revascularisation

This is reserved for symptomatic patients.

Revascularisation is a rapidly developing multi-disciplinary speciality that requires the input of radiologists, vascular surgeons, cardiologists, lipidologists, secondary prevention nurses, exercise training personnel and staff experienced in smoking cessation.

Percutaneous angioplasty and (where appropriate) stenting, aided by intravascular ultrasound, are now performed for a wide variety of lesions in peripheral, renal and carotid artery disease.

Surgery is used in cases where these techniques are currently not appropriate.

Advice for patients

- The symptoms of claudication are due to a build-up of fat in the arteries which supply blood and oxygen to the leg muscles. It is part of a generalised furring-up process which may affect other arteries. Patients with peripheral vascular disease are at increased risk of stroke and heart attack.
- If you have pain in your toes or you experience pain in your feet at night, come to see us as soon as possible.
- If left untreated, claudication may progress to severe pain and restriction of activities, and in very severe cases to amputation of the leg.
- You can do a lot to help yourself by stopping smoking, losing weight, taking daily regular exercise for 30 minutes at a time, making sure that your blood pressure is normal and your cholesterol level is low, and checking that you do not have diabetes. If you do have diabetes, this needs very tight control.
- You will be prescribed various tablets, including aspirin, an angiotensin-converting-enzyme (ACE) inhibitor and a statin.
- We will refer you to a vascular surgeon who will do some tests to see why you have claudication, where the arterial blockages are, and whether you would benefit from a ballooning procedure or a bypass operation to improve the blood supply to your legs and feet. These tests include an ultrasound scan and an angiogram. The ultrasound scan is painless and quick, and a probe is placed over the arteries of the legs to detect blockages in the flow of blood. The angiogram involves your lying on an X-ray table, and a needle is inserted into the artery in the groin of the affected leg and radio-opaque fluid is injected into the artery. Pictures are then taken to locate and assess the severity of the arterial narrowings.
- Take the condition seriously, remember to take all your tablets, and let us know immediately if your symptoms deteriorate or you develop a painful white foot. If you do, you should go to hospital immediately.

Answers to case studies

1   Although this patient may have peripheral vascular disease, his symptoms are not consistent with claudication. They may be due to sciatica or lumbar canal stenosis. If he has good pulses, claudication is unlikely and he should be referred to a back surgeon for evaluation. He should be advised to stop smoking, and should be offered bupropion and all other appropriate cardiovascular prevention advice.

2   Advise this patient that chelation therapy is not helpful and that it is expensive. Make sure that she has full cardiovascular secondary prevention, and check her

medication and that she is taking it. Her diabetes must be tightly controlled. She should be referred to the vascular surgeon (or referred again if she has already been seen) for investigation to see whether angioplasty would help her.

3   It is possible that this patient has had an embolus. He must be referred as an emergency to hospital for a diagnosis and treatment to save the leg. Possible causes include a thrombotic embolus due to atrial fibrillation, trauma to the leg arteries and (rarely) an atrial myxoma or a blood disorder. He will need urgent ultrasound scanning and angiography and appropriate treatment. Depending on the cause, he may need long-term anticoagulation therapy.

4   There appears to be no prospect of further revascularisation. Aggressive secondary prevention, including aspirin, possibly with clopidogrel, high-dose statins and angiotensin-converting-enzyme (ACE) inhibitors, and stopping or reducing β-blockers are important. Make sure that he is not diabetic or smoking. He should be strongly encouraged to do at least daily energetic exercise training on a treadmill or cycle in the hope that this will improve his symptoms. The long-term prognosis is not good, but it is important to encourage the patient and support him.

Further reading

- Burns P, Gough S and Bradbury AW (2003) Management of peripheral arterial disease in primary care. *BMJ*. **326**: 584–8.
- CAPRIE Steering Committee (1996) A randomised, blinded trial of clopidogrel versus aspirin in patients at risk of ischaemic events (CAPRIE). *Lancet*. **348**: 1329–39.
- Gardener AW and Poehlman ET (1995) Exercise rehabilitation programs for the treatment of claudication pain. A meta-analysis. *JAMA*. **274**: 975–80.
- Hiatt WR (2001) Medical treatment of peripheral arterial disease and claudication. *NEJM*. **344**: 1608–21.
- Hirsch AT, Treat-Jacobson D, Lando HA *et al.* (1997) The role of tobacco cessation, antiplatelet and lipid-lowering therapies in the treatment of peripheral arterial disease. *Vasc Med*. **2**: 243–51.
- Leng GC, Lee AJ, Fowkes FGR *et al.* (1996) Incidence, natural history and cardiovascular events in symptomatic and asymptomatic peripheral arterial disease in the general population. *Int J Epidemiol*. **25**: 1172–81.
- Perkins JM, Collin J, Creasy TS *et al.* (1996) Exercise training versus angioplasty for stable claudication. Long and medium term results of a prospective, randomised trial. *Eur J Vasc Endovasc Surg*. **11**: 409–13.
- Stewart KJ, Hiatt WR and Regenstein JG (2002) Exercise training for claudication. *NEJM*. **347**: 1941–51.

CHAPTER 12

Hypertension

Case studies

1 A 40-year-old symptom-free man who is moderately overweight has a blood sugar level of 7 mmol/l and is worried about his blood pressure, which he checks himself frequently and he records as 150/100 mmHg. What would you do?

2 A 75-year-old known hypertensive man comes to see you with headache, and you record his blood pressure as 190/150 mmHg. What would you do?

3 A 34-year-old woman is 28 weeks into her second pregnancy, having been diagnosed as having borderline hypertension during her first uncomplicated pregnancy 4 years ago. She feels well, but the nurse in the hospital antenatal clinic has found her blood pressure to be 145/95 mmHg. What would you do?

4 A fit 86-year-old woman has a blood pressure of 175/80 mmHg, but because she feels fine, can do the crossword and does a lot of voluntary work at the home for the elderly, is not keen to take any tablets. What would you advise her to do?

5 A 67-year-old obese woman with type 2 diabetes, hyperlipidaemia and mild claudication has a blood pressure of 165/95 mmHg, despite a thiazide diuretic and an angiotensin-converting-enzyme (ACE) inhibitor. How would you manage her?

The management of hypertension in primary care

Screening for and the continual monitoring, treatment and control of hypertension as part of a comprehensive or global strategy of cardiovascular prevention constitutes a major part of the workload in primary care, and it has a significant impact on the health of the population.

Despite improved management, surveys have shown that several difficult issues remain unresolved.

- The cause of hypertension is unknown in over 90% of patients.
- Hypertension remains under-diagnosed. Many patients with 'mild' hypertension are untreated, and the majority of those with 'severe' hypertension are under-treated or not taking the prescribed medication. Thus large numbers of people are at unnecessarily high risk of coronary heart disease and stroke.
- Less than 10% of hypertensive patients have 'target' levels.
- There is a reluctance to treat elderly patients with 'mild hypertension' and isolated systolic hypertension.
- Some patients who are treated for hypertension might not need medication if they adhered to non-pharmacological measures.

- 'White-coat hypertension' as a potentially confusing phenomenon is recognised by clinicians and patients, but its prognostic implications and the need for treatment remain unclear.
- The roles of ambulatory blood pressure recordings and self-monitored recordings as useful diagnostic and monitoring tools, and their use in treatment as well as diagnosis are becoming clearer.
- The importance of diet, weight loss, exercise and other non-pharmacological measures in cardiovascular prevention and in the treatment of patients with borderline and established hypertension is now accepted, although patients generally find these self-administered interventions difficult to implement. Primary care clinicians are well placed to encourage and activate these aspects of treatment.
- Some drug treatments for hypertension (e.g. β-blockers and ACE inhibitors) have other synergistic beneficial cardiovascular effects.
- Most patients with hypertension will require more than one type of drug to reduce the blood pressure to the target level.
- Consensus guidelines have recommended lower target blood pressure levels for patients with a high absolute cardiovascular risk, including diabetics, smokers and those with coronary artery disease or target organ damage, particularly left ventricular hypertrophy. It is important that these groups of high-risk patients are identified and treated effectively.
- Compliance with drug and non-pharmacological treatment can be improved by explaining to patients the nature of hypertension, its complications and potential drug side-effects, and by continual clinical monitoring and checks on tablet intake.

Haemodynamic changes in hypertension

Hypertension occurs when excessive vasoconstriction and/or volume is not compensated for by adequate pressure natriuresis or suppression of the renin–aldosterone system.

The importance of hypertension as a cardiovascular risk factor

Hypertension is the commonest cause of stroke, the most common reversible cause of heart failure, and an important cause of coronary heart disease in diabetics.

The relationship between blood pressure and cardiovascular disease is continuous and graded, and there is no cut-off value which separates those patients who will and those who will not have a cardiovascular event. The risk of an individual developing cardiovascular disease depends on the level of the blood pressure and coexistent risk factors, including age, male sex, family history, raised cholesterol level, smoking, diabetes, obesity, sedentary lifestyle and left ventricular hypertrophy. An understanding of absolute and relative risk is important when deciding on treatment for patients with hypertension.

New epidemiological and clinical trial information has reshaped treatment guidelines. An understanding of absolute and relative risk (*see* Chapter 4) is essential when making treatment decisions for individual patients. Grading hypertension as mild, moderate or severe may be misleading. For example, a blood pressure recording of 150/95 mmHg has different implications for a 70-year-old man and a 35-year-old man. The 75-year-old has a higher absolute cardiovascular risk, but the 35-year-old is at higher relative risk compared with normal men of his age.

> Treatment decisions should be based on formal estimation of the 10-year coronary heart disease risk using the 'Cardiac Risk Assessor' program or the coronary heart disease risk chart issued by the Joint British Societies.

Isolated systolic hypertension vs. diastolic blood pressure

In patients over 50 years of age, elevation of systolic blood pressure predicts the risk of cardiovascular disease better than increases in diastolic blood pressure. In patients under 50 years, diastolic blood pressure is a stronger predictor of fatal and non-fatal coronary artery disease. After the age of 60 years, diastolic pressure is inversely related to coronary risk, so that pulse pressure is a better predictor of cardiovascular events than systolic blood pressure. The increasing systolic blood pressure increases left ventricular work and the risk of hypertrophy. The lowering of the diastolic blood pressure compromises coronary blood flow. Thus a blood pressure of 150/85 mmHg carries a higher risk than a blood pressure of 150/95 mmHg in patients over 60 years of age. A wide pulse pressure is an important risk factor, and lowering of the systolic blood pressure alone is a primary objective of treatment of hypertension, although it is difficult to achieve.

Isolated systolic blood pressure is defined as a systolic blood pressure of ≥ 140 mmHg with a normal diastolic pressure. It is the commonest form of hypertension, occurring in over two-thirds of people aged over 65 years and three-quarters of those aged over 75 years.

Lowering systolic blood pressure to less than 150 mmHg is associated with reductions of 40% in stroke, 16% in coronary events, 50% in heart failure and 15% in mortality. Observational studies suggest that the lower the blood pressure the better, although this notion is not confirmed by individual outcome trials, except in diabetics.

Reducing systolic blood pressure is difficult, and even with multiple optimal drug combinations it is only achieved in 60% of patients.

Recording devices

Health and safety regulations have relegated the mercury sphygmomanometer to history in hospitals, which now mainly use automated, semi-automated and aneroid devices.

Measurement of blood pressure

Blood pressure is often measured inaccurately, and cardiologists may be especially culpable! Blood pressure is a very labile haemodynamic parameter, varying with each heart beat, hour of the day, season of the year, activity and position of the individual.

Accurate recordings are inexpensive, easily obtained, non-invasive determinants of cardiovascular status and cardiovascular events.

- Blood pressure should be measured with the patient sitting (and standing if they are elderly or diabetic, or if orthostatic hypotension is suspected).
- Current guidelines recommend that recordings should be taken in all patients at least every 5 years, but the frequency of recordings will be determined by the patient's clinical state. Patients with borderline recordings and those with hypertension which is difficult to control will require more frequent recordings and clinical assessments.
- The recording device should be validated, calibrated and regularly maintained. The blood pressure cuff must be of an appropriate size for the patient's arm, which should be at the level of the heart, and the cuff must be deflated slowly enough to aim to measure the blood pressure to the nearest 2 mmHg.
- The cuff should be inflated above the systolic level by feeling the brachial artery pulsation disappear as the cuff is inflated, and then applying the stethoscope over the brachial artery as the cuff is gradually and slowly deflated.
- The systolic pressure should be recorded as the level when the pulse sounds reappear with cuff deflation. The diastolic level should be recorded as the level at which the pulse sounds disappear (Korotkov phase 5).
- Because of the weighting given to blood pressure in cardiovascular risk assessment, use the average recording from several visits when estimating the 10-year risk.

Self-measurement of blood pressure

This is popular with patients who like to record their blood pressure for a variety of reasons. Those with hypertension may be anxious and wish to monitor their condition. Individuals with 'white-coat' syndrome may wish to record their blood pressure from time to time or when they 'feel hypertensive', and they need to be told that anxiety and stress may raise their blood pressure but this does not mean that they have hypertension. Patients may become obsessed with their blood pressure measurements, and this is obviously undesirable. If there is any question that their blood pressure is not controlled, then a 24-hour ambulatory recording may be helpful and hopefully reassuring. Individuals with a family history of hypertension, stroke or premature coronary heart disease may feel vulnerable and want to know if they are also at risk.

There are several blood pressure machines available for self-recording. In general, arm recorders are more accurate than wrist recorders. It is useful for patients to check their device and the accuracy of their self-recording against a simultaneous recording taken in the surgery.

Ambulatory blood pressure recording

This is a very useful and accurate method of non-invasive measurement of the blood pressure during normal daily activities over a 24-hour period, and it should be available in every GP surgery. It provides blood pressure data when the patient is asleep, driving, working or engaged in activities that would be expected to have a significant effect on blood pressure, and when self-recordings or clinic recordings would be difficult to obtain.

Many GP surgeries now have their own machines and computer software for analysing the data, and this greatly improves the quality of care for patients with established or suspected hypertension.

Ambulatory blood pressure recordings are a much stronger predictor of cardiovascular morbidity and mortality than conventional blood pressure recordings, and should be available to all patients with known or suspected hypertension.

Ambulatory blood pressure recordings have shown the natural circadian variation in blood pressure, with an early-morning surge, high levels associated with stress, and low levels when the patient is asleep or resting. It provides a full 24-hour 'panorama' of the patient's blood pressure, rather than a 'snapshot' measurement taken when the patient (and possibly the GP or nurse) is stressed in a busy clinic.

Ambulatory blood pressure recordings and 'white-coat' syndrome

Ambulatory blood pressure recording is particularly useful for evaluating the possibility of 'white-coat' syndrome, which is present in around 25% of people who appear to have hypertension. This condition may be defined as high clinic readings (above 140/90 mmHg) but normal ambulatory blood pressure recordings except for the first stressful and unfamiliar hour of the ambulatory recording. Patients with this common condition do not appear to benefit from antihypertensive treatment. Patients with raised clinic recordings but with an average 24-hour blood pressure level of < 130/80 mmHg are no more likely than normotensive individuals to have a cardiovascular event. They do not need medication and would therefore avoid the associated side-effects. In addition, the exclusion of hypertension has important employment and insurance benefits for the patient, and reduces healthcare costs. In contrast, some individuals with 'normal' self-monitored blood pressure recordings may have high 24-hour ambulatory recordings and would benefit from medication.

Ambulatory blood pressure recordings are a better predictor of cardiovascular out-comes than isolated clinic recordings in patients with treated hypertension. High ambulatory recordings (a mean blood pressure of > 135/85 mmHg) are also a reliable predictor of cardiovascular events. Patients with raised clinic blood pressure recordings should be considered for ambulatory recordings.

Guidelines for the use of 24-hour ambulatory blood pressure recording
- For diagnosis of 'white-coat' syndrome.
- For deciding the diagnosis in patients with borderline clinic readings.
- For clarifying unusual variability of clinic recordings.
- For resistant hypertension (> 150/90 mmHg despite three or more drugs).
- For cases of suspected hypotension.
- For patients with a blood pressure of > 160/100 mmHg with no target organ damage and an estimated 10-year cardiovascular risk of < 15%. If the average ambulatory blood pressure recording is normal, medication may not be necessary.
- For deciding treatment in elderly patients with isolated systolic hypertension.
- For hypertension in pregnancy.
- When a previous ambulatory blood pressure recording is normal, but the patient has borderline hypertension or is at significant cardiovascular risk for other reasons.
- For evaluating the efficacy of treatment.

Interpreting the results of ambulatory blood pressure recordings
The decision to treat should be based on the average daytime readings, not the average 24-hour recording. The threshold for starting treatment should be 12/7 mmHg lower than the clinic readings, because blood pressure recordings are systematically lower with ambulatory recordings. Thus an average ambulatory recording of 148/83 mmHg which equates to a clinic blood pressure of 160/90 mmHg may require treatment.

> An average ambulatory blood pressure of 135/85 mmHg is normal in low-risk individuals, but a level of 130/80 mmHg is optimal in diabetics.

Ambulatory 24-hour blood pressure recordings identify patients whose blood pressure does not fall normally at night ('non-dippers'), who are probably at high risk.

Initial evaluation of the hypertensive patient

The principles of management are as follows.

1 Confirm the diagnosis of hypertension.
2 Evaluate and treat contributing comorbidities and risk factors.
3 Assess the presence of end-organ damage.
4 Consider and screen for possible secondary causes of hypertension.
5 Plan and discuss long-term management with the patient.

Causes of hypertension

> The commonest cause of hypertension is 'essential hypertension' which accounts for at least 94% of cases.

Secondary causes of hypertension

Renovascular causes
Reduced blood flow to either or both kidneys due to renal artery stenosis results in activation of the renin–angiotensin system with increased renin levels and fluid retention. There are two causes of renal artery stenosis.

- *Fibromuscular dysplasia* (25% of cases) typically occurs in young women who present with hypertension and no family history of hypertension.
- *Atherosclerotic stenosis* (70% of cases) is usually bilateral, although one artery is often more affected, and is a progressive disease. It should be considered in patients with resistant hypertension and those who have evidence or a high probability of vascular disease (those who have smoked, those with peripheral vascular, cerebrovascular or coronary artery disease, and those who develop increasing renal impairment when

treated with ACE inhibitors or angiotensin-II antagonists). Bilateral renal artery stenosis may cause 'flash pulmonary oedema' with normal left ventricular failure.

Diagnosis and management

Patients with suspected renal artery stenosis should be referred for a specialist opinion. Duplex ultrasound, computerised tomography (CT) and magnetic resonance imaging (MRI) can be used to select patients for arteriography and revascularisation with angioplasty and stenting (which can be performed at the same time as arteriography), or for surgical reconstruction of the affected arteries.

- Angioplasty and stenting is useful in patients with *fibromuscular renal artery stenosis*. Renal angioplasty may be complicated by local problems, initial proteinuria following a sudden increase in renal artery pressure after dilatation of the stenosis, radiographic contrast agent-induced renal damage, cholesterol emboli (in atherosclerotic disease) and re-stenosis (50% of patients).
- In patients with *atherosclerotic renal artery stenosis*, renal angioplasty is no more effective for control of blood pressure than antihypertensive drug therapy alone. It is therefore no longer necessary to screen all hypertensive patients for renal artery stenosis with a view to angioplasty. However, it should be considered for those with uncontrolled hypertension, high serum creatinine levels, bilateral renal artery stenosis and flash pulmonary oedema and severe unilateral renal artery stenosis.

All classes of antihypertensive drugs may be used. ACE inhibitors may be used in unilateral renal artery stenosis, but are contraindicated in severe bilateral disease. All patients on ACE inhibitors need to have regular renal function tests. Increases in serum creatinine levels are usually reversed when the ACE inhibitor is stopped. In patients on maximal medical treatment but who have resistant severe hypertension, the risk of continuing ACE inhibitors must be weighed against the dangers of uncontrolled hypertension. These patients require specialist assessment.

Renal disease

Hypertension may result from acute renal failure of any cause, including acute glomerulonephritis, vasculitis or acute obstruction, or chronic renal failure due to diabetic nephropathy or chronic glomerulonephritis.

Management

The threshold for treatment in patients with renal disease is > 140/90 mmHg, and the target is < 130/85 mmHg. These patients should be referred to a specialist to plan and monitor the long-term management of the underlying renal disease and to choose the most appropriate combination of tablets. Thiazide diuretics (e.g. bendrofluazide, indapamide, hydrochlorothiazide) may be ineffective, and high-dose loop diuretics (frusemide) may be required. Aggressive lowering of the blood pressure may slow progression of the renal disease. Salt reduction is important in patients with impaired renal function. The use of aspirin and statins should be considered.

Aortic coarctation

This is a narrowing of the aorta, usually distal to the left subclavian artery, and it may be associated with a bicuspid aortic valve and other heart defects. Affected patients may have a heart murmur, hypertension and decreased leg pulses. The resulting hypertension usually resolves if the coarctation is resected during childhood. Hypertension usually persists if surgery is performed in a patient over 40 years of age. Affected patients are vulnerable to hypertensive complications at a younger age.

Management
These patients should be referred for investigation and consideration of surgery or angioplasty. Even after correction of the coarctation, patients require follow-up for hypertension and its complications.

Cushing's syndrome
The diagnosis can be made on the basis of the typical physical appearances. Around 70% of these patients have hypertension.

Management
These patients should be referred for investigation and management of Cushing's syndrome, but they also require effective treatment for hypertension.

Conn's syndrome (primary hyperaldosteronism)
This is most commonly due to a benign, unilateral, autonomous adenoma of the adrenal gland secreting aldosterone. It results in low renin levels, increased sodium and low potassium levels, particularly in patients who are taking diuretics. Importantly, most patients have normal plasma electrolytes at presentation.

Management
These patients should be referred for confirmation and categorisation of the diagnosis, and guidance on the most appropriate medical treatment if necessary. The diagnosis is made by measuring 24-hour urinary aldosterone levels or the plasma aldosterone to plasma renin ratio after withdrawing antihypertensive treatment for 2 weeks.

Aldosterone-secreting adenomata should be localised by either CT or MRI scanning and removed, as this leads to resolution of hypertension in 70% of cases.

Phaeochromocytoma
These are catecholamine-secreting tumours that are usually unilateral and limited to the adrenal glands. They may present incidentally as a first hypertensive episode perioperatively, or as episodic hypertension, headache, palpitation with or without tachycardia and sweating. Other symptoms that reflect catecholamine excess include anxiety, tremor, nausea, chest or abdominal pain, weight loss and fatigue. There may be dramatic increases in blood pressure.

The diagnosis should be suspected in patients with suggestive symptoms, resistant hypertension or severe hypertension during pregnancy (when the uterus may press on the adrenal gland).

Management
The diagnosis can be made by measuring the levels of catecholamine breakdown products in the urine over a 24-hour collection period. A negative assay has a 98% predictive value for excluding the condition in a primary care population, and the test may be arranged with the local pathology department, which will be able to provide instructions on what food and medication the patient can take before and during the collection.

The patient should be referred to a specialist, who may wish to perform further tests (including localisation of the tumour by MRI or CT scanning). Surgical removal of the tumour(s) usually results in normalisation of the blood pressure, but 25% of patients may have persistent hypertension.

Drug causes of hypertension

The following drugs may cause hypertension:

- oestrogens
- β-agonists (bronchodilators, stimulant abuse, over-the-counter 'cold cures')
- steroids
- liquorice
- non-steroidal anti-inflammatory drugs.

Correctable factors that contribute to hypertension

These include the following:

- overweight
- excess alcohol consumption (> 3 units per day)
- excess salt intake
- lack of exercise.

Complications and target organ damage associated with hypertension

These include the following:

- stroke
- multi-infarct dementia
- left ventricular hypertrophy
- heart failure
- coronary artery disease
- peripheral vascular disease
- retinal hypertensive changes
- proteinuria
- renal impairment.

British Hypertension Society guidelines

The following initial investigations are recommended in the British Hypertension Society guidelines:

- urinalysis for protein and blood
- serum creatinine and electrolytes
- blood glucose
- serum total:HDL-cholesterol
- ECG.

Echocardiography is valuable for assessing the presence of left ventricular hypertrophy.

Treatment of hypertension

The following recommendations have been made by the British Hypertension Society.

> The aim of treatment is to lower blood pressure sufficiently to prevent cardiovascular complications with no drug-induced adverse effects. The choice of drug is of secondary importance.

> The response to treatment is mainly determined by the patient's age.

Patient education

One of the major problems in treating hypertension is that most patients are symptom-free and do not like taking tablets. It is important that the patient understands what hypertension is, what the possible complications may be, what general measures they can and should instigate and maintain for themselves, what tablets they should take, and how they should be monitored. They should be told both their current blood pressure and their target level.

Although the prevention of cardiovascular complications is the primary aim and (hopefully) result of treatment, antihypertensive treatment also prevents dementia, which suggests that it improves both mental and physical quality of life in symptom-free patients.

> After a diagnosis of hypertension has been established, the patient needs to understand that treatment and lifestyle measures are for life. Medication may need to be adjusted or changed depending on the response or the development of side-effects.

Blood pressure targets

> In general, the lower the blood pressure the better, particularly in diabetics.
> - The target for all patients of all ages is < 140/90 mmHg.
> - The target for patients with target-organ damage or cardiovascular disease is 130/85 mmHg.

There is less evidence for this principle in patients with left ventricular damage, renovascular disease, or cardiovascular or cerebrovascular disease.

Targets are helpful to clinicians but are difficult to achieve, even in fully compliant patients. The blood pressure levels suggested as 'audit standards' in the current guidelines are higher than the recommended targets.

Because blood pressure increases with age, life events and other factors, the recommended targets become increasingly difficult to achieve. Reduction of blood pressure, particularly systolic pressure levels in people over 60 years of age, is important for decreasing the incidence of cardiovascular events.

When the target blood pressure is not achieved

Patients may become very anxious if they feel that they have 'failed' by not achieving their target blood pressure. They should be told that this is unfortunately not uncommon, even with perfect compliance and the best medication. Occasionally this anxiety and frustration may lead to a preoccupation with their blood pressure levels, making control even more difficult. When starting drug therapy, it can be helpful to advise the patient that it may not be possible to achieve the target blood pressure despite perfect compliance and the best medication. Further emphasis on non-pharmacological measures often helps to raise the patient's morale.

Target achievers

Some responders may feel that the diagnosis was wrong, and may stop or ask to stop taking their tablets. If hypertensive patients stop taking their tablets, their blood pressure will inevitably increase within a few weeks, but it may occasionally be necessary to go through this exercise to satisfy doubtful patients.

Target achievers should be congratulated on achieving their targets and reassured that the reason their blood pressure is 'low' is because of the medication they are taking and the other measures they are adopting.

Table 12.1:   Target blood pressures during antihypertensive treatment (both the systolic and diastolic blood pressure targets should be achieved)

	Clinic BP (mmHg)		Mean daytime ABPM or home BP (mmHg)	
	No diabetes	Diabetes	No diabetes	Diabetes
Optimal BP	< 140/85	< 140/80	< 130/80	< 130/75
Audit standard	< 150/90	< 140/85	< 140/85	< 140/80

BP, blood pressure; ABPM, ambulatory blood pressure monitoring.

The audit standard referred to in Table 12.1 is the minimum recommended level of blood pressure control, recognising that only 10% of patients have target blood levels.

Non-pharmacological measures

Primary prevention of hypertension

Quite often it is found that overweight, stressed, inactive individuals with high clinic blood pressure readings respond, at least initially, to the following measures, which are effective in primary prevention and may render drug treatment unnecessary or at least reduce the number of different drugs needed by enhancing their antihypertensive effect:

- weight loss (*see* Chapter 7)
- reduction of salt intake to less than 5 g (1 teaspoonful) per day
- low-fat diet (*see* Chapter 7)
- modest alcohol consumption (< 21 units per week for men and < 14 units per week for women)
- cardiovascular exercise (*see* Chapter 9) (e.g. 20 minutes of fast walking per day) and avoidance of isometric exercise
- plenty of fruit and vegetables (*see* Chapter 7)
- stopping smoking (*see* Chapter 8)
- optimisation of lipids, with drugs if necessary (*see* Chapter 5).

The importance of these measures should be emphasised and continually reiterated with enthusiasm by the practice nurse and GP, who should show patience with the patient and their family. These measures are an integral part of the initial and long-term treatment of all patients with hypertension. Drug treatment may need to be started without delay in patients with severe hypertension.

Treatment thresholds

These are based on an estimation of coronary heart disease risk (*see* Chapter 4).

> Effective antihypertensive treatment results in a relative risk reduction of 38% for stroke, and a 16% reduction in coronary events.

The benefits and drawbacks of drug treatment must be explained to patients who reach the treatment thresholds. Ultimately it is the responsibility of the patient to comply with the advice given, but additional consultations are helpful in addressing concerns that they or their family may have.

The main thresholds for antihypertensive treatment are as follows:

- A target of < 140/85 mmHg is recommended for most patients.
- The target for diabetic patients is < 140/80 mmHg.
- Patients with accelerated (malignant) hypertension (papilloedema, fundal haemorrhages or exudates) should be referred and admitted to hospital for immediate treatment, but treatment should be started in the surgery if there is a delay.
- Treatment should be started immediately in patients with a blood pressure of > 220/120 mmHg.
- Drug therapy should be started in all patients with sustained (monitored over a 4-week period) systolic blood pressure of > 160 mmHg or sustained diastolic blood pressure of > 100 mmHg despite non-pharmacological measures.
- Drug therapy should be started in patients with sustained systolic blood pressure of > 140 mmHg or diastolic blood pressure of > 90 mmHg only if:
  - target-organ damage is present, or
  - there is evidence of cardiovascular disease and/or diabetes, or

  – the 10-year coronary heart disease risk is > 15%.
Otherwise, patients with a blood pressure of < 160/100 mmHg and *no* target-organ damage or cardiovascular complications, no diabetes and a 10-year coronary heart disease risk of < 15% do not need drug treatment, but should be given advice about non-pharmacological measures and be monitored monthly.

• Patients with a blood pressure of < 135/85 mmHg should be reassessed every 5 years.

Choice of antihypertensive drug

The British Hypertension Society indications and contraindications for different classes of antihypertensive drugs are useful, and are presented in Table 12.2.

Factors that influence the choice of antihypertensive drug

Table 12.2 provides useful clinical pointers when selecting an antihypertensive drug. The 'AB/CD rule' is helpful when choosing drug combinations in hypertension, and refers to the first letter of the four main classes of drugs used (see below).

Table 12.2:   British Hypertension Society indications and contraindications for different classes of antihypertensive drugs

Class of drug	Indications	Contraindications
α-Blockers	Prostatism	Postural hypotension
	Dyslipidaemias	Urinary incontinence
ACE inhibitors	Heart failure	Pregnancy
	Left ventricular dysfunction	Renovascular disease
	Diabetic nephropathy	Peripheral vascular
	Chronic renal disease[a]	disease[b]
β-Blockers	Myocardial infarction	Asthma/COAD
	Angina	Heart block
	Heart failure[c]	Bradycardia
		Severe claudication
Calcium blockers	Elderly with ISH	—
(dihydropyridines)	Angina	
Calcium blockers	Angina	Heart block
(rate-limiting)	Uncontrolled atrial fibrillation	Bradycardia
	Heart failure	
Thiazides	Elderly	Gout

[a]ACE inhibitors may be beneficial in chronic renal failure but should be used with caution, monitoring of renal function, and with specialist advice if the patient has severe renal impairment.
[b]Peripheral vascular disease is a possible contraindication to the use of ACE inhibitors because of its association with renal artery stenosis and renovascular disease.
[c]Use carefully (low dose to start with, and increase slowly) in patients with significant left ventricular impairment or a history of heart failure.
COAD, chronic obstructive airways disease; ISH, isolated systolic hypertension.

Renin levels and hypertension

The recognition that younger (< 55 years), white patients are more likely to have vasoconstrictor, high-renin hypertension (type 1), while Afro-Caribbean and older white patients tend to have volume-dependent, low-renin hypertension (type 2), provides a pathophysiological rationale when choosing antihypertensive drugs.

- The high-renin, type 1 hypertensive patient should be treated with ACE inhibitors or angiotensin II antagonists (A), or β-blockers (B).
- Patients with low renin levels (e.g. Afro-Caribbean patients) are best treated with a calcium antagonist (C) or a diuretic (D), and should have a low-salt diet. β-blockers and ACE inhibitors may be ineffective as monotherapy, although these drugs may be used when combined with a drug that activates the renin–angiotensin system (e.g. diuretics, calcium antagonists or α-blockers).
- For both types of hypertension, dietary measures are important, but compared with patients with type 2 hypertension, salt restriction in patients with type 1 hypertension may not be as effective in reducing blood pressure.

Drug combinations

Drugs from different classes have additive effects when combined. Sub-maximal doses of two drugs may avoid or reduce the side-effects of maximal doses of a single drug. The A or B plus C or D rule applies.

Rational drug combinations include the following:

- a diuretic (D) plus either a β-blocker (B) or an ACE inhibitor (A), or
- a calcium antagonist (C) plus either a β-blocker (B) or an ACE inhibitor or angiotensin II antagonist

- if a third antihypertensive drug is necessary, a calcium antagonist (C) can be added to a diuretic and an ACE inhibitor (A), or to a diuretic (D) and a β-blocker (B).

> Less than half of all hypertensives will be controlled on one drug, and one-third of patients will require three or more drugs.

Initial drug treatment in hypertension

- Use a low-dose diuretic as first-line treatment unless there is a contraindication or a compelling indication for using another drug.
- An ACE inhibitor would be appropriate for patients with diabetes and/or vascular disease.
- For patients with cardiac failure, use a combination of a diuretic and an ACE inhibitor plus a β-blocker if appropriate.
- Dihydropyridine calcium antagonists can be used as an alternative to a diuretic in cases of isolated systolic hypertension in the elderly, and have been shown to prevent strokes.

Inappropriate drug combinations

The following combinations are not recommended:

- β-blocker plus verapamil or diltiazem (bradycardia)
- ACE inhibitor plus angiotensin II antagonist (renal failure and hyperkalaemia)
- potassium-sparing diuretic plus ACE inhibitor.

Compliance

> Drugs do not work if they are not taken.

> Treatment failure – is it due to the drug or the patient?

However good and rational the choice of antihypertensive drugs, there is little chance of lowering blood pressure if the patient does not take their medication as prescribed. It is essential that they understand why, despite feeling well, they need to take tablets as prescribed for life, and that the dose of their medication may need to be increased or additional drugs prescribed if their blood pressure remains high.

Non-compliance is an important cause of failure to achieve blood pressure targets. Lack of recognition of this leads to the clinician prescribing a higher dose of the prescribed medication, or alternative additional tablets. Most patients take approximately 75% of doses as prescribed across a variety of medical disorders. Compliance does not correlate with intelligence, personality, age, level of education or the number of drugs prescribed, but is probably increased just before and after surgery appointments. Whether it is affected by the healthcare professional whom the patient sees (GP or practice nurse) is unclear.

> Non-compliance should be suspected and explored as the first reason for persistent hypertension.

There are several reasons for non-compliance which may be viewed as 'part of human nature'.

- Non-compliance is more likely with frequent dosing during the day, and can be improved with once daily dosing.
- Non-compliance may develop in previously compliant patients if they feel that the medication is not necessary or they become relaxed about their condition.
- Patients, particularly the elderly or the very busy, may simply forget to take their tablets at the prescribed times.

Potential dangers of non-compliance

Omission of short-acting drugs (e.g. calcium antagonists, β-blockers or vasodilators such as doxazocin) may result in blood pressure surges, with the risk of vascular events.

Improving drug compliance

Try to select drugs which can be given together, preferably once a day and at a time the patient will remember and schedule as part of their daily routine. Ask the patient what time of day they would prefer and would be more likely to remember their tablets. This depends on the patient having some order to their day. For example, it may be with their first cup of tea, with breakfast, when they arrive at work, or with their lunch. Competent patients have to take responsibility for taking their medication.

Combination tablets that are prescribed once a day improve compliance. Check compliance whenever the patient comes to the surgery. Patients who travel frequently for work or social purposes need to establish a routine for taking their tablets.

Aspirin in hypertension

Treating a hypertensive patient with aspirin decreases cardiovascular events by 15% and myocardial infarction by 36%, but the benefit depends on the individual's absolute cardiovascular risk. The number of aspirin-related bleeds is similar to the number of cardiovascular events prevented by aspirin. Mortality is unaffected. Therefore aspirin confers only a marginal benefit. Hypertension must be controlled before starting aspirin, which is recommended in primary and secondary prevention as follows.

1   In primary prevention to:

- patients aged > 50 years with target organ damage (left ventricular hypertrophy, proteinuria or renal impairment) with no contraindication *and* a blood pressure of < 150/90 mmHg, or
- a 10-year coronary heart disease risk of > 15% (antihypertensive treatment reduces this risk by 25%, and aspirin will reduce this risk by a further 15%), or
- type 2 diabetics.
  The numbers needed to treat analysis for aspirin:
  - 60 hypertensive patients will need to be treated with aspirin for 5 years in order to prevent one cardiovascular complication
  - 90 hypertensive patients will need to be treated with aspirin for 5 years in order to prevent one myocardial infarction.

2   In secondary prevention.

Treating hypertension in diabetics

Hypertension is present in 70% of patients with type 2 diabetes, but its prevalence is not increased in patients with type 1 diabetes without nephropathy (microalbuminuria or proteinuria).

- Type 1 diabetes without nephropathy – threshold for drug intervention is > 140/90 mmHg, and optimal blood pressure is < 140/80 mmHg.

- Type 1 diabetes with nephropathy – blood pressure reduction and ACE inhibitors slow the rate of decline in renal function and delay progression to nephropathy.

> ACE inhibitors are the first-line treatment in diabetics, and should be given and titrated up to the maximum recommended and tolerated dose, even in patients who are normotensive.

Patients should be given an angiotensin II blocker if they cannot tolerate an ACE inhibitor. The blood pressure target is 130/80 mmHg, and 125/75 mmHg if there is proteinuria. Treatment with aspirin and a statin should be considered.

Type 2 diabetes

Hypertension is common, is related to obesity and is predictive of cardiovascular events.

> - Hypertension control in diabetics is more important than glycaemic control in improving survival. It reduces cardiovascular events by 50%.
> - The recommended threshold for intervention with antihypertensive drugs in type 2 diabetes is < 140/90 mmHg, and the target blood pressure is <140/80 mmHg.

The choice of drugs (apart from using an ACE inhibitor) does not appear to matter.

Patients with type 2 diabetes and nephropathy are at high risk of cardiovascular events, and all of their risk factors need vigorous attention. They should be taking aspirin. The target blood pressure is 130/75 mmHg.

Hypertension after myocardial infarction

β-blockers are recommended for all patients without contraindications after myocardial infarction, and ACE inhibitors for patients with left ventricular systolic impairment and for diabetics. All vascular risk factors should be treated.

Hypertension in pregnancy

Hypertension occurs in 10% of pregnancies, and is an important cause of maternal and fetal morbidity and mortality. It is associated with abruptio placentae and cerebral haemorrhage in the mother, and with fetal prematurity, stillbirth and neonatal death.

Hypertension may be the first sign of pre-eclampsia, which further increases the maternal and fetal risk, and is characterised by significant proteinuria (oedema is no longer a diagnostic criterion). The mechanism of eclampsia remains unclear. It may lead to intrauterine growth restriction. Both the mother and the baby should be monitored carefully and may need referral to hospital if the blood pressure is not optimally controlled, if the baby is not growing or if there is proteinuria.

Hypertensive patients who become pregnant and those who develop hypertension during pregnancy must be referred to a cardiologist who should liaise with obstetric colleagues to optimise management during pregnancy, delivery and postpartum.

Treatment thresholds during pregnancy

In the absence of evidence from randomised trials, treatment guidelines are based on observational studies, experience and a reluctance to use drugs which could result in teratogenicity.

Blood pressure levels fall during pregnancy, so it may be possible to reduce or withdraw medication in patients with mild hypertension, although frequent monitoring is essential.

Drug treatment is essential at a blood pressure of > 170/110 mmHg, but is justified at > 140/90 mmHg. The blood pressure should be measured and the urine checked for protein every week. If either of these are unsatisfactory, the patient should be referred to hospital.

All women with hypertension during pregnancy should be monitored after delivery to determine whether they need long-term treatment or further investigations.

'White-coat' hypertension occurs in 30% of pregnant women. Ambulatory blood pressure recordings are very useful, and the confirmation of a normal or only slightly raised blood pressure can mean the avoidance of unnecessary anxiety, treatment and hospital admissions in this large group of women.

Pre-eclampsia

Patients are usually symptom-free, and 30% of pre-eclamptic fits occur in the absence of a raised blood pressure or proteinuria.

The diagnostic criteria are as follows:

- a rise in diastolic blood pressure of 15 mmHg or in systolic blood pressure of > 30 mmHg from early pregnancy, or
- a diastolic blood pressure of > 90 mmHg on two occasions 4 hours apart or of > 110 mmHg on one occasion and proteinuria.

Pre-eclampsia resolves with delivery, which must be timed carefully to optimise fetal maturation.

Risk factors for pre-eclampsia include first pregnancy, change of partner, previous pre-eclampsia, family history of pre-eclampsia, idiopathic hypertension, chronic renal disease, diabetes, multiple pregnancy and obesity. Antihypertensive treatment has not been shown to improve fetal outcome.

> Patients with pre-eclampsia need urgent referral and treatment.

Choice of antihypertensive treatment in pregnancy

Methyldopa (750 mg to 4 g daily in three or four divided doses) remains the drug of choice because of its relatively low risk of side-effects, and long experience of its use. Other acceptable drugs include calcium antagonists, hydralazine and labetalol. Diuretics reduce plasma volume and may theoretically increase the risk of pre-eclampsia. ACE inhibitors are contraindicated because of the risk of renal malformation.

Hypertensive women who become or plan to become pregnant should switch to a drug regime that is recommended as safe during pregnancy, and switch back to their usual medication after delivery.

Oral contraceptives in patients with hypertension

The combined oral contraceptive pill has a small and unpredictable adverse effect on blood pressure. Blood pressure should be measured before starting oral contraceptives and 6-monthly thereafter. Although the combined oral contraceptive pill is not absolutely contraindicated in hypertensive women, non-hormonal forms of contraception or switching to a progestogen-only pill are recommended for patients with other cardiovascular risk factors. The latter should be addressed and treated.

Chronic hypertension

This is hypertension which occurs before 20 weeks' gestation, and although it is usually idiopathic, other secondary causes should be considered and excluded. Most physicians recommend drug intervention at a blood pressure level of > 140/90 mmHg.

Hormone replacement therapy in hypertension

This is not contraindicated in controlled hypertension, which should be monitored frequently during the first few months and then 6-monthly. It may need to be temporarily stopped in patients with resistant hypertension.

Resistant hypertension

This can be defined as a blood pressure above target levels despite an optimal combination of drugs – for example, (A or B) + (C or D). Assuming that there is drug compliance, alcohol is the commonest cause. It may also be due to a 'white-coat' phenomenon.

Treatment of resistant hypertension

Compliance must first be checked, contributing factors should be addressed, and secondary causes of hypertension, particularly phaeochromocytoma, hyperaldosteronism (Conn's syndrome) and renal artery stenosis must be excluded. Patients with a high aldosterone:renin ratio may respond to treatment with spironolactone.

For patients who are already on four or five drugs, minoxidil, a powerful vasodilator, is effective. Its side-effects include hirsutism (which may be welcomed by bald men).

A combination of a diuretic (D), a calcium antagonist (C), an ACE inhibitor (A) and/or an α-blocker is effective.

The 'white-coat' effect is the term used to describe the rise in blood pressure that occurs in a medical setting regardless of the ambulatory blood pressure recording. As many as 75% of treated hypertensive patients may have clinic recordings which exceed the average of their ambulatory 24-hour recording by 20/10 mmHg, due to this effect rather than to resistant hypertension.

Hypertension in the elderly

Isolated systolic hypertension is common in elderly patients, but may be overestimated by clinic readings, leading to excessive treatment and possible side-effects, including drug-related hypotension and falls. Ambulatory blood pressure recordings are helpful when evaluating this group of patients. Management of the elderly hypertensive is dealt with in Chapter 23.

Emergency treatment of hypertension

This is indicated for the following:

- hypertensive encephalopathy (most often due to eclampsia)
- left ventricular failure
- dissecting aortic aneurysm.

Intravenous nitrate alone or with labetalol is useful for lowering blood pressure in cases of acute aortic dissection. Nitroprusside (for a maximum of a few days only, due to cyanide toxicity) can be used for the other two conditions.

Answers to case studies

1   If a 24-hour blood pressure recording shows an average blood pressure of $\leq 135/85$ mmHg, then this patient can be reassured and encouraged to exercise and lose weight. His blood sugar level will need review. If the 24-hour blood pressure recording is > 140/90 mmHg, he should be encouraged to pay serious attention to all of his modifiable risk factors and have another 24-hour blood pressure recording after he has lost weight. If his blood pressure remains > 135/85 mmHg and a formal cardiovascular risk estimation indicates that he is at greater than 15% risk, he should be treated with either a thiazide or a β-blocker or, if he is diagnosed as diabetic or cannot tolerate a β-blocker, with an ACE inhibitor.

2   Treatment must be started immediately and the patient should be referred to hospital for further investigation.

3   If there is doubt about this patient's true daily blood pressure recordings, check her 24-hour recordings. If these show a sustained rise in diastolic pressure of > 15 mmHg or a rise in systolic pressure of > 30 mmHg, the patient fulfils the criteria for pre-eclampsia and should be referred to hospital for treatment and control. Treatment should be started if the blood pressure is > 170/110 mmHg, but many physicians would start treatment at a level of > 140/90 mmHg. Even if the result of the 24-hour recording is satisfactory, the patient's blood pressure should be monitored continually during pregnancy and after delivery, as it is likely that she will require treatment at some stage.

4   Explain to this patient the potential advantages of blood pressure control in reducing stroke, cardiovascular events, heart failure and dementia, and try her on a thiazide diuretic. Reducing her blood pressure is likely to prolong her active

life. The target blood pressure level is 140/90 mmHg, and she may need an additional drug (e.g. an ACE inhibitor).

5 The target blood pressure for patients with type 2 diabetes is < 140/80 mmHg, and at this level there is a 50% reduction in cardiovascular events. This patient should be gently reminded that she has a 30% risk of a cardiovascular event within 10 years. Combinations of an ACE inhibitor, β-blockers, dihydropyridine calcium-channel blockers, thiazide diuretics and α-blockers are all suitable. It is important to pay attention to all cardiovascular risk factors. It is clearly going to be difficult for this patient to achieve her blood pressure targets, and she will need help, encouragement and regular monitoring.

Further reading

- ALLHAT Officers and Co-ordinators for the ALLHAT Collaborative Research Group (2002) Major outcomes in high-risk patients randomized to angiotensin-converting-enzyme inhibitor or calcium-channel blocker vs diuretic. The Antihypertensive and Lipid-Lowering Treatment to Prevent Heart Attack Trial (ALLHAT). *JAMA*. **288**: 2981–97.
- August P (2003) Initial treatment of hypertension. *NEJM*. **348**: 610–17.
- Benetos A, Thomas F, Bean K *et al.* (2002) Prognostic value of systolic and diastolic blood pressure in treated hypertensive men. *Arch Intern Med*. **162**: 577–81.
- Blood Pressure Lowering Treatment Trialists Collaboration (2000) Effects of angiotensin-converting-enzyme inhibitors, calcium antagonists and other blood pressure-lowering drugs on mortality and major cardiovascular morbidity. *Lancet*. **356**: 1955–64.
- Brown MJ (2001) Matching the right drug to the right patient in essential hypertension. *Heart*. **86**: 113–20.
- Brown MJ, Palmer CR, Castaigne A *et al.* (2000) Morbidity and mortality in patients randomised to double-blind treatment with once daily calcium-channel blockade or diuretic in the International Nifedipine GITS Study: intervention as a goal in hypertension treatment (INSIGHT). *Lancet*. **356**: 366–42.
- Clement DL, De Buyzere ML, De Bacquer DA *et al.* (2003) Prognostic value of ambulatory blood-pressure recordings in patients with treated hypertension. *NEJM*. **348**: 2407–15.
- Franklin SS, Khan SA, Wong ND *et al.* (1999) Is pulse pressure useful in predicting risk for coronary heart disease? The Framingham Heart Study. *Circulation*. **100**: 354–60.
- Heart Outcomes Prevention Evaluation Study Investigators (2000) Effects of Ramipril on cardiovascular and microvascular outcomes in people with diabetes mellitus: results of the HOPE study and MICRO-HOPE substudy. *Lancet*. **355**: 253–9.
- O'Brien E (2003) Ambulatory blood pressure monitoring in the management of hypertension. *Heart*. **89**: 571–6.
- Pickering T (1988) How common is white coat hypertension? *JAMA*. **259**: 225–8.
- Ramsay LE, Williams B, Johnston GD *et al.* (1999) BHS guidelines. Guidelines for the management of hypertension: report of the third working party of the British Hypertension Society. *J Hum Hypertens*. **13**: 569–92.
- Van Jaarsveld BC, Krijnen P, Pieterman H *et al.* (2000) The effect of balloon angioplasty on hypertension in atherosclerotic renal-artery stenosis. *NEJM*. **342**: 1007–14.
- Wing LMH, Reid CM, Ryan P *et al.* (2003) A comparison of outcomes with angiotensin-converting-enzyme inhibitors and diuretics for hypertension in the elderly. *NEJM*. **348**: 583–92.

CHAPTER 13

Heart failure

Case studies

1 An 81-year-old hypertensive woman complains of exertional breathlessness and ankle swelling, but has normal left ventricular function on echocardiography. What would you do?
2 A 68-year-old man develops a dry unpleasant cough 6 months after starting an angiotensin-converting-enzyme (ACE) inhibitor? What would you do?
3 A 76-year-old man with heart failure develops dizziness and breathlessness after starting a β-blocker. What would you do?
4 The creatinine concentration increases to twice the normal level in a 71-year-old man with peripheral vascular disease and hypertension shortly after increasing the dose of an ACE inhibitor. What would you do?
5 A 73-year-old man with a dilated cardiomyopathy requires repeated hospital treatment for deteriorating heart failure. What would you do?
6 A 69-year-old woman develops hyperkalaemia. What would you do?

Importance of heart failure in primary care

The incidence and prevalence of heart failure are increasing due to a combination of factors. There are nearly one million people with heart failure in the UK. People are living longer, partly due to improved living standards, cancer screening and treatment, widespread public recognition of the importance of lifestyle changes, and improved management of cardiovascular risk factors and treatment of hypertension and myocardial infarction. Because domiciliary management plays an important role in reducing hospital admissions, and most patients with stable or compensated heart failure will be managed in primary care, primary care clinicians need to be familiar with the modern management of this condition.

Heart failure treatment and hospitalisations account for 2% of UK health expenditure. Most patients with heart failure will attend their GP surgery at least 10 times per year.

The National Service Framework for Coronary Heart Disease emphasises the importance of heart failure in primary care. It involves producing a register of patients with coronary heart disease and left ventricular impairment – the major cause of heart failure in the UK.

Treatment complexities in managing heart failure

A greater proportion of patients with heart failure will be older and more likely to have coexisting morbidity (e.g. memory impairment and difficulty with medication compliance, immobility for various reasons, valve disease, widespread vascular disease, diabetes and renal impairment) which can complicate management. Most patients with heart failure also have vascular disease and are taking several different drugs. These conditions pose significant management challenges.

Factors that improve the community management of heart failure

Most GPs will have responsibility for the management of at least 20 patients with heart failure, and this figure will probably increase.

More patients can and should be diagnosed, treated and monitored in the community by well-trained, experienced and energetic multi-disciplinary teams that are familiar with all aspects of heart failure management and aware of the potential medical and psychological problems involved. They should be alert to situations where specialist referral is advisable. The management of heart failure in the community is improved by good communication between secondary and primary care, accessible and prompt echocardiography, and links to expert sub-specialty cardiology services that offer the electrophysiological expertise of arrhythmia management, biventricular pacing and cardiac defibrillators, cardiac surgery and specialist nurse services.

Specialist nurses can provide the following:

- medical and lifestyle advice and information regarding fluid and food intake, smoking cessation, blood pressure control, diet, weight control, exercise and cardiovascular risk factor management
- psychological support and identification of patients who require assessment for antidepressants or other forms of therapy and support
- supporting and educating carers about heart failure management
- advice on contraception and vaccination. It is recommended that patients with heart failure should be offered an annual vaccination against flu and the single vaccination against pneumococcal disease
- domiciliary visits to check the clinical status, heart rhythm and fluid status of the patient to measure their weight, ensure drug compliance and recognise any clinical deterioration that necessitates a change in medication or specialist review.

What is heart failure?

> Heart failure is a syndrome that results from any structural or functional disorder which affects the heart.

Although the long-term prognosis of heart failure remains poor despite advances in medical and non-pharmacological therapy, much may be done to reduce its incidence and progression and to improve the quality of life of the growing proportion of the population who have this common condition.

The commonest type is *systolic heart failure*, which is usually due to impaired left ventricular contraction. This occurs in all age groups, mainly affects males, and is often due to myocardial infarction and hypertension. The left ventricle is usually dilated and the ejection fraction is reduced.

Diastolic heart failure with preserved left ventricular function, occurs in around 40% of patients, and is due to abnormal filling of the ventricles. The haemodynamic and clinical consequences are similar to those for systolic heart failure. Patients with diastolic heart failure are typically elderly, female, obese, hypertensive and diabetic, and in contrast to patients with systolic heart failure, they have preserved or normal left ventricular size, systolic function and ejection fraction. The diagnosis is made by finding clinical features of heart failure but normal systolic function on echocardiography, which may also show signs of abnormal ventricular filling.

Diagnostic criteria for heart failure

The European Society of Cardiology criteria for the diagnosis of heart failure are as follows:

- appropriate symptoms and/or signs of heart failure
- objective evidence of cardiac dysfunction on echocardiography and electro-cardiography
- appropriate response to treatment.

Clinical features of heart failure

Symptoms include the following:

- shortness of breath on exercise and at rest in severe cases
- fatigue
- fluid retention.

Signs include the following:

- tachycardia
- raised jugular venous pressure
- added heart sounds
- pulmonary crackles
- ankle swelling.

Diagnosis of heart failure

Heart failure should be suspected if a patient has relevant symptoms and/or signs. However, the sensitivity of clinical features in diagnosis is poor. For example, oedema and orthopnoea have a sensitivity of only 20%, and their specificity is 80%.

Chronic airways disease should be excluded on clinical grounds and by chest X-ray and spirometry.

Figure 13.1 shows the algorithm for diagnosing heart failure based on guidelines from the European Society of Cardiology.

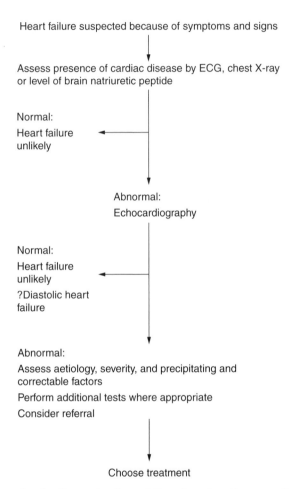

Heart failure suspected because of symptoms and signs

Assess presence of cardiac disease by ECG, chest X-ray or level of brain natriuretic peptide

Normal:
Heart failure unlikely

Abnormal:
Echocardiography

Normal:
Heart failure unlikely
?Diastolic heart failure

Abnormal:
Assess aetiology, severity, and precipitating and correctable factors
Perform additional tests where appropriate
Consider referral

Choose treatment

Figure 13.1:   Algorithm for diagnosing heart failure, based on European Society of Cardiology guidelines.

Classification of heart failure

Until recently, patients with heart failure were classified according to their functional limitation using the New York Heart Association (NYHA) classification (*see* Chapter 2). This classification does not take into account their risk factors for heart failure. Patients in NYHA class IV may after treatment revert to stage III, although their underlying pathology remains unchanged.

A new classification published by the American College of Cardiology and the American Heart Association emphasises the evolution and progression of heart failure, highlights prevention strategies and superimposes treatment strategies. Four stages have been described.

- Stage A – the patient is at high risk of developing heart failure, but has no structural heart abnormality.
- Stage B – the patient has a structural heart abnormality, but has never had symptoms of heart failure.
- Stage C – the patient has a structural heart abnormality and current or previous symptoms of heart failure.
- Stage D – the patient has end-stage heart failure that is refractory to standard treatment and requires special intervention.

Although patients may show an improvement in their NYHA class, patients can only deteriorate in class using the new staging classification which is analogous to staging of cancer.

Investigations

The most important and useful investigation is *echocardiography*, which may show either global (e.g. in a dilated cardiomyopathy) or regional (e.g. after myocardial infarction) ventricular wall movement abnormality. Systolic heart failure can be excluded if the echocardiogram is normal.

- Cardiac chamber size measurement is useful for evaluating severity and prognosis, and it provides a baseline. Mitral and/or aortic valve disease should be excluded. Occasionally heart failure may be caused by infective endocarditis, which may be difficult to diagnose clinically.
- A *12-lead electrocardiogram* is usually normal in patients with stage A heart failure, but is rarely normal in patients with stages B, C or D heart failure. It may show atrial fibrillation or ectopic beats, signs of myocardial infarction, left ventricular hypertrophy and ST and T-wave changes, conduction abnormalities or bundle branch block. These findings are important both diagnostically and prognostically. Patients who have left bundle branch block and stages C and D heart failure should be considered for cardiac resynchronisation therapy.
- A *chest X-ray* may show an enlarged heart shadow, signs of pulmonary oedema and pleural effusions. Heart failure may develop in susceptible patients as a result of a chest infection or pneumonia.
- *Blood tests* – check the renal function, glucose, blood count, thyroid function, liver function and blood lipids.
- *Urinalysis* – check for protein and glucose.
- *Brain natriuretic peptide (BNP)* is a hormone that is released from the cardiac ventricles in response to stretch and dilatation, and its levels are increased in patients with right or left systolic or diastolic heart failure of any cause. BNP levels rise with age.

    BNP can now be measured in primary care. This facility for 'point of care' testing' would reduce the number of patients referred for a consultation or for

echocardiography with suspected heart failure, and it would also provide rapid results, allowing equally rapid changes in therapy.
- The widely accepted cut-off value for BNP is 100 pg/l.
- Heart failure can be ruled out in a patient with symptoms that suggest heart failure, if the BNP level is normal.
- If the BNP concentration is raised, there is a strong possibility that the patient has heart failure, for which they should undergo investigations with echocardiography.

   A raised BNP level in a patient with normal ventricular function on echo-cardiography is compatible with diastolic heart failure, left ventricular hypertrophy, unstable angina or pulmonary hypertension.

   BNP measurements are helpful for confirming the diagnosis of heart failure, for triaging patients with suggestive symptoms for echocardiography, and for screening patients at risk of heart failure. BNP levels decrease after effective treatment of heart failure.

Note: The severity, cause, precipitating factors, risk factors, type of cardiac dysfunction and underlying cardiac structural abnormality should be defined.

Other tests (e.g. coronary angiography) may be required. The stage of heart failure is then classified, and treatment is started.

Causes of heart failure

The common causes of heart failure in the UK, accounting for over 90% of cases, are coronary heart disease (ischaemia and myocardial infarction) and hypertension. Congestive heart failure is a term used to describe combined right and left heart failure. Primary right heart failure due to chronic obstructive airways disease is also common.

Box 13.1:   Causes of heart failure

Causes of primary left heart failure
Hypertension
Coronary heart disease (ischaemia, infarction)
Cardiomyopathy
  Dilated
  Hypertrophic
  Viral myocarditis
Valvular heart disease
  Mitral valve disease
  Aortic valve disease
Congenital heart disease
  Atrial septal defect
  Ventricular septal defect
Arrhythmias
  Chronic persistent atrial fibrillation
  Chronic bradycardia (complete heart block)

Chronic excessive alcohol consumption
Drugs that depress contraction of a weak heart (β-blockers, verapamil)

Causes of right heart failure due to pulmonary artery hypertension
Chronic airways disease (cor pulmonale)
Chronic repeated pulmonary emboli
Pulmonary arterial hypertension
Any cause of left heart failure

Risk factors for heart failure

Effective management of hypertension and vascular risk factors is both important and effective in preventing heart failure.

Hypertension
Even moderate hypertension increases the risk of developing heart failure, and lowering blood pressure reduces the risk. Effective treatment of hypertension decreases the occurrence of left ventricular hypertrophy and cardiovascular mortality, and reduces the incidence of heart failure by 30–50%. Diastolic blood pressure should be reduced below 80 mmHg in individuals at risk, particularly diabetics.

Left ventricular hypertrophy
This is independent of hypertension, and it predicts the risk of developing heart failure.

Smoking
This is an independent and strong predictor of heart failure.

Hyperlipidaemia
A raised triglyceride level or a high ratio of total cholesterol to HDL-cholesterol is associated with an increased incidence of heart failure. Lipid lowering with statins reduces the risk of developing heart failure.

Diabetes mellitus
This is an independent risk factor for heart failure, and it occurs in around 20% of patients. It predicts death in high-risk patients who have a left ventricular ejection fraction of < 35%.

Microalbuminuria
Patients with an albumin:creatinine ratio of > 2 mg of microalbumin/mmol of creatinine have a higher risk of developing heart failure than those with a normal albumin: creatinine ratio.

Obesity
This is an independent risk factor for heart failure, and weight loss reduces the risk and helps to correct lipid abnormalities and associated hypertension.

Asymptomatic left ventricular dysfunction

This is an independent risk factor for heart failure and death, and it occurs in around 1–5% of the adult population, depending on their risk profile. This highlights the interest in early diagnosis with echocardiography, although as yet there is no evidence that screening and treatment (except perhaps in high-risk individuals) are beneficial.

Age spectrum of patients with heart failure

The median age at presentation is 74 years. Heart failure is rare in young people, and its prevalence increases with age. The prevalence is around 1 in 35 in people aged 65–74 years, 1 in 15 in those aged 75–84 years, and 1 in 7 in people aged over 85 years.

Prognosis of heart failure

The prognosis remains poor mainly because most of the patients affected are elderly and they may have one or more coexisting medical conditions which themselves affect the prognosis. Other factors that affect the prognosis include the severity of left ventricular function and the haemodynamic, neuroendocrine, renal and biochemical consequences of the poor cardiac output (*see* Boxes 13.2 and 13.3).

Prompt intervention and correction of treatable, mechanical causes of heart failure improve the prognosis (e.g. valve surgery in severe aortic stenosis).

Box 13.2: Non-cardiac factors that affect the prognosis in patients with heart failure

Age
Genetic background
Gender
Coexisting conditions
    Vascular disease
    Diabetes mellitus
    Hypertension
    Renal impairment
    Coronary artery disease
    Anaemia
    Obesity
    Sleep apnoea
    Depression
    Lung disease
Lifestyle
    Smoking
    Alcohol consumption

Recognition and haemodynamic resuscitation of patients with the uncommon condition of heart failure due to acute viral myocarditis may be life-saving.

Patients with *chronic heart failure* have a poorer prognosis than patients with breast, prostate or colon cancer, with percentage survival rates at 1, 2 and 3 years of 67%, 41% and 24%, respectively.

Box 13.3:   Cardiac factors that affect the prognosis in patients with heart failure

Degree of left and/or right ventricular damage (ejection fraction)
Left ventricular hypertrophy
Extent of myocardial ischaemia
Hibernating myocardium
Severity of coronary artery disease
Valvular disease
   Mitral regurgitation
   Aortic stenosis

Effects of interventions in heart failure

The prognosis and quality of life of patients with heart failure remain poor, but have improved somewhat with new pharmacological and non-pharmacological treatments.

The prognosis of patients with heart failure enrolled in trials differs from that of patients observed in the community, probably because patients in clinical trials are monitored very carefully, are prescribed effective medication and their compliance is checked. Clinical trials of ACE inhibitors, angiotensin-receptor antagonists, spironolactone, biventricular pacing, coronary artery surgery and multi-disciplinary teams have been shown to decrease the rate of hospital admissions and to reduce mortality or improve functional ability. However, data from large epidemiological surveys (e.g. the Framingham study) have not shown that the death rate from heart failure has changed significantly. This difference may be explained by the way in which patients in clinical trials are selected and the way in which their medication, compliance and clinical state are carefully monitored.

Economic benefits of reducing hospital care for patients with heart failure

It is estimated that heart failure, with all of its management and treatment components both in hospital and in the community, accounts for 2% of all health expenditure in the UK. This figure may be much higher in future, with the introduction of expensive electrophysiological assessment techniques and interventions, including pacing and cardiac surgery. Heart failure is the cause of approximately 20% of all hospital admissions, and consequently it is a major drain on healthcare resources.

Improving the effectiveness of care in the community reduces the necessity for and frequency of hospital readmissions, can shorten hospital stay, and is important for improving the morale and self-confidence of patients, as well as reducing healthcare costs. A number of organisational factors have been shown to be effective and to allow a larger proportion of patients to be treated comfortably and safely at home. These include the following:

- providing GPs and nurses with education and training in cardiovascular medicine and heart failure
- open-access hospital echocardiography and portable domiciliary echocardiography
- increasing confidence among primary care clinicians in diagnosing heart failure and initiating treatment when appropriate with β-blockers, ACE inhibitors and spironolactone
- the establishment of hospital-based and primary care nurse-led clinics and multi-disciplinary teams that provide domiciliary services to monitor patients' response to treatment
- careful and detailed continuing review of patients' drug treatment and non-pharmacological treatment
- recognising when patients need admission to hospital or domiciliary visits by trained nurses.

Treatment of heart failure patients at home

Patients should be treated at home if this is safe and clinically appropriate and there is adequate social support. Bed rest is helpful for relieving symptoms by reducing heart rate and workload, but prolonged periods of bed rest, particularly in elderly patients, increase the risk of venous thrombosis and embolism, pressure sores, chest infection, depression and weakness of the arms and legs, making rehabilitation difficult.

Patients should be given subcutaneous fractionated heparin to reduce the thrombotic risk. Warfarin is used for patients in atrial fibrillation. The other medical treatments are discussed below.

However, a large proportion of patients with severe, refractory heart failure with co-morbidity will need to be readmitted to hospital for intense medical treatment (*see* Box 13.4).

Box 13.4:   Reasons why patients with heart failure may require readmission to hospital

Haemodynamic decompensation with pulmonary oedema or leg swelling
   Deterioration in cardiac function
   New myocardial infarct
   Myocardial ischaemia
   Arrhythmia
   New or increasing mitral regurgitation
   Heart block

Right heart decompensation
    Chest infection
    Pulmonary emboli
    Arrhythmia
Failure to take prescribed medication
Renal impairment
Physical deterioration
    Falls
    Weakness
    Stroke
    Inadequate social support at home
Other coexisting medical problems
Depression, fear and anxiety

Principles of hospital management

Acute heart failure

This condition is usually due to acute myocardial infarction. The prognosis depends on the severity of left ventricular damage. Over 90% of patients with cardiogenic shock – that is, the triad of low cardiac output, hypotension (systolic blood pressure < 90 mmHg) and oliguria – die in hospital. In contrast, the mortality rate of patients with myocardial infarction but no signs of heart failure is around 5%. Other causes of acute heart failure include acute decompensation of chronic heart failure.

The principles of management of patients with heart failure are as follows:

- to relieve symptoms and improve myocardial and tissue oxygenation with oxygen (nasal continuous positive airway pressure – CPAP), relieve symptoms and improve haemodynamics with diamorphine and intravenous diuretics
- to treat significant arrhythmias
- to maintain the circulation with inotropes, and with intra-aortic balloon pumping in severe cases
- to improve the cardiac output by improving myocardial blood flow and oxygenation with thrombolysis or, if possible, primary coronary angioplasty.

The medical management of these patients will need to be reviewed with the aim of improving their symptoms, quality of life and prognosis. The reasons for the patient's deterioration should be investigated, together with a re-evaluation of renal and cardiac function. Expert opinions may need to be sought for patients who might benefit from angioplasty, cardiac surgery and electrophysiological evaluation with a view to bi-ventricular pacing and implantable defibrillators. Suitable patients with stage D heart failure require evaluation at a specialised centre for cardiac transplantation. Although this treatment option is restricted to a small fraction of the heart failure population because of the limited number of donor hearts, the long-term results of the procedure are good.

The patient's social circumstances will need to be reviewed with the primary care team, and this is another example of the importance of good communication and co-operation between the hospital and primary care teams, providing seamless, co-ordinated care with the aim of getting the patient back to their home safely and with the necessary support. Patients, their families and carers should be educated about the condition, and the reason for their deterioration should be explained. Advice should be given about lifestyle (*see* below).

Pathological processes associated with hypertension, and the rationale of heart failure treatment

Rational treatment of the syndrome of heart failure requires an understanding of its complex and interrelated biochemical, neuroendocrine, structural and haemodynamic consequences. Drugs and pacing are used to target several pathological processes that result from heart failure.

- *β-Blockers* are used to block the production by the sympathetic nervous system of the cathecholamines (adrenaline and noradrenaline) and other vasoactive substances that trigger vasoconstriction, tachycardia and deleterious ventricular remodelling and dilatation.
- *Diuretics* reduce fluid accumulation.
- *Digoxin* is a weak inotrope that slows the ventricular rate in atrial fibrillation.
- *ACE inhibitors* and *angiotensin receptor antagonists* are powerful vasodilators. They block the renin–angiotensin–aldosterone system, reduce salt retention by decreasing aldosterone levels (in common with the aldosterone antagonist, spironolactone), prevent the deleterious vasoconstriction and myocardial hypertrophy induced by angiotensin II, and prevent the degradation of bradykinin (which is a vasodilator and increases fluid excretion).
- *Hydralazine* and *isosorbide* decrease the afterload and preload, thereby reducing cardiac work.
- *Cardiac resynchronisation* using biventricular pacing improves left ventricular function.
- *Exercise* improves peripheral blood flow and skeletal muscle physiology.
- *Anaemia* is common, and is associated with decreased functional activity, worsening symptoms and increased mortality. It results from renal insufficiency due to plasma volume overload. Treatment with *erythropoietin* results in improved symptoms and left ventricular ejection fraction.

Structural and electrical consequences of heart failure

Myocardial remodelling

This is the term used to describe the dilatation and change in shape of the heart, which leads to impaired myocardial function due to fibrosis, hypertrophy and loss of myocytes. The commonest condition is myocardial infarction resulting in ventricular scarring, but remodelling also occurs in cardiomyopathy, hypertension and valvular heart disease. It is important because interventions which result in reverse remodelling and a return to a more normal heart shape and size improve cardiac function, symptoms and prognosis. Examples include ACE inhibitors, β-blockers and cardiac resynchronisation with biventricular pacing (*see* below).

Mitral regurgitation

Mitral regurgitation is another consequence of left ventricular dilatation, and it results in further cardiac enlargement due to volume overload. Correction of primary mitral regurgitation by valve repair or replacement can be beneficial in selected patients.

Arrhythmias and bundle branch block

Myocardial ischaemia, fibrosis and atrial dilatation may result in atrial fibrillation, which can precipitate heart failure and stroke. It is important to diagnose this promptly and treat patients with warfarin to reduce the risk of stroke.

Left bundle branch block is caused by ischaemia and fibrosis of the conducting tissue, and is a major predictor of sudden death due to ventricular arrhythmias. It occurs in at least 30% of patients with heart failure. It results in abnormal and unco-ordinated cardiac contraction and relaxation, with delayed opening and closure of the mitral and aortic valves. This leads to a reduced ejection fraction, decreased cardiac output and a reduction in blood pressure. Biventricular pacing is used to restore synchronous ventricular contraction, improve ventricular function and exercise capacity and reduce the need for hospital readmissions (*see* below).

Management of patients with heart failure (*see* Figure 13.1 and Box 13.1)

Treatment of patients with stage A heart failure

The aim is to prevent ventricular remodelling. The interventions and principles discussed below should be used for patients with all stages of heart failure.

Risk factor control

Active and effective management of risk factors for heart failure is very important, and should be continually emphasised to patients and their families. Both the prognosis and quality of life can be improved by the following:

- weight loss
- individually prescribed exercise
- control of hypertension
- treatment of hyperlipidaemia
- smoking cessation
- a low-salt diet
- tight diabetic control.

Alcohol should be consumed only in moderation because it increases weight and can be arrhythmogenic in patients with more advanced stages of heart failure and structural heart disease. It should be avoided in patients with alcoholic cardiomyopathy.

Angiotensin-converting-enzyme (ACE) inhibitors

ACE inhibitors improve survival and reduce by around 20% the incidence of myocardial infarction and stroke in asymptomatic, high-risk patients with diabetes or vascular disease and no history of heart failure.

There is probably no significant difference between the different types of ACE inhibitor. They act by decreasing the conversion of angiotensin I to angiotensin II. The latter has deleterious effects which include vasoconstriction, salt retention and induction of cardiac hypertrophy.

ACE inhibitors also potentiate the effects of bradykinin, which is a vasodilator and causes water loss via the kidneys. ACE inhibitors have several beneficial effects in patients with chronic heart failure or with heart failure complicating myocardial infarction.

- They improve survival by 20%.
- They reduce progression to heart failure.
- They reduce the frequency of readmission to hospital by 33%.
- They improve symptoms.
- They improve cardiac performance.
- They reverse remodelling.

ACE inhibitors should therefore be given to patients with all stages of heart failure. Contraindications to their use include anuric renal failure, very low systolic blood pressure, very elevated creatinine levels, hyperkalaemia and bilateral renal artery stenosis.

The commonest side-effect is a dry cough (in around 20% of patients), thought to be due to increased levels of bradykinin. Occasionally the cough may resolve if the ACE inhibitor is stopped and another one is substituted, although the use of an angiotensin receptor antagonist instead is usually well tolerated. Other adverse effects include hypotension, renal failure, hyperkalaemia and angio-oedema. These adverse effects may be avoided if the ACE inhibitor is started at a low dose and gradually titrated upward. Because ACE inhibitors are so useful, it is important to make sure that the patient's symptoms are genuine side-effects of the drug.

ACE inhibitors should be started at a low dose, which should be doubled every 2 weeks. The highest tolerated dose of ACE inhibitor should be used. High-dose is superior to low-dose ACE inhibition in reducing the combined end-point of death and hospital re-admission, although there is no reliable evidence that ACE inhibitors reduce the rate of sudden death.

ACE inhibitors can usually be started safely by GPs and 'first-dose' hypotension avoided if the first dose is low and is started when the patient goes to bed and is not over-diuresed and dehydrated.

Angiotensin II receptor antagonists

These very useful drugs block the effects of angiotensin II at the receptor, and are currently recommended for patients who cannot tolerate ACE inhibitors, usually because of a cough, or less commonly because of angioneurotic oedema. They may be used in conjunction with ACE inhibitors.

They are of similar benefit to ACE inhibitors, and may act synergistically with the latter in reducing death and cardiovascular events. However, this benefit of combined treatment may not extend to patients who are taking β-blockers. Angiotensin II antagonists are recommended for patients with stage B heart failure (symptom-free patients with hypertensive heart disease), in whom they reduce cardiovascular mortality and morbidity.

Candesartan has recently been shown to reduce cardiovascular death and readmissions to hospital for heart failure by 23% in patients with left ventricular impairment. These benefits apply to its use either alone or with β-blockers in patients who cannot tolerate ACE inhibitors. When added to ACE inhibitors (with or without β-blockers), candesartan results in a further 15% reduction in cardiovascular death and heart failure.

Patients should be monitored closely for hypotension, hyperkalaemia and renal impairment, which may necessitate withdrawal of the drug. A total of 23 patients need to be treated with candesartan for 3 years to prevent one cardiovascular death or hospital readmission for heart failure.

Patients who cannot tolerate ACE inhibitors or angiotensin II receptor blockers
This is unusual, but elderly patients and those with renal impairment may be tried on a combination of hydralazine and isosorbide dinitrate. They should also be prescribed a diuretic and a β-blocker.

Patient education

This is of fundamental importance to patients with all stages and types of heart failure. It is a primary function of community heart failure clinics.

Most patients are frightened when told that they have heart failure. Patients and carers will need a careful, sympathetic and gentle explanation of what this means, and patients should be taught the basic reasons for their symptoms and what they can and should do to mitigate and control their condition. This includes careful attention to correctable risk factors. They should be educated about their medication, what the tablets are for, what they look like, when they should be taken and what they should do if they forget to take their medication. They should be warned about the common side-effects and advised to report any worsening of their symptoms. It is useful for patients to have the name of a clinician whom they can contact for advice, and this may reduce the number of unnecessary clinic visits.

Some GP practices have arranged specialist outreach clinics where a consultant cardiologist visits the surgery to see patients with known or suspected heart failure, and where 'point of care' echocardiography can be performed to either confirm or exclude the diagnosis. Primary care trusts may wish to support these initiatives, which reduce hospital outpatient waiting times and improve the quality of primary care services. This model of care is supported by the National Institute for Clinical Excellence.

Advice may need to be given about the level and type of exercise that is appropriate, employment and work, sex, contraception and vaccination.

Drug compliance

Compliance with drug treatment and lifestyle advice is crucial. Some elderly patients who for any reason have difficulty taking their medication may need help from a domiciliary nurse specialist with this. Medication should be prescribed in such a way as to increase the likelihood of compliance. Methods that simplify drug administration and reduce its frequency will improve compliance and thereby reduce the likelihood of cardiac decompensation and the need for readmission to hospital.

Diet

This is part of patient education, and it is a very important component of the management of patients with all stages of heart failure.

Patients who are overweight should lose weight and aim to achieve their optimal body mass index (*see* Chapter 7).

A low-salt diet of around 2 g of sodium per day is desirable. A 'low sodium' salt preparation is preferable. A minimal amount of salt should be used for cooking, and patients should be advised not to add salt to their food. Ready-to-cook meals and convenience meals (e.g. Pot Noodles) generally contain a large amount of salt, which increases the tendency for fluid accumulation and the need to increase the dose of diuretic. Foods which have a high salt content include crisps and salted nuts, sausages and meat pies, Chinese and Indian meals, cheese, bacon, ham and tinned meats, smoked fish, chocolate and most tinned foods (including soups and vegetables). Patients should be advised that these foods contain high levels of salt, and they should be mindful of this and read the contents of any processed or packaged food.

Fluid

Strict fluid restriction is very unpleasant for patients, who should be told to try to avoid salty and sweet food in order to reduce their thirst.

A diet rich in fresh fruit, vegetables, fish and eggs (in moderation) is low in salt and is highly recommended.

Daily weight measurement

A reliable set of scales is essential. Patients should be advised to be vigilant about foot swelling, and the diuretic dosage or route of administration may need to be changed if body weight increases by > 2 kg over 2 days. The usual reason is congestion of the gut mucosa and impaired absorption of the medication.

Patients with severe heart failure may require additional nutrition, vitamins and a formal nutritional assessment because they may have a poor appetite and an increased metabolic rate.

Treatment of patients with stage B, C or D heart failure

The aims of treatment for patients with a low ejection fraction are to improve survival, slow the progression of disease, alleviate symptoms and minimise risk factors.

Non-steroidal anti-inflammatory drugs may result in cardiac decompensation and new heart failure.

Diuretics

These are the mainstay of treatment for patients with symptoms of pulmonary oedema or peripheral oedema, and in these conditions they should be combined with an ACE inhibitor and/or a β-blocker.

The synergistic effect of combining a loop diuretic (e.g. frusemide or bumetanide) with a thiazide diuretic (e.g. bendrofluazide, hydrochlorothiazide or metolazone) is very effective in severe resistant cases of heart failure, particularly if the patient has peripheral oedema and right heart failure. The loop diuretic should be given intravenously if the patient is likely to have decreased and unpredictable absorption through a congested oedematous gut. The diuretic dose should be gradually increased until the oedema resolves. The most appropriate maintenance dose of loop diuretic is then prescribed, if necessary together with an intermittent dose (e.g. once or twice a week) of a thiazide diuretic.

It is very important to monitor the patient carefully both clinically (including daily weighing at the same time of day and at the same interval after drug administration) and by checking renal function and electrolytes. Sodium levels may be lowered and potassium levels may increase if an ACE inhibitor is used in conjunction with a potassium-sparing diuretic (e.g. spironolactone or amiloride).

β-Blockers

β-Blockers blunt the effects of the sympathetic nervous system and reduce heart rate, force of cardiac contraction and blood pressure. They have been used for many years to treat patients with hypertension, angina and arrhythmias, but only recently to treat heart failure.

β-Blockers improve survival, morbidity, left ventricular ejection fraction, exercise capacity, remodelling, quality of life, need for hospitalisation and the incidence of sudden death. There are no comparative trial data showing clear superiority of one β-blocker over the others. The selective β_1-adrenergic blockers metoprolol and bisoprolol and the inexpensive and commonly used atenolol (for which there is little evidence) appear to be as effective as the more expensive, non-selective carvedilol.

β-Blockers should be used in carefully selected patients and can be started in primary care. Patients may deteriorate initially, but can be continued on the drug unless they are unwell. Treatment should not be started in patients with pulmonary oedema or signs of congestive heart failure. β-Blockers should be started only after fluid overload has been corrected, and the lowest doses should be used (bisoprolol 1.25 mg every morning, metoprolol 6.25 mg twice a day, carvedilol 3.125 mg every morning, atenolol 12.5 mg every morning). The dose should be increased gradually every 2 to 3 weeks and the patient must be carefully monitored for signs of decompensation and hypotension. The patient should stop the drug if it results in haemodynamic decompensation, and they may need to be referred to hospital, but this is rare if patients are carefully selected and monitored.

The dose may need to be reduced if the patient develops side-effects (bradycardia < 50 beats/minute), but not for asymptomatic hypotension.

Contraindications include asthma and chronic airways disease, bradyarrhythmias and heart block in patients who do not have a pacemaker, and diabetics who have frequent attacks of hypoglycaemia.

Digoxin

This has weak positive inotropic actions and slows the heart rate through vagal stimulation. Its main indication is for lowering the ventricular rate in patients with atrial fibrillation. It is also indicated for worsening systolic heart failure in patients who are already on other treatment.

Digoxin does not reduce mortality. Although it has only marginal benefits in patients who are in sinus rhythm, it reduces the need for hospital readmission, and it is reasonable to continue its use in patients with persistent symptoms despite other medication.

The usual dose of 0.25 mg every morning may need to be reduced in elderly patients, those with renal impairment and those taking amiodarone. Side-effects including nausea, anorexia and arrhythmias may occur with 'normal' drug levels (which are rarely needed diagnostically or to control the dose), and are more likely to develop in elderly patients with renal impairment and hypokalaemia. A low drug level is as effective as a higher dose in reducing cardiovascular events, and is less likely to result in side-effects.

Additional treatment for patients with stage C or D heart failure

Spironolactone

In severe heart failure, aldosterone levels are raised as a result of high angiotensin II levels and decreased clearance by the liver. Aldosterone stimulates salt retention, myocardial hypertrophy and potassium excretion. Spironolactone, an aldosterone antagonist, has been shown to reduce mortality in patients with severe systolic heart failure, and may (by the same mechanisms) confer similar benefits on patients with other types and stages of heart failure, although as yet there are no data available to support this.

The addition of spironolactone (25–50 mg daily) to standard treatment reduces mortality in patients with severe congestive heart failure.

Spironolactone should not be given to patients with hyperkalaemia (potassium concentration > 5.0 mmol/l) or renal failure (creatinine concentration > 220 μmol/l) because the combination of spironolactone and either an ACE inhibitor or an angiotensin II receptor antagonist blocks the renal excretion of potassium. Severe hyperkalaemia (potassium concentration > 6.0 mmol/l) may occasionally occur in patients who are elderly or have diabetes, even without renal impairment. Serum electrolytes and creatinine levels should be checked as part of the clinical assessment soon after starting treatment and regularly thereafter.

Atrial fibrillation in patients with heart failure

Atrial fibrillation is an important precipitant of heart failure, and results in worsening symptoms and left ventricular function. Rate control and anticoagulation are important, although rhythm control may obviate the need for negatively inotropic anti-arrhythmic drugs and the practical difficulties of anticoagulation control.

Cardiac resynchronisation therapy using biventricular pacemakers

This is a new and technically difficult treatment for patients with severe heart failure and left bundle branch block, which occurs in around 30% of patients. This results in asynchronous and unco-ordinated cardiac contraction and further impairment of cardiac contraction and function. The pacemaker is implanted to correct specific electrical abnormalities resulting from abnormal activation of the heart. It does not improve the force of myocardial contraction, so patients must be carefully selected, and this evolving therapy should not at present be applied to all patients with stage C or D heart failure. Not all patients with severe symptomatic heart failure improve as a result of biventricular pacing, but certain criteria help to select those patients who should be referred to a centre with the necessary expertise.

Patients with any of the following should be referred for biventricular pacing:

- systolic heart failure
- severe symptoms despite optimal medical treatment
- left bundle branch block
- significant mitral regurgitation.

The method involves the use of three (rather than the usual one or two) pacing electrodes which are inserted into the right heart via the cephalic and subclavian veins. Two electrodes are positioned in the right atrium and right ventricle, and the third electrode is positioned via the right atrium and coronary sinus into a left ventricular cardiac vein to pace the left ventricle and restore cardiac synchrony.

> Biventricular pacing improves exercise capacity and quality of life and, importantly, it reduces the rate of hospital readmission. There is no evidence that it improves survival.

Implantable cardiac defibrillators

Serious ventricular arrhythmias (ventricular tachycardia or ventricular fibrillation) are common in patients with impaired left ventricular impairment, and are the cause of death in most patients. Implantable cardiac defibrillators are implanted like a pacemaker, and have been shown to reduce mortality by around 30% in survivors of sudden cardiac death and patients with ventricular arrhythmias and severe left ventricular impairment. The use of these devices will probably increase, and currently they are indicated for survivors of sudden death or significant ventricular arrhythmias. Biventricular pacemakers now have a defibrillator facility. They reduce all-cause mortality and readmission to hospital. Although these devices are expensive, the indications for their use are becoming clearer and expanding, and patients with severe heart failure and dizzy turns or loss of consciousness should be investigated for ventricular arrhythmias and heart block and referred to a specialist centre.

Cardiac surgery

Severe left ventricular impairment increases the risk of both coronary angioplasty and cardiac surgery. Patients with angina should be referred for investigation, including coronary angiography, which may show suitable lesions for coronary angioplasty or bypass surgery.

Theoretically, myocardial revascularisation using either or both (hybrid) coronary angioplasty and coronary artery surgery should improve function in 'hibernating' (ischaemic but potentially recoverable heart muscle), but it is not yet clear whether myocardial revascularisation improves survival. Hibernating myocardium is a presumed diagnosis that is made in patients in whom the heart muscle, when visualised by echocardiography, shows increased contractility to intravenous dobutamine. Therefore patients with severe heart failure which is probably due to coronary artery disease should be referred for assessment of underlying myocardial ischaemia and hibernating myocardium. If the latter are present, coronary angiography should be performed with a view to revascularisation.

Mitral valve repair or replacement
This may be helpful in the 10% of patients whose heart failure results from severe mitral regurgitation or aortic stenosis disease. Surgery is not indicated if mitral regurgitation is a consequence of cardiac dilatation (as in dilated cardiomyopathy).

Resection of localised left ventricular aneurysms that result in or contribute significantly to heart failure
Such aneurysms may be suitable for resection, and the procedure has been combined in a few centres with mitral valve repair (the Batista procedure), but the results (except in experienced centres) are poor, although this might reflect the high-risk patients (transplant candidates) who have been studied.

Intra-aortic balloon pumps
These are inserted percutaneously into the aorta via a femoral artery. They augment diastolic blood pressure and are used as a short-term haemodynamic support measure in patients with severe acute heart failure after infarction, or with haemodynamic impairment following heart surgery.

Left ventricular assist devices
These are mechanical electrically powered pumps which may be either implanted into the left ventricle or connected to the heart, but are carried outside the body. The increasing incidence of end-stage heart failure and the shortage of donor hearts for transplantation has fuelled considerable interest in developing these devices, which allow the patient to go home and lead a fairly active life.

Left ventricular assist devices improve 1-year survival in patients with end-stage heart failure who are awaiting cardiac surgery or transplantation. The 1- and 2-year survival rates for patients with a left ventricular assist device compared with medical treatment are 50% vs. 25% and 23% vs. 8%, respectively.

These devices are of most benefit in the uncommon situation where recovery is possible (e.g. peripartum cardiomyopathy or myocarditis). They suck blood out of the left ventricle and pump it into the aorta, allowing the left ventricle to rest. They were used initially as a bridge to heart transplantation. New data suggest that they can be used to rest an 'end-stage heart' which may recover. Although the complications of bleeding, malfunction of the device and infection are serious, these devices can improve survival and quality of life in patients with end-stage heart failure who are unable to have or who are not candidates for a heart transplant.

Cardiac transplantation

This is an effective operation, but the availability of donor hearts is insufficient to meet the demand. The operative mortality rate is 10% and the survival rates at 1, 5 and 10 years are 92%, 75% and 60%, respectively. This compares with a 1-year survival rate of less than 50% for patients with stage C or D heart failure who are given optimal medical treatment. There are a few national transplant centres, and patients are usually referred by their cardiologist.

The main indication for cardiac transplantation is stage D heart failure in patients with NYHA class 4 symptoms. Contraindications include active and significant malignancy (which would in itself shorten life expectancy), active infection or systemic disease (which would significantly increase the risk of the transplant or shorten life expectancy), and pulmonary hypertension or other causes of increased pulmonary vascular resistance (which would result in failure of the transplanted right heart). Transplants should not be performed if the patient is psychologically unsuitable or socially unsupported. Most transplant centres offer donor hearts preferentially to younger patients.

Accelerated small-vessel coronary artery disease is a major problem for patients after transplantation. Although the mechanism is unclear, it appears to be related to the anti-rejection immunotherapy.

Palliative care

Modern treatment has resulted in an increasing number of elderly patients surviving longer but eventually developing symptoms that are refractory to medical treatment, who are not candidates for specialised treatments. Palliative care similar to that provided for patients with cancer, either at home or in a hospice, should be offered to these patients, who may have severe breathlessness at rest, mental disturbances and pain.

Patients who should be referred to a specialist

These include the following:

- those for whom the diagnosis is in doubt
- patients who remain symptomatic despite conventional medical treatment
- cases where there is a suspicion of severe valvular disease (murmurs, echocardiographic features)

- patients with angina and those in whom revascularisation may be indicated (e.g. triple-vessel coronary artery disease and hibernating myocardium)
- patients with conditions that make pharmacological vasodilatation (ACE inhibition) risky (e.g. severe hypotension and left ventricular impairment, possible renal artery stenosis)
- those with arrhythmia (e.g. atrial fibrillation that is difficult to control)
- those with bradycardia and heart block that will require pacing
- those with significant renal impairment or other difficult coexisting medical problems
- patients who wish to see a specialist.

Answers to case studies

1 This patient may have diastolic heart failure, but other causes (including mitral and aortic valve disease, chronic obstructive airways disease, anaemia and hypothyroidism) should be excluded. The principles of managing diastolic heart failure in the absence of evidence from clinical trials are control of blood pressure, heart rate, myocardial ischaemia and other risk factors.

2 Exclude pulmonary oedema with a chest X-ray, and review the patient to ensure that there has not been a significant clinical deterioration. Stop the ACE inhibitor, and if the cough resolves quickly (within a few days) either re-challenge the patient with another ACE inhibitor after explaining that this, too, might result in similar side-effects, or simply change the treatment to an angiotensin II blocker and ask the patient to let you know how he gets on. Take the opportunity to review all the medication, ask about compliance, and check blood tests if they have not been checked recently.

3 This patient may be hypotensive or he may have developed heart failure or bradycardia due to the β-blocker. Ask the patient and any available witnesses about loss of consciousness and symptoms of pulmonary oedema. Examine the patient and check his lying and standing blood pressure, state of hydration, heart rate and rhythm, also checking for signs of cardiac decompensation. Perform an ECG to check the heart rate and rhythm, and to look for signs of conduction abnormality, heart block and new myocardial infarction. The β-blocker may need to be stopped if there is heart block or profound bradycardia (< 40 beats/minute), but otherwise the dose can be reduced and the patient monitored, the situation explained and the potential benefits of β-blockade reiterated. It may be possible to gradually increase the dose again. If the patient is difficult to control, discuss the case with or refer him to the cardiologist.

4 This patient may have important bilateral renal artery stenosis which will need to be excluded by magnetic resonance imaging or Duplex ultrasound and referral to hospital. ACE inhibitors and angiotensin receptor antagonists are contraindicated in patients with bilateral renal artery stenosis. The diuretic dosage may need to be reduced.

5 The causes of repeated hospitalisations are listed above, and need careful review with a multi-disciplinary perspective and solution, and close collaboration with the hospital team.

6 Check the patient's diet and medication. Potassium-sparing diuretics (e.g. amiloride, spironolactone) may need to be reduced or stopped, and the doses of ACE inhibitors and angiotensin II blockers may need to be reduced. Avoid hypovolaemia. Use low doses of spironolactone, ACE inhibitors and angiotensin II blockers in patients with renal impairment, and monitor their renal function.

Further reading

Reviews

- Gomberg-Maitland M, Baran DA and Fuster V (2001) Treatment of congestive heart failure: guidelines for the primary care physician and the heart failure specialist. *Arch Intern Med.* **161**: 342–52.
- Jessup M and Brozena S (2003) Heart failure. *NEJM.* **348**: 2007–18.
- McMurray J and Pfeffer MA (2002) New therapeutic options in congestive heart failure. *Circulation.* **105**: 2099–106, 2223–8.
- Remme WJ and Swedberg K (2001) Guidelines for the diagnosis and treatment of chronic heart failure. *Eur Heart J.* **22**: 1527–60.

Medical treatment

- Brater DC (1998) Diuretic therapy. *NEJM.* **339**: 387–95.
- Brenner BM, Cooper ME, de Zeeuw D *et al.* (2001) Effects of Losartan on renal and cardiovascular outcomes in patients with type II diabetes and nephropathy. *NEJM.* **345**: 861–9.
- McMurray JJL, Östergren J, Swedberg K *et al.* for the CHARM Investigators and Committees (2003) Effects of candesartan in patients with chronic heart failure and reduced left ventricular systolic function taking angiotensin-correcting-enzyme inhibitors: the CHARM added trial. *Lancet.* **362**: 767–71.
- Digitalis Investigation Group (1997) The effect of digoxin on mortality and morbidity in patients with heart failure. *NEJM.* **336**: 525–33.
- Foody JM, Farrell MH and Krumholz HM (2002) Beta-blocker therapy in heart failure: scientific review. *JAMA.* **287**: 883–9.
- Garg R and Yusuf S (1995) Overview of randomised trials of the effect of angiotensin-converting-enzyme inhibitors on mortality and morbidity in patients with heart failure. *JAMA.* **273**: 1450–6 (erratum: *JAMA.* **274**: 462).
- Heart Outcomes Prevention Evaluation Study Investigators (2000) Effects of an angiotensin-converting-enzyme inhibitor, ramipril, on cardiovascular events in high-risk patients. *NEJM.* **342**: 145–53 (erratum: *NEJM.* **342**: 748, 1376).
- Pitt B, Zannad F, Remme WJ *et al.* (1999) The effect of spironolactone on morbidity and mortality in patients with severe heart failure. *NEJM.* **341**: 709–17.

Biventricular pacing

- Chow AWC, Lane RE and Cowie MR (2003) New pacing technologies for heart failure. *BMJ.* **326**: 1073–7.

Exercise training

- Hambrecht R, Gielen S, Linke A *et al.* (2000) Effects of exercise training on left ventricular function and peripheral resistance in patients with chronic heart failure: a randomized trial. *JAMA.* **283**: 3095–101.

Surgery

- Bitran D, Merin O, Klutstein MW *et al.* (2001) Mitral valve repair in severe ischaemic cardiomyopathy. *J Cardiothorac Surg.* **16**: 79–82.

Guidelines

- Department of Health (2000) *National Framework for Coronary Heart Disease.* The Stationery Office, London.
- National Institute for Clinical Excellence (2003) *Chronic Heart Failure: management of chronic heart failure in adults in primary and secondary care. A clinical guideline for the NHS in England and Wales.* National Institute for Clinical Excellence, London.

Brain natriuretic peptide

- de Lemos JA, McGuire DK and Drazner MH (2003) β-type natriuretic peptide in cardiovascular disease. *Lancet.* **362**: 316–22.

CHAPTER 14

Management of angina

Case studies

1 A 70-year-old man presents with typical angina 4 months after coronary angioplasty performed for single-vessel left anterior descending coronary artery disease. What would you do?
2 A 30-year-old woman, who exercises regularly and has no risk factors for coronary artery disease, complains of localised left inframammary chest pain and wants reassurance that the pain is not related to her heart. What would you do?
3 A 68-year-old man with a history of cancer of the prostate comes to see you because of breathlessness and chest pain. What would you do?
4 A 65-year-old obese hypertensive woman with disabling arthritis of the knees and a long history of typical angina notices an increase in the frequency of her symptoms. What would you do?
5 A 55-year-old diabetic man with treated hyperlipidaemia develops mild chest discomfort which is not consistently related to exercise. What would you do?
6 A 58-year-old man with type 2 diabetes and angina asks you for advice about impotence. What would you do?

Pathology of angina

Virtually all patients with angina have atherosclerotic obstructive coronary artery disease which leads to an imbalance between myocardial blood and oxygen supply and demand. Occasionally patients may have angina but normal epicardial coronary arteries. Other unusual causes of angina include microvascular angina, vasculitis and syndrome X (which is a combination of angina, normal coronary arteries on angiography and exercise-induced ST depression).

Identification of patients with angina in primary care

Patients with exertional chest pain and/or breathlessness usually present initially to their GP, who makes the diagnosis and initiates treatment and specialist referral. Patients with angina require prompt identification because symptoms are an unreliable guide to the severity of underlying coronary artery disease. Management is determined largely by the severity of symptoms and the coronary artery anatomy.

Patients with chronic stable angina may be managed in primary care, but those with acute coronary syndromes and suspected myocardial infarction need urgent referral to hospital. Patients with non-cardiac-related symptoms require appropriate investigation and treatment.

The role of the primary care clinician in the management of patients with coronary artery disease is as follows:

- to distinguish patients with angina and acute coronary syndromes from those with non-cardiac chest symptoms (*see* Chapter 2)
- to treat and monitor cardiovascular risk factors
- to treat patients who have angina with aspirin and anti-anginal medication
- to identify those patients with acute myocardial infarction or acute coronary syndromes who need to be seen urgently in hospital
- to identify patients who should be referred for exercise testing or other non-invasive tests for myocardial ischaemia
- to refer patients with important symptoms and/or those who need further investigations and possible myocardial revascularisation.

Diagnosis of angina

Angina is a clinical diagnosis made solely on the grounds of the history and the probability of coronary artery disease based on the patient's age, gender and risk-factor profile.

- Angina is characterised by exercise- or stress-related tightness, discomfort or an unpleasant feeling of constriction or breathlessness in the chest that is typically relieved by rest or glyceryl trinitrate (GTN).
- Patients may describe symptoms in the arm, jaw, shoulder and back. Angina may be precipitated or exacerbated by cold weather, which increases peripheral vasoconstriction and cardiac work, or by a meal, which diverts blood away from the heart to the gut.

Likelihood of angina according to age and gender

The patient's age and risk-factor profile are very helpful in making or excluding a diagnosis of angina (*see* Table 14.1). For example, in a 30-year-old woman with no cardiovascular risk factors it is very unlikely (12% probability) that coronary artery disease will account for symptoms of severe chest pain. However, mild chest discomfort in a 70-year-old man who smokes, is hypertensive and has hyperlipidaemia is highly likely (94%) to represent angina, and even if he complained only of exertional arm or neck discomfort the probability of coronary artery disease would be 72%.

Table 14.1: The probability of coronary artery disease measured as a narrowing (percentage occlusion) of at least one coronary artery

Age (years)	Non-anginal chest pain		Atypical angina		Typical angina	
	Men	Women	Men	Women	Men	Women
30–39	4	2	34	12	76	26
40–49	13	3	51	22	87	55
50–59	20	7	65	31	93	73
60–69	27	14	72	51	94	86

Source: American College of Cardiology (ACC)/American Heart Association (AHA) guidelines on the management of stable angina.

Clinical assessment of patients with suspected angina in primary care

The history and examination are dealt with in Chapters 2 and 3.

Investigations to be performed in patients with stable angina in primary care

These are as follows:

1 haemoglobin
2 fasting glucose
3 fasting lipid profile (including total, HDL- and calculated LDL-cholesterol and triglyceride levels)
4 ECG at rest and during chest pain if possible. This does not exclude coronary artery disease. Q-waves, ST and/or T-wave changes and voltage criteria of left ventricular hypertrophy increase the probability of coronary artery disease
5 chest X-ray in patients with signs of heart failure or valvular disease. This is not useful as a routine test
6 exercise testing in patients with an intermediate probability of having coronary artery disease
7 atherosclerosis imaging using electron beam computed axial tomography (EBCAT) is not indicated in patients with either a low or high probability of coronary artery disease.

Principles of management of patients with suspected angina

The aim is to relieve symptoms and reduce mortality and cardiovascular events so that the patient may have a full and active life.

1 Patients with acute coronary syndromes and myocardial infarction need to be referred urgently to hospital for specialist evaluation and exclusion of myocardial infarction.
2 If the probability of angina and coronary artery disease is low, other non-cardiac diagnoses should be investigated and the patient should be referred to the appropriate specialist.
3 The prognosis of a patient with angina depends on the characteristics of the presenting symptoms, the patient's age, their clinical characteristics and risk profile, left ventricular function and extent of coronary artery disease, their functional capacity and the extent of inducible ischaemia on exercise.
4 Exclude associated conditions which may cause or exacerbate angina:
   • severe anaemia
   • hyperthyroidism
   • uncontrolled hypertension
   • tachyarrhythmias and bradyarrhythmias
   • valvular conditions (aortic stenosis)
   • left ventricular hypertrophy and hypertrophic cardiomyopathy.
5 Patient education about all aspects of the condition and its long-term management is very important.
6 The **ABCDE** mnemonic is useful for remembering the ten most important aspects of treatment for patients with stable angina, which together reduce the risk of cardiovascular events.
   • **A**spirin and **A**nti-anginal treatment.
   • **B**eta-blockers and **B**lood pressure control.
   • **C**holesterol reduction and **C**igarette cessation.
   • **D**iet and weight advice and **D**iabetes control.
   • **E**ducation and **E**xercise.

Management of patients with angina

Patients with a high probability of unstable angina or myocardial infarction

These patients should be treated with aspirin 300 mg and, if they are in severe pain, with diamorphine 5 mg intravenously, maxalon 10 mg intravenously and oxygen and sent urgently by ambulance to the nearest hospital Accident and Emergency department that can deal with this problem. Ideally, patients with acute ST-elevation myocardial infarction should be sent to a hospital that has the facilities and staff necessary to perform coronary angioplasty with cardiac surgery on site.

Patients with a high probability of stable angina who do not require urgent hospital admission

Investigations
Exclude aggravating or precipitating factors, including severe anaemia and hypothyroidism, and for patients with a heart murmur use echocardiography. Exercise testing should be used for patients with an intermediate probability of coronary artery disease.

Treatment

The following treatments reduce the risk of death and cardiac events and/or relieve symptoms:

- aspirin 75 mg every morning or clopidogrel 75 mg if aspirin is contraindicated
- liberal prophylactic glyceryl trinitrate to abort attacks
- β-blockers (they are all equally effective) or slow-release diltiazem if the patient cannot tolerate β-blockers. This combination may result in bradycardia and is not recommended
- angiotensin-converting-enzyme (ACE) inhibitors for patients with vascular disease and/or diabetes and/or left ventricular impairment
- add in or substitute slow-release and long-acting dihydropyridine calcium antagonists for patients who cannot tolerate β-blockers
- statins to lower total and LDL-cholesterol levels to recommended targets
- if anginal symptoms persist despite treatment, add in or substitute long-acting nitrates. Review the patient's treatment and compliance and their cardiovascular risk factors. Further stress testing may be helpful, but specialist referral and coronary angiography with a view to myocardial revascularisation are the next step.

Revascularisation for chronic stable angina

There is an expanding choice of revascularisation approaches. The widespread and increasing use of intracoronary stents, coated stents and other interventional devices, including atherectomy, cutting balloons and rotablation, has increased the choice of revascularisation method and allowed the use of angioplasty in patients who would previously have been considered unsuitable (e.g. those with multi-vessel disease, left main stem disease or bypass graft disease).

There are a number of possible treatment options:

1 medical treatment
2 coronary artery surgery:
   - open-heart approach on either a conventional bypass or a 'beating heart'
   - minimally invasive approach
   - robotic approach for isolated left anterior descending coronary artery disease
3 coronary angioplasty and other interventional techniques
4 combined angioplasty and coronary artery surgery.

Making the choice

Patients should be offered the views of a number of experts, who should review the clinical and investigational data (including the angiograms) of any patient who is being considered for revascularisation.

There are a number of situations in which one form of myocardial revascularisation has an advantage over another, and other circumstances where although there is no evidence for the superiority of one approach, technical, convenience and cost considerations influence the decision. Ultimately, the choice of approach depends on the experience, results, views and opinions of the cardiologist, the cardiac surgeon and the patient, and is dictated by assessment of the risks and benefits of each possible approach in the individual patient. Where one approach is clearly the most appropriate, this should be recommended to the patient. In situations where either coronary artery surgery or coronary angioplasty would be appropriate, it is the responsibility of the cardiologist to discuss the merits and potential drawbacks of each approach with the patient, and to allow the patient to come to their own decision. These aspects will be discussed in Chapter 16.

Revascularisation should be performed in symptom-free patients only when there is evidence that the procedure would result in prognostic benefit.

Indications for revascularisation using coronary artery surgery
- Patients with left main stem coronary disease.
- Patients with three-vessel coronary artery disease and severe left ventricular impairment.
- Patients with coronary artery disease that is unsuitable for coronary angioplasty.
- Repeat coronary artery surgery for patients with multiple saphenous vein graft stenoses, particularly supplying the left anterior descending coronary artery.

Indications for coronary angioplasty
- Symptomatic one-, two- or three-vessel proximal coronary artery disease that is suitable for angioplasty, with satisfactory left ventricular function and no diabetes.
- Symptomatic coronary artery disease in patients with previous angioplasty or coronary artery surgery to the previously treated artery or a different artery.
- Patients with coronary artery lesions that are suitable for angioplasty but unsuitable for coronary artery surgery
- Patients in whom coronary artery surgery is too risky.

Indications for coronary artery surgery or coronary angioplasty
- Patients with two-vessel coronary artery disease involving the proximal left anterior descending coronary artery with either abnormal left ventricular function or ischaemia shown on non-invasive stress testing.

Treatments for which there is no evidence of benefit, or where harm may result

See Chapter 5 on cardiovascular risk factors. There is widespread public interest in alternative medical treatments, but no evidence that any of the following have any beneficial effect in patients with angina and coronary heart disease:

- chelation
- homeopathic and other treatments, including aromatherapy, reflexology, massage, hypnosis, acupuncture or other non-conventional treatments
- hormone replacement therapy
- vitamin C and E supplementation
- garlic
- stress reduction.

New invasive treatments for refractory angina

These have been generally disappointing. There is no consistent evidence from randomised placebo-controlled trials that laser revascularisation, neurostimulation using spinal cord stimulation or angiogenesis improve either the symptoms or the prognosis in this increasingly large group of patients who continue to experience significant angina despite medical treatment, and in whom revascularisation is not an option. It is not understood why some patients with chronic angina develop a collateral circulation, and various explanations (including exercise) have been proposed.

Considerations when requesting exercise tests

Before requesting an exercise test, it is important to appreciate the value and limitations of an exercise test result based on an understanding of Bayes' theorem and how the test result will influence management.

Patient's ability to exercise

The patient must be willing and able to exercise. The test procedure should be explained to them before requesting the test, and patients with musculoskeletal, neurological or psychological conditions which would make the test impossible or unhelpful should not be referred.

Cycle or treadmill?

Most hospitals in the UK and the USA use treadmills, although European centres favour cycles. Many patients find it easier and less psychologically stressful to cycle.

Analysis of exercise test results

Bayes' theorem helps to explain the fairly common occurrence of a false-positive exercise test result (i.e. exercise-induced ST depression but normal coronary arteries) in low-risk individuals, and this has implications for the screening of 'healthy' individuals.

Bayes' theorem states that test results cannot be interpreted adequately without knowing the prevalence of disease in the population under study.

The *pre-test likelihood* is the probability of disease in a patient to be tested

$$= \frac{\text{number of patients with disease in the test population}}{\text{total number of patients in the test population}}.$$

The *post-test likelihood* is the probability of disease in a patient showing an abnormal test result

$$= \frac{\text{number of patients with disease showing an abnormal test result}}{\text{total number of patients with an abnormal test result}}.$$

The *sensitivity* of a test is the probability that a patient with disease will be correctly identified by having an abnormal test result

$$= \frac{\text{number of patients with disease with an abnormal test result}}{\text{total number of patients with disease tested}}$$

$$= \frac{\text{true positives}}{\text{true positives} + \text{false negatives}}.$$

The *specificity* of a test is the probability that an individual without disease will be correctly identified by having a normal test result

$$= \frac{\text{number of individuals with a normal test result}}{\text{number of normal individuals tested}}$$

$$= \frac{\text{true negatives}}{\text{true negatives} + \text{false positives}}.$$

The *predictive value of a positive (abnormal) test* result is the probability that a positive (abnormal) test result will correctly indicate that the patient has disease

$$= \frac{\text{number of patients with disease}}{\text{total number of patients with a positive test result}}$$

$$= \frac{\text{true positives}}{\text{true positives} + \text{false positives}}.$$

The *predictive value of a negative (normal) test* result is the probability that a negative (normal) test result will correctly indicate that the individual does not have disease

$$= \frac{\text{number of individuals without disease}}{\text{total number of individuals with a negative test result}}$$

$$= \frac{\text{true negatives}}{\text{true negatives} + \text{false negatives}}.$$

- If the prevalence of coronary heart disease in a population of patients similar to the patient tested is high, as in the case of a population of patients with typical angina, then both the pre-test and post-test probabilities of disease will be high.
- Conversely, if the prevalence of disease in a population of patients similar to the patient tested is low, as in the case of a population of young patients without angina and with no cardiovascular risk factors, then both the pre-test and post-test probabilities of coronary heart disease will be low.

Sensitivity, specificity and false-positive and false-negative exercise test results

Patients are generally aware that exercise testing is not a perfect test. It has a sensitivity of around 75% and a specificity of around 85%.

Consider the case of a 30-year-old woman with non-anginal chest pain. It can be seen from Table 14.1 that her pre-test probability of coronary heart disease is 2%. If a decision is made to refer her for an exercise test, what is the probability that a 'positive' test result showing ST depression truly indicates coronary heart disease?

The exercise test will detect only 75% of the true positives ($=1.5$). The total number of patients with a positive test result will be 75% of the true positives (i.e. 1.5) plus 15% of the true negatives (i.e. 14.7)

$$= \frac{2.25}{16.2}$$

$$= 14\%.$$

Therefore the predictive accuracy of a positive test in an individual with a low pre-test probability of having coronary artery disease is low. However, the predictive accuracy of a negative test result in this individual is high

$$= \frac{85\% \times 98}{25\% \times 2 + 85\% \times 98}$$

$$= 99\%.$$

In the case of a 70-year-old man with typical angina, the predictive value of a positive test result is 99%, whereas the predictive value of a negative test result is 18%.

> Therefore exercise testing in both high- and low-risk patients adds very little diagnostic information. Exercise testing is of greatest diagnostic value in patients with an intermediate risk of having coronary artery disease.

Indications for exercise testing

- To diagnose obstructive coronary artery disease in patients with an intermediate pre-test probability of coronary artery disease, including those with right bundle branch block.
- For risk assessment and prognosis in patients undergoing initial evaluation.
- To guide prognosis and exercise capacity in patients with an abnormal resting ECG and those with known coronary artery disease.
- To assess new symptoms in patients with significant cardiovascular risk factors.
- To evaluate the response to treatment (stress imaging may be performed in patients after coronary artery surgery).
- To evaluate the blood pressure response in patients with suspected hypertension.
- To evaluate functional capacity in patients with impaired cardiac function.

Non-invasive stress tests assess the effects of obstructive coronary artery disease on myocardial blood flow which, if impaired, may be revealed by an abnormal test result. In the most commonly used test, namely exercise testing, the hallmark of exercise-induced myocardial ischaemia is ST depression, but there are other markers of ischaemia (*see* Table 14.2).

Table 14.2: Exercise test variables used in risk stratification

Exercise test variable	High risk	Low risk
Exercise time	< 3 minutes	> 12 minutes
Time to angina	< 3 minutes	No angina
Time to 1 mm ST depression	< 3 minutes	No ST depression
Extent of ST depression	> 2.5 mm	< 1 mm
Duration of ST depression[a]	> 5 minutes	Immediate resolution
Blood pressure response[b]	Abnormal	Normal
Heart rate response[c]	> 70% APMHR	< 70% APMHR
Ventricular ectopics and tachycardia	Present	No arrhythmias
ST elevation[d]	Present	Not present

[a] An adverse prognosis and multi-vessel coronary artery disease are associated with widespread, pronounced ST depression lasting for more than 5 minutes after the end of exercise.

[b] During maximal, symptom-limited exercise, the systolic blood pressure should increase by at least 20 mmHg, reflecting normal left ventricular systolic function, myocardial blood supply and cardiovascular reflexes. If it does not rise, or if it falls at any stage during exercise, particularly below the resting level, this suggests impaired left ventricular function and/or blood supply and a poor prognosis.

[c] The age-predicted maximal heart rate (APMHR) is estimated by deducting an individual's age from 220. For example, the age-predicted maximal heart rate of a 70-year-old man is 150 beats/minute. Some exercise ECG centres use 70% of the age-predicted heart rate as an exercise end-point, but patients on β-blockers would have a blunted heart rate and blood pressure response. However, it is potentially dangerous to stop β-blockers suddenly, and neither practicable nor necessary to stop them prior to an exercise test, even though the sensitivity of the test may be reduced.

[d] ST elevation occurring in Q-wave-bearing leads in patients after myocardial infarction is associated with a poor prognosis and is related to left ventricular impairment.

Exercise testing will add very little diagnostic information in the case of a patient with typical symptoms of angina, although certain features of the exercise test will aid prognostic risk stratification (identifying patients at high and low risk of cardiovascular events), and these features are used to identify patients for coronary angiography and revascularisation.

Exercise test scoring systems used to assess prognosis

All of the exercise test variables listed in Table 14.2 are useful for predicting prognosis.

Various scoring systems have been developed, but these are not commonly used in routine clinical practice. One of the strongest prognostic markers is maximum exercise capacity, so it is important to request a symptom-limited exercise test.

The Duke University score combines exercise time on the treadmill, the extent of ST depression and the severity of angina to produce a score which identifies young patients at risk of cardiovascular death, ranging from low (0.25%) to high (5.25%) risk. It is not commonly used in UK hospitals. The score was derived from data obtained in patients with a mean age of 49 years, and is unreliable for predicting events in patients aged over 75 years.

Other tests used to assess myocardial ischaemia and angina

Stress echocardiography

This test is not widely available. It is used to evaluate ischaemia in patients who cannot exercise or who have resting ECG abnormalities, and after myocardial revascularisation. Interpretation of the results is very subjective. The test has a high specificity and provides information about cardiac anatomy. It is used to differentiate infarcted (dead) heart muscle from hibernating and ischaemic heart muscle which might improve after revascularisation. It is reviewed in Chapter 25.

Stress perfusion imaging

This test involves the injection of radioactive material and imaging of the left ventricle both at rest and after stress (which may be induced by either exercise or dobutamine). It is expensive, and is only available in a few centres in the UK (*see* Chapter 25).

Coronary angiography

This is the 'gold standard' that provides the most accurate information about coronary anatomy and left ventricular function. It shows the location, severity and extent of atherosclerotic disease (the most powerful predictors of prognosis), and identifies patients with normal arteries. The procedure is described in Chapter 25.

Indications for coronary angiography

- Patients with chronic stable angina despite medical treatment.
- Patients identified as being at high risk on the basis of clinical criteria or non-invasive tests.
- Survivors of sudden death (resuscitated or spontaneous conversion from ventricular tachycardia).
- Patients with angina and signs of heart failure.
- Patients with suspected coronary artery disease but indeterminate non-invasive test results.
- Patients who are unable to have or unsuitable for non-invasive tests.
- Patients with inadequate prognostic information.

Many GPs are now familiar with the limitations of non-invasive testing for ischaemia and refer patients for direct coronary angiography. This includes patients with a high risk of severe coronary artery disease, those who cannot exercise, those with recurrent symptoms after revascularisation or infarction, and occasionally those in whom coronary artery disease needs to be excluded for occupational or insurance reasons.

Coronary angiography provides essential information for deciding on management with regard to revascularisation using angioplasty, coronary artery surgery or both (hybrid procedure), or medical treatment. No other investigation can provide this information with sufficient accuracy at present.

Answers to case studies

1 The most likely diagnosis is restenosis in the left anterior descending coronary artery, which may occur in up to 30% of cases after angioplasty, usually within 6 months of the procedure. It is less frequent after stenting (20%), and even less frequent if a drug-eluting stent has been implanted (10%). Restenosis is due to fibromuscular hypertrophy occurring as a result of trauma to the vessel wall during dilatation, and this is more likely than new atheroma occurring in the two other apparently normal arteries. Exercise testing or other non-invasive tests for reversible ischaemia will add little to management, and are unnecessary in view of the symptoms, which are the same as those the patient experienced before angioplasty. Review all of his cardiovascular risk factors and his treatment (he should be on aspirin 75 mg every morning, a β-blocker, prophylactic GTN and other anti-anginal medication. Because the artery may have an important stenosis and an anatomical diagnosis is required, the patient should be seen quickly, ideally by the cardiologist who performed the angioplasty, and a repeat angiogram should be performed and followed, if appropriate, by repeat intervention. This patient may not be suitable for repeat percutaneous intervention and so may need coronary artery surgery.

2 It is highly unlikely that this patient has coronary heart disease (pre-test probability < 3%), so exercise testing would not provide any useful diagnostic information. If she is very anxious, an exercise test showing a good exercise tolerance and no ST depression, together (if she wished) with a cardiology opinion, might reassure her.

3 The question is whether this patient's chest pain and breathlessness are due to prostatic secondaries or other possible causes, or due to cardiac problems including angina and/or heart failure. Before embarking on cardiac tests, investigations are needed for his prostate and chest, and it might be easier for the patient and his family if he were admitted to hospital under the care of his urologist, who should liaise with the cardiologist. If he is reluctant to go into hospital, some of the preliminary tests could be performed as an outpatient in consultation with both specialists.

4 This patient's arthritis would probably preclude her from exercise testing. Left ventricular hypertrophy and obesity complicate the interpretation of both nuclear perfusion scanning and stress echocardiography. If her symptoms are disabling, coronary angiography would be the most accurate and useful investigation, and would provide the opportunity to perform angioplasty at the same time. You should contact the appropriate cardiologist to discuss this. As in all cases of vascular disease, the patient's cardiovascular risk factors and treatment should be checked. Cardiac revascularisation may be necessary prior to orthopaedic surgery.

5 This patient is at intermediate cardiac risk on the basis of risk factors and the questionable history, so symptom-limited exercise testing would be diagnostically useful. If there are signs of exercise-induced reversible ischaemia, or the test is equivocal, or as in this case the possibility of coronary artery disease needs to be excluded, coronary angiography is indicated.

6 Erectile dysfunction is particularly common for a number of reasons in men of this age who have diabetes and vascular disease. It should be identified by direct questioning in primary care because of its psychosocial effects on the patient and his partner, and because it is often a marker for vascular disease. The patient's cardiovascular risk factors should be reviewed and treated, and if he is on a β-blocker, this should be discussed with him and withdrawn slowly, and an alternative anti-anginal drug prescribed. Drug treatment with sildenafil (Viagra) would probably improve his symptoms, but he should be told not to take either long- or short-acting nitrates because of hypotension, and he should be warned about the possible side-effects of headache and facial flushing.

Further reading

- Charlson ME and Isom OW (2003) Care after coronary-artery bypass surgery. *NEJM*. **348**: 1456–63.
- Gruentzig AR, Senning A and Siegenthaler WE (1979) Nonoperative dilatation of coronary artery stenosis: percutaneous transluminal coronary angioplasty. *NEJM*. **301**: 61–8.
- Patil CV, Nikolsky E, Boulos M *et al.* (2001) Multivessel coronary artery disease: current revascularisation strategies. *Eur Heart J*. **22**: 1183–97.
- Pocock SJ, Henderson RA, Seed P *et al.* (1996) Quality of life, employment status and anginal symptoms after coronary angioplasty or bypass surgery: 3-year follow-up in the Randomized Intervention Treatment of Angina (RITA) Trial. *Circulation*. **94**: 135–42.
- Schofield PM (2003) Indications for percutaneous and surgical intervention: how far does the evidence base guide us? *Heart*. **89**: 565–70.

CHAPTER 15

Myocardial infarction and other acute coronary syndromes

Importance of prompt diagnosis and hospital referral of patients with acute coronary syndromes

Patients with acute coronary syndromes may present or be referred directly to the hospital, where cardiac investigations are performed, the diagnosis is made and treatment is started.

However, for a variety of reasons, some patients present to primary care. These individuals may not recognise that their new chest pain could be related to their heart. Some may suspect that it might be, but hope that it will not be necessary for them to go to hospital. Patients with known chronic angina which becomes unstable may think that they only need extra tablets. The reasons for patients presenting to hospital late with acute myocardial infarction are complex.

Delayed presentation delays treatment. Thrombolytic drugs and/or direct coronary intervention improve the prognosis by restoring blood flow to the heart if administered very soon after coronary thrombosis and occlusion.

Role of primary care clinicians in the management of acute coronary syndromes

Primary care clinicians therefore play a major role in diagnosing acute coronary syndromes and educating patients at risk about what to do if they develop suspicious symptoms.

Acute coronary syndromes are not managed in primary care, but GPs need to know the current principles of management after patients have left hospital.

Which patients are at risk of developing an acute coronary syndrome?

All patients with vascular or coronary artery disease, angina or a high cardiovascular risk are at risk of developing an acute coronary syndrome.

Definition of acute coronary syndrome

The diagnosis of acute coronary syndrome refers to one of the following acute ischaemic states:

- unstable angina (defined as angina at rest lasting for > 20 minutes, new-onset severe angina, or angina that is occurring more frequently and lasting longer, without ECG changes or a rise in enzymes)
- non-ST-segment-elevation myocardial infarction
- ST-segment-elevation myocardial infarction.

Patients with unstable angina and non-ST-elevation myocardial infarction present in a similar manner. It may not be possible to distinguish between them until hours or days after presentation, when ECG changes develop or when levels of biochemical markers of myocardial necrosis become raised. Both conditions may progress to ST-elevation myocardial infarction with new Q-wave formation, which is associated with more extensive myocardial damage and a poorer prognosis. This highlights the necessity for early diagnosis of the condition and prompt referral.

Pathology of acute coronary syndromes

Various triggers that cause an increase in heart rate and blood pressure may lead to the complex sequence of reactions that results in acute coronary syndromes. Thrombosis occurs at the site of mild or moderate stenosis (usually < 70% narrowed) in a coronary artery due to rupture of an atheromatous plaque. Plaques that contain a lot of fat are more likely to rupture than stable plaques, which characteristically contain very little fat and have a firm fibrous cap. Platelets and inflammatory cells, together with thrombin and fibrin, are deposited at the ruptured plaque and form a thrombus.

There is a fine balance between thrombosis and spontaneous thrombolysis, which allows some ruptured plaques to heal but leaves a potentially unstable, high-risk lesion. Some of these lesions become quiescent with aggressive medical management and plaque stabilisation with statins and antiplatelet agents.

Myocardial infarction is caused by complete coronary artery occlusion, whereas unstable angina or non-Q-wave infarction is caused by incomplete coronary artery occlusion.

Diagnosis of acute coronary syndromes

Symptoms

There is prolonged ischaemic chest pain and/or breathlessness lasting for more than 20 minutes, associated with sweating, faintness, loss of consciousness and numbness or tingling in the arms (more commonly the left arm).

The symptoms of myocardial infarction are usually more severe, and include nausea, vomiting, fear, prolonged left arm pain and shortness of breath. The differential diagnosis includes aortic dissection (diagnosed by high-quality echocardiography, magnetic resonance imaging and/or spiral CT scanning), which may cause acute myocardial infarction, pericarditis (diagnosed with the ECG and normal cardiac markers), pneumonia (diagnosed by the history and chest X-ray), cholecystitis (a diagnosis suggested by exclusion of infarction, abdominal ultrasound scanning and liver function tests) and pancreatitis (diagnosed by serum amylase levels and abdominal ultrasound scanning).

Signs

There are signs of sympathetic nervous system overactivity, including sweating, pallor, tachycardia, hypertension (or hypotension in patients with shock), added heart sounds and mitral regurgitation (papillary muscle infarction), and signs of left or right ventricular failure.

ECG

This should be recorded as soon as possible. A normal ECG in a patient presenting with chest pain which started more than 30 minutes earlier, makes a diagnosis of infarction unlikely, although ECG changes may develop later. Therefore ECGs are recorded serially in patients if the diagnosis is in doubt.

Acute myocardial infarction

The ECG should be examined for new Q-waves, ST elevation, peaked T-waves and left bundle branch block. Occasionally, in patients with coronary artery spasm, ST elevation resolves with sublingual GTN.

Non-ST-elevation myocardial infarction

There is ST-segment depression and/or T-wave inversion. Patients with ischaemic chest pain and ST-segment depression are at high risk of developing Q-wave myocardial infarction.

Blood markers of myocardial necrosis

Creatinine kinase and its cardiac subform (CK-MB) have been superseded by cardiac troponins as biochemical markers of myocardial necrosis. Troponins are part of the contractile protein of cardiac muscle cells. Whereas creatine kinase levels may remain normal for several hours after the onset of coronary artery occlusion, troponin levels become elevated shortly after the onset of myocardial cell necrosis and may be elevated in conditions other than acute myocardial infarction. Troponin data are available within minutes, and this allows patients to be triaged in hospital Accident and Emergency departments.

Troponin levels can be measured at the bedside and also in the GP surgery by means of a simple test. A raised troponin level identifies patients with myocardial infarction, and also aids risk stratification when patients first present. Thus patients whose symptoms have resolved and who have a normal ECG and troponin level are at very low risk and may be allowed home. Patients at intermediate risk and those with myocardial infarction are monitored and treated in hospital.

Management of acute coronary syndromes

The rationale for aggressive cardiovascular prevention is to reduce the risk of acute plaque rupture. Patients should be referred to hospital as an emergency for diagnosis, risk stratification and monitoring for complications.

The management of this spectrum of disorders has changed considerably recently, with a more invasive and interventional approach for patients at high risk, and aggressive antiplatelet and anti-ischaemic treatments, secondary prevention and long-term use of antiplatelet and anti-anginal drugs. Patients are investigated as inpatients if they have persistent symptoms or unstable ECG changes. However, most patients 'cool off' on medical treatment and can be investigated as outpatients with stress testing and coronary angiography if necessary.

Acute myocardial infarction

Diagnosis

The diagnosis is made by the combination of symptoms, new Q-waves or ST-segment elevation and diagnostic elevation of troponin levels.

Management

Initial treatment
Patients are treated with oxygen, diamorphine and intravenous nitrates if there is continuing ischaemic pain. Treatment for heart failure and for arrhythmias is started simultaneously. The earlier the occluded artery is opened, the more heart muscle is saved. Hospitals now audit their 'pain to needle time' as a measure of the quality of service provided for patients with acute myocardial infarction. Most patients in the UK who present with ST-elevation acute myocardial infarction are treated with thrombolysis.

Drug treatment
Oral aspirin and β-blockers are started as soon as possible. Angiotensin-converting-enzyme (ACE) inhibitors are started soon after admission and the dose is titrated upward gradually. ACE inhibitors have been shown to reduce the incidence of heart failure and death after infarction, and should be continued long term. Renal function should be monitored. Most patients are prescribed a statin to reduce the cholesterol and LDL-cholesterol levels and to stabilise atheromatous plaques.

Invasive and interventional treatment
A minority of patients may have primary angioplasty. This is only possible in hospitals that have the appropriate facilities and staff. Coronary angiography shows the coronary anatomy and the occluded artery ('culprit lesion'). Some patients may have no important

coronary artery lesion. This may be explained by spontaneous thrombolysis of a ruptured plaque. Angioplasty provides mechanical rather than pharmacological thrombolysis. Angioplasty and stenting, if performed quickly after coronary artery occlusion, result in a better outcome than thrombolysis, and allow the patient to leave hospital earlier because the risk of further ischaemia is reduced.

Patients who present to hospitals that have facilities for coronary angiography and who are under the care of a cardiologist trained in intervention are likely to undergo angiography. This provides accurate diagnostic and prognostic information quickly and safely, together with the possibility of opening up the occluded or narrowed artery.

Patients with persistent pain, new ECG changes, heart failure or cardiogenic shock should be transferred to a centre with facilities for angioplasty and coronary artery surgery.

After the infarct
The prognosis after infarction depends largely on the degree of heart damage. This can be assessed at several stages after the infarct. Patients who present with heart failure have a poorer prognosis than those without clinical features or X-ray findings. Echocardiography does not reliably diagnose acute myocardial infarction, but is useful for evaluating left ventricular function, which may change after infarction. Exercise testing is useful for identifying patients at low risk for subsequent cardiac events after infarction. Patients enjoy the test, and it gives the patient and their family confidence and reassurance. Patients with angina or ischaemia after infarction should be referred for coronary angiography.

Many patients enjoy and benefit from a cardiac rehabilitation course. Information may have been given to the patient while they were in hospital, or it can be obtained from the hospital.

Non-ST-elevation myocardial infarction and unstable angina

Patients are treated with antithrombotic drugs (aspirin, glycoprotein IIb/IIIa inhibitors, low-molecular-weight heparin) and β-blockers with or without nitrates and calcium-channel blockers.

High-risk patients

An early invasive strategy results in a better outcome in patients at high risk (older patients, and those with persistent or recurrent angina, widespread ST-segment depression, high troponin levels or haemodynamic instability). Coronary angioplasty and stenting is generally the preferred approach, and usually the most pragmatic one, too, as it follows immediately after the angiogram. Alternatively, off-pump coronary artery bypass surgery may be offered to patients with triple-vessel coronary artery disease, occluded vessels, a left main stem lesion or complex disease that is not suitable for angioplasty, and those with valvular disease. Some patients will be treated medically if they are unsuitable for either form of revascularisation.

Patients at high risk are treated with aspirin, low-molecular-weight heparin, β-blockers, clopidogrel, an ACE inhibitor and a glycoprotein IIb/IIIa inhibitor.

Low-risk patients

These represent 80% of patients who present with unstable angina. They tend to be younger, with no previous history of angina, their symptoms usually resolve within a day or two, and their ECG may remain normal or show transient, minor T-wave changes. The troponin levels remain normal. Patients at low risk may be treated medically and considered for coronary angiography if they develop ischaemia on exercise testing. They should remain on aspirin long term, and most patients should have a statin and a comprehensive secondary prevention evaluation.

Aspirin

Aspirin blocks platelet cyclo-oxygenase activity and platelet aggregation. It reduces the risk of death from cardiac causes and fatal and non-fatal myocardial infarction by around 60% in patients presenting with unstable angina. The initial dose for newly diagnosed acute coronary syndromes is 300 mg, and 75 mg daily thereafter on an indefinite basis.

Clopidogrel

This is a thienopyridine which affects the ADP-dependent activation of the glycoprotein IIb/IIIa complex and thereby inhibits platelet aggregation. It is given initially at a dose of 300 mg and thereafter at 75 mg daily for patients with acute coronary syndromes. It is also used in conjunction with aspirin on a long-term basis to reduce the risk of thrombosis occurring within coronary artery stents.

Glycoprotein IIb/IIIa inhibitors

GPs may not initiate treatment with these new and powerful drugs, but should be aware of their use in hospital. They inhibit the final common pathway involved in platelet inhibition, activation and aggregation. There are three classes, namely an antibody form (abciximab) that is used intravenously with aspirin and heparin during coronary angioplasty in patients who have or are at high risk of developing intracoronary thrombus, a synthetic peptide form (e.g. eptifibatide) and a non-synthetic form (e.g. tirofiban).

Warfarin

Before the use of antiplatelet drugs, warfarin was given to patients for secondary prevention of myocardial infarction. Warfarin has been shown to reduce the incidence of death, stroke and reinfarctions, and is at least as effective as aspirin, but the logistics and costs of controlling the international normalised ratio (INR) and the threefold higher risk of bleeding make it less attractive. It is not used in the UK except in a few situations, including patients with extensive intravascular or left ventricular thrombus or with atrial fibrillation, patients who are already taking warfarin, and those with aspirin resistance.

Heparin

Most hospitals now use subcutaneous, low-molecular-weight heparin rather than unfractionated heparin, because it has a lower side-effect profile, a longer half-life and a more predictable dose–response curve, so clotting does not need to be monitored. The dose is determined by the patient's weight. Enoxaparin, a low-molecular-weight heparin, is superior to unfractionated heparin in reducing the incidence of myocardial infarction and the need for emergency revascularisation in patients with unstable angina. It is not yet clear whether low-molecular-weight heparins should be given with glycoprotein IIb/IIIa inhibitors to all patients with acute coronary syndromes, or just those at high risk (old age, heart failure, low blood pressure).

Thrombolysis

Thrombolytic drugs are given as soon as possible, and preferably within 6 hours, to patients with ST-elevation myocardial infarction, and those with left bundle branch block and symptoms consistent with infarction. These drugs are not used for patients with unstable angina or non-Q-wave myocardial infarction, because they increase the incidence of death and myocardial infarction. Thrombolytics are contraindicated in patients with a recent history of bleeding, stroke, recent surgery, prolonged resuscitation or possible aortic dissection.

Streptokinase was the first thrombolytic agent to be used for acute myocardial infarction. It is given as an infusion followed by an infusion of heparin. Recombinant-DNA-manufactured tissue plasminogen activators given as a single bolus offer the advantages of simplicity and speed of administration, greater efficacy in arterial recanalisation and myocardial perfusion, and do not stimulate antibody production (which meant that streptokinase could be given to the same patient only once). Hospitals vary in their choice of thrombolytic agent.

β-Blockers

These are well-established and effective agents for the treatment of hypertension, angina and heart failure. They reduce mortality in acute myocardial infarction, and are used (with a smaller evidence base) in patients with acute coronary syndromes. Small doses of short-acting β-blockers are used initially. Patients are often discharged from hospital on β-blockers.

Nitrates

These are used in acute coronary syndromes, although there is little evidence that they reduce mortality or the rate of new myocardial infarction. Intravenous nitroglycerin is used rather than oral long-acting nitrates because of its ease of administration and titration, and the rapid resolution of side-effects when the infusion is discontinued. Patients may be discharged on oral, long-acting or short-acting (sublingual) nitrates. Nitrate tolerance developing after 24 hours of administration is a disadvantage of continuous nitrates. It may be avoided by switching to an oral or transdermal form and allowing an 8-hour nitrate-free period.

Calcium-channel blockers

Both dihydropyridines (e.g. nifedipine, amlodipine) and non-dihydropyridines (e.g. diltiazem, verapamil) dilate coronary arteries and reduce blood pressure, and are useful for the symptomatic treatment of angina. Neither group of drugs reduces mortality or the incidence of myocardial infarction. Dihydropyridines should not be given without β-blockers because of the increased risk of myocardial infarction and recurrent angina. Diltiazem is the preferred calcium antagonist because it slows the heart rate and unlike verapamil does not lower the blood pressure. It is recommended for patients who cannot tolerate β-blockers and for patients who have refractory symptoms despite nitrates and β-blockers.

Myocardial revascularisation

There is accumulating evidence that patients with acute myocardial infarction should be treated with 'primary' angioplasty. This results in a better outcome because it provides a greater chance of arterial recanalisation, myocardial perfusion and salvage of jeopardised heart muscle. The seemingly insoluble problem of enabling widespread patient access to hospitals that provide this service, which necessitates a team of highly skilled personnel, limits its use at present to only a few centres (which operate a service during normal daily working hours).

Advice for patients

- Heart attacks are due to blockage of a heart artery with a clot. The clot forms on fatty material in the wall of the artery. Patients with certain lifestyle factors or habits are more likely than others to have deposition of this fatty material. Stopping smoking, controlling high blood pressure, diabetes and high cholesterol levels, reducing weight and taking daily exercise are helpful in preventing heart attacks, and play an important part in reducing the likelihood of a second heart attack.
- If you experience chest discomfort or breathlessness, arm pain or symptoms that occur with exercise or stress, come to see us. If you have had a heart attack, heart bypass surgery or angioplasty and you develop similar symptoms again, come to see us as soon as possible. Do not ignore worrying symptoms. At certain times it may be safest to dial 999 and go directly to the Accident and Emergency department to have an ECG and blood tests. GPs usually advise patients with prolonged angina (more than 15 minutes) to go directly to hospital in case they are having a heart attack.
- You will be given tablets to take after the heart attack, and you may need to continue on some of these long term. Please come to see us so that we can monitor your progress and decide which tablets need to be taken and at what dose.
- Some patients benefit from attending the hospital rehabilitation course. You may already have enrolled on this while you were in hospital.
- After the heart attack you will have tests to see how much, if any, of the heart muscle has been damaged and what further tests you will need. Some patients have an X-ray of the heart arteries called an angiogram, and may have

---

balloon or opening of the arteries (angioplasty). Occasionally, coronary artery bypass is necessary.

- Most patients understandably feel anxious, depressed and lose their self-confidence after the heart attack. Your confidence will improve as you do more exercise, and the doctors and nurses may have given you advice about how much to do. Fears of dying or of having another heart attack are common. If you are worried, please come to see us and we can help by arranging an exercise test or, if necessary, arranging for you to go to a rehabilitation course or to see the cardiologist.
- The tablets that have been given to you together with the suggested changes to your lifestyle will reduce the likelihood of your having another heart attack. Try to stay optimistic and confident.
- You should not drive or do any heavy lifting for a month. Inform your insurance company about your heart attack.
- Inform the DVLA if you have an HGV or public carriage vehicle (PCV) licence. You will need tests before they let you know whether you can keep your licence.
- If you have done well during an exercise test after the heart attack, this is good news and means that you are at low risk and can start to exercise without fear. Regular fast walking is good for you. If you feel tired, then rest. If you feel in the mood to exercise, walk – progressively longer and faster each day. Only you know how much you can do. If you can exercise without chest pain or breathlessness, keep going but be sensible! Stairs are good exercise, as are gentle treadmill, cycling, swimming, housework and gentle gardening.
- Most people can return to work 6 weeks after the heart attack. If you have a heavy job, start slowly with reduced duties and hours. Talk to your employers, and we can also help by writing a letter (with your permission).
- Sex is good exercise unless it results in chest pain or undue breathlessness. If you can walk upstairs quickly or fairly long distances easily, it is safe to have sex. Men may become impotent after a recent heart attack, and this may be due to fear, depression or some of the tablets that have been prescribed. Speak to us about this. The problem usually improves.
- Avoid too much alcohol, but a small amount (a glass or two of red or white wine, or a glass of spirits) will make you feel better and more relaxed. Everything in moderation!
- It is safe to fly 10 days after a heart attack. Make sure that you have travel insurance and you take enough tablets with you, and avoid going to places where the hospital facilities are not of a high standard. Avoid stressful journeys.

Further reading

- Braunwald E, Antman EM, Beasley JW *et al.* (2002) ACC/AHA 2002 guideline update for the management of patients with unstable angina and non-ST-segment elevation myocardial infarction: a report of the American College of Cardiology/American Heart Association task force on practice guidelines. *J Am Coll Cardiol.* **40**: 1366–74.
- Yeghiazarians Y, Braustein JB, Askari A *et al.* (2000) Unstable angina. *NEJM.* **342**: 101–14.

CHAPTER 16

Myocardial revascularisation

Case studies

1　A 68-year-old licensed cab driver who had coronary artery surgery 6 weeks previously comes to see you feeling fit and well, and wants to start work. He has stopped all his medication apart from aspirin. What advice would you give him?

2　An 81-year-old woman with angina comes to see you because she has been told that she needs coronary angioplasty. She does not really understand what this means, and she is scared. How would you help her?

3　The wife of a patient of yours who is in hospital waiting for bypass surgery for a left main stem stenosis comes to see you because she wants to know if the operation is really necessary, and whether the arteries could be ballooned instead. What would you tell her?

4　A 48-year-old man who was discharged 3 days ago after angioplasty and coronary artery surgery experiences abdominal pain. What would you do?

5　Your practice nurse tells you that she is with a patient who is complaining of a throbbing painful lump in the right groin which developed over the last few days since his angioplasty. What would you do?

Role of primary care in the management of patients before and after myocardial revascularisation

Coronary heart disease in all its presentations is common, and the average age of patients undergoing coronary angioplasty and coronary artery surgery is increasing. Therefore primary care clinicians are responsible for the care of a large number of patients at various stages of this chronic condition.

Primary care clinicians are involved in nearly all aspects of the care of patients with coronary heart disease, from primary and secondary prevention to diagnosing acute coronary syndromes, referring patients with angina for specialist advice after initiating investigations and treatment, and managing patients after myocardial infarction and revascularisation.

Myocardial revascularisation is not a cure for coronary artery disease but, together with medical therapy, it is a useful treatment option performed for symptomatic and prognostic reasons at certain stages of the condition.

Patients return home increasingly soon after the revascularisation procedure to primary care, where they are monitored to ensure that all relevant secondary prevention measures are activated and recurrent symptoms identified.

Patients and their families often ask the GP for further advice or clarification of what they have been told after a hospital visit to the cardiologist or cardiac surgeon. It is usually easier and quicker to ask the GP for information about a planned procedure than to obtain another outpatient appointment to see the cardiac surgeon, who nowadays may meet the patient for the first time when they are admitted to hospital for cardiac surgery. This is because pre-operative consultations and investigations for patients with coronary heart disease are undertaken by the GP and cardiologists, who then refer the patient to cardiac surgeons after a joint cardiology/cardiothoracic meeting held in the absence of the patient. However, cardiac surgeons do see patients with complex clinical conditions in the clinic to discuss various aspects of surgery.

Patients may ask whether they really need to undergo a procedure at all, what it entails, its risks and benefits, how long they will have to wait, how long the procedure takes and how long they will be in hospital, what tablets they will need to take and for how long afterwards, and the implications of the procedure for their lifestyle and whether and when they will be able to return to work.

Historical perspective of revascularisation and changing attitudes to coronary heart disease management

Coronary artery bypass surgery and percutaneous coronary intervention improve the supply of blood and oxygen to heart muscle, and are commonly used either separately or together (hybrid procedure), sometimes more than once in the treatment of patients with coronary heart disease. Whereas coronary artery surgery bypasses arterial narrowing, coronary angioplasty targets the narrowing directly.

Coronary artery bypass surgery was first performed in 1964. It is a major operation with appreciable risks. The complications largely depend on the patient's risk profile. The duration of inpatient stay and the time for recovery and resumption of normal activities have decreased with recent advances, including less invasive approaches, avoidance of cardiopulmonary bypass ('off-pump' technique), and 'robotic' surgery.

Balloon coronary angioplasty (now termed *coronary intervention*, to include all percutaneous treatments for coronary heart disease) was first performed by Dr Gruentzig in 1979 in a patient with a narrowing in one artery. Until then, patients with angina were treated with anti-anginal tablets and coronary artery bypass surgery.

Both angioplasty and coronary artery surgery are being performed in older patients with comorbidity and complex coronary arterial disease. This is due to more aggressive and effective primary and secondary prevention strategies and new, more effective drugs. These include aspirin, β-blockers, angiotensin-converting-enzyme (ACE) inhibitors and statins. Survival after revascularisation has also improved with new angioplasty technology and surgical and anaesthetic techniques.

Impact of coronary angiography and coronary angioplasty on management of coronary heart disease

Coronary angioplasty has stimulated a more direct and interventional approach to the management of patients with all presentations of coronary heart disease, from stable angina to acute myocardial infarction.

Until fairly recently, patients with angina were treated with tablets and may not have been referred for a specialist opinion. The results of trials showing the safety and benefits of angioplasty and coronary artery surgery together with the availability of coronary angiography have provided GPs with a reason to refer patients for a cardiological opinion with a view to myocardial revascularisation.

In some centres diagnosis and treatment of coronary artery disease is a hospital outpatient procedure. Coronary angioplasty performed at the same time as coronary angiography offers patients immediate treatment (avoiding cardiac events on the waiting list), the need for only one arterial puncture, reduced radiation and radiographic contrast medium, and reduced disposable costs. However, the patient who is expecting immediate treatment may become depressed if the angioplasty is unsuccessful.

Percutaneous coronary intervention

This term is used to incorporate balloon coronary angioplasty and stent implantation and all of the other therapeutic treatments that are used percutaneously in the management of coronary heart disease.

It has become the preferred form of myocardial revascularisation because it avoids the adverse consequences of coronary artery bypass surgery (*see* below). In selected patients it is associated with a lower mortality and morbidity, greater accessibility and convenience, lower short-term costs, and shorter duration of hospital stay, recovery time and time off work. It is used in a wide variety of patients of all ages with both single- and multi-vessel coronary artery disease, as well as in those thought to be at too high a risk for coronary artery bypass grafting.

The practice of angioplasty is progressing rapidly in the search for techniques and treatment to reduce the risk of the artery narrowing down (restenosis) or thrombosing after dilatation, and to treat blocked arteries and heavily diseased vein grafts. Recent advances include the following:

- stents coated with drugs which diffuse into the arterial wall and reduce restenosis created by scar formation at the site of balloon dilatation
- radiofrequency guidewires to improve the success rate of opening up blocked arteries
- intravascular ultrasound scanning to image and characterise the lesion
- distal protection devices that trap material released during balloon dilatation and prevent it from embolising down the artery or vein graft and blocking blood flow to the heart muscle
- brachytherapy to treat restenosis
- antiplatelet drugs to reduce thrombosis

- aggressive comprehensive secondary prevention treatment, including statins and ACE inhibitors.

These advances have widened the application of angioplasty to patients who would until recently have needed coronary artery bypass surgery. Angioplasty is now used to treat patients with multi-vessel coronary artery disease, those with impaired left ventricular function, elderly patients, those who have had previous coronary artery surgery or angioplasty, and patients with comorbidity. The associated risk for either form of myocardial revascularisation or any surgical operation is correspondingly greater in these higher-risk patients.

Indications for percutaneous coronary intervention

- Patients with angina and/or important ischaemia and suitable coronary artery disease.
- Patients with acute coronary syndromes.

Risk assessment for patients undergoing percutaneous coronary intervention

A 'suitable' lesion may be defined as one which the interventional cardiologist feels competent to dilate satisfactorily with a low risk of complications. Interventional cardiologists differ in their opinion about what they consider to be low- or high-risk lesions. Nevertheless, most agree that certain clinical features and angiographic appearances identify patients at high and low risk of procedure-related complications. Angioplasty review sessions provide a useful forum where the clinical and angiographic features of each case are discussed and a strategy is agreed.

Low-risk characteristics
- Age < 80 years.
- Single-vessel, non-calcified, discrete, mid-vessel lesion with no thrombus.
- Stable angina.
- Normal left ventricular function.
- No other vascular disease (cerebral, renal or peripheral).
- No comorbidity.
- Low cardiovascular risk.

Approximate complication rates of low-risk angioplasty
- Death: < 1 in 1000.
- Ten-year survival: 90%.
- Symptomatic outcome: 80%, 10 years post procedure.
- Procedural success: > 95%.
- Myocardial infarction, need for urgent coronary artery surgery, stroke – combined risk: 2%.
- Local arterial problem: 1%.
- Restenosis: 30% (< 10% with stent); most occur within 6 months.

High-risk characteristics

- Age > 80 years.
- Unstable coronary syndrome with thrombus in the artery.
- Multi-vessel coronary artery disease.
- Severe eccentric calcified long lesion in a small-calibre tortuous artery involving a side-branch.
- Diffuse distal coronary artery disease.
- Lesion involving or near to the left main stem.
- Long chronically occluded artery.
- Bulky disease in a coronary artery vein graft.
- Severe left ventricular impairment.
- Important renal impairment.
- Widespread vascular disease.
- Significant renal impairment.
- Diabetes.
- High cardiovascular risk.

Approximate complication rates for patients at high risk for percutaneous intervention

- Mortality: 5%.
- Mortality associated with treatment of cardiogenic shock: 50%.
- Myocardial infarction, need for urgent coronary artery surgery, stroke – combined risk: around 10%.
- Procedural success: 70–80% for non-occluded vessels and 50% for chronic occlusions.
- Restenosis: 50%.

Restenosis

This remains the major defect of angioplasty, and it occurs in a significant minority of patients. Restenosis is the growth of scar tissue resulting from stretching and cracking of the inside of the arterial wall during angioplasty.

It is more likely to occur after angioplasty to occluded arteries, long lesions, small-calibre arteries and patients with uncontrolled cardiovascular risk factors (e.g. diabetes, smoking, hyperlipidaemia).

No drugs have been shown to reduce the incidence of restenosis.

Brachytherapy uses intravascular radiation and reduces the risk of recurrent restenosis within a stent from 50% to 15%. It is available in only a few major centres in the UK.

Stents

These are made of a stainless steel mesh and reduce the risk of restenosis from 30% (without a stent) to 20%. They are mounted on a conventional balloon catheter. The dilated balloon impacts the dilated stent against the inner wall of the artery. The stent acts as scaffolding, sticking back dissected intima against the vessel wall. After being coated with cells, stents become part of the structure of the arterial wall within a few weeks. They increase the diameter of the arterial lumen, reduce elastic recoil and prevent torn areas of the inner arterial wall from blocking off blood flow down the artery. Stents have improved procedural success rates and reduced the need for urgent coronary artery bypass surgery, so that selected low-risk cases are now performed in hospitals without the ideal and secure back-up of on-site standby coronary artery surgery.

Drug-eluting stents are coated with drugs which further reduce the risk of restenosis to less than 10%. They are expensive and increase the cost of consumables, and may not be available to all patients. Their cost is balanced by the reduced need for further interventions.

The angioplasty procedure

Outpatients are admitted to hospital starved for at least 5 hours, having had the procedure explained to them in the clinic.

Antiplatelet agents, usually clopidogrel, and aspirin should ideally have been given before the procedure. Other medication (apart from metformin, which increases the risk of renal impairment when patients are dehydrated and given radio-opaque contrast medium) should be continued.

The procedure is performed using local anaesthetic (which stings) for the groin puncture site and light sedation. The patient's ECG, oxygen saturation and direct arterial blood pressure (through the sheath side-arm) are recorded continuously during the procedure.

Sheaths are inserted into the femoral artery and vein. Depending on the time interval since the last angiogram and the clinical circumstances, coronary angiography may be performed first to make sure that the coronary anatomy has not changed. Coronary artery disease may in some patients progress rapidly, but in others improve because the lesion seen in the original angiogram may have been composed of thrombus which may disperse.

A catheter is then introduced through the sheath and engaged in the mouth of the artery to be treated under X-ray guidance. Heparin is given to avoid thrombus formation. A thin, steerable guidewire is then manipulated down the artery past the target lesion. A deflated balloon catheter with a lumen through its shaft, radio-opaque markers and filled with contrast is threaded over the guidewire. The balloon is positioned at the site of the lesion under X-ray guidance and inflated to varying pressures, usually for less than 60 seconds, until the arterial narrowing has been obliterated and the lumen is wide open. The balloon is then deflated and removed from the coronary artery and the cardiologist takes X-ray pictures to ensure that the artery has been dilated sufficiently and without complications (e.g. dissection, perforation, embolisation).

A coronary artery stent may be implanted at the time of the first balloon inflation (primary stenting) or after the artery has been inflated (predilatation). Angiography is performed throughout the procedure to check the appearance of the arteries being treated. Some patients (e.g. those with or at risk of coronary artery thrombus) may be given intravenous antiplatelet treatment during and after the procedure. The patient is monitored carefully on the cardiac care ward and the sheaths are removed when the clotting status is satisfactory. Cardiac enzymes and ECGs are recorded. If there are no complications, the patient leaves hospital the day after the procedure, although in some centres they could be allowed home the same evening.

The patient is reviewed by the cardiologist and/or the GP within a few weeks to ensure that all secondary preventive measures are taken, and is followed up to monitor their progress and drug compliance, to address any questions they may have, and to check on recurrent angina with exercise testing as appropriate.

Adjunctive antiplatelet treatment

Glycoprotein IIa/IIIb inhibitors given before and on a long-term basis after coronary angioplasty and stent implantation, together with aspirin, reduce both short- and long-term thrombosis. The risk of bleeding is slightly increased, and these drugs may be contraindicated in patients at higher risk of bleeding.

Advice for patients having coronary angioplasty

- This procedure is generally very safe and effective in relieving angina.
- The artery may narrow down again in around 10% of cases, usually within a year.
- Most patients stay in hospital overnight.
- The procedure is performed under local anaesthesia and mild sedation.
- You might experience a stinging sensation with the local anaesthesia, and chest pain when the balloon is inflated to widen the artery.
- You will have to sign a consent form allowing the doctors to perform the angioplasty and implant a stent, and allowing them to perform urgent coronary artery bypass surgery if the artery blocks off during the procedure. This is necessary in around 2% of cases. Death is very unlikely, occurring in around 1 in 1000 cases.
- The procedure takes around 30 to 60 minutes and is similar to a coronary angiogram.
- Stents are made of stainless steel. They remain in the artery and do not move or fall out and cannot be removed because after a few weeks they become coated with your own cells to form part of the wall of the heart artery. Most patients will have a stent implanted if the artery is suitable.
- You will need to continue with aspirin and another tablet long term to reduce the likelihood of the artery clotting off.
- You will have to lie flat in bed for several hours after the procedure before the tubes are removed from your groin, and then for another few hours to allow the groin to heal before you sit up, and this might give you backache. Men may find it difficult to pass urine while lying flat, and might need a urinary catheter during this period.
- Tell the doctor or nurse if you feel sweaty or experience chest pain. This may occur in around 5% of cases, and is rarely serious, but it may mean that you require further tests and need to stay in hospital for another day.

- Most patients have bruising and a lump (haematoma) in the groin for several days after the procedure. This settles quickly, but your leg may be bruised for a week or two.
- You are not allowed to drive for 1 week after the procedure. PCV and HGV drivers are not allowed to drive for 6 weeks after the procedure, and need further tests before they can drive again.
- You should not do any heavy lifting or gardening until the groin feels comfortable. If you notice a painful throbbing lump, see your doctor immediately because you may need an ultrasound test to determine whether you have a 'blow-out' or aneurysm of the groin artery.

Coronary artery bypass surgery

Coronary angioplasty has not yet replaced the need for coronary artery surgery, which for the foreseeable future will remain a very useful and commonly performed treatment for angina.

It improves the prognosis in patients with left main stem stenosis and its equivalent (severe proximal disease in both branches of the left coronary artery) and in patients with triple-vessel coronary artery disease and impaired left ventricular function. It is combined with aortic and mitral valve replacements in patients with valvular heart disease and coronary artery disease.

It is a form of myocardial revascularisation for selected patients who are not suitable for percutaneous intervention or who, for prognostic reasons, are best revascularised by surgery. Most patients will have either surgery or angioplasty, but some may be offered a hybrid procedure using each form of revascularisation to different arteries. A large proportion of patients will have both forms of revascularisation, but at different times, because of progressive disease.

Conventional coronary artery surgery

This is performed through a median sternotomy extending along most of the sternum, which is cut and separated. The circulation is maintained by bypassing blood away from the right side of the heart, oxygenating it and pumping it back into the aorta. The heart is stopped and the coronary artery blood flow is interrupted by cross-clamping the aorta. The heart muscle is supplied by infusing fluids into the coronary arteries. This traditional method provides a bloodless, motionless, wide field of view for dissecting out and pulling down the left internal mammary artery, sewing on grafts, and palpating and examining the distal coronary arteries.

Peri-operative risks of coronary artery bypass surgery

Conventional coronary artery surgery is associated with a mortality rate of 1–3% and a complication rate of 15%. Patients stay in hospital for a week after uncomplicated bypass surgery, and full recovery takes at least 6 weeks or more, depending on the patient's age and pre-operative fitness.

Some of the major morbidity and mortality relates to cardiopulmonary bypass, aortic manipulation causing micro-embolisation, and sternotomy problems.

Complications are more commonly found in association with the following factors:

- elderly patients
- diabetes
- chronic lung disease
- obesity
- renal impairment
- widespread vascular disease
- impaired left ventricular function
- immobility
- previous deep vein thrombosis or pulmonary emboli.

Complications include the following:

- chest infection (20%)
- myocardial infarction (< 5%)
- atrial fibrillation (30%)
- infection of the saphenous vein donor site (< 10%)
- sternal incision problems (infection, prolonged pain and non-union of the sternum).

These result in significant delay in recovery as well as psychological distress to the patient and their family.

A considerable proportion of patients, particularly those with widespread vascular disease, develop minor neurocognitive impairment, including loss of memory, depression, decreased concentration and loss of mental acuity, which may persist in 20% of patients. A small number of patients develop strokes of varying severity. About 18% of patients develop new depression after surgery.

Minimally invasive coronary artery surgery

The incision is smaller, and grafting to all three arteries is possible without a pump oxygenator or aortic manipulation.

Laparoscopic robotic surgery is being evaluated in highly selected patients to treat isolated disease in the left anterior descending artery. It may be combined with angioplasty and stenting to posterior arteries (hybrid procedure). The operation time is longer.

'Off-pump' coronary artery surgery

This is becoming widely used, but demands additional technical expertise because grafting is performed on a beating heart, using a clamp to stabilise the coronary arteries. As yet there is no convincing evidence that the incidence of cardiopulmonary bypass complications is lower with the off-pump technique, but hospital stay and other costs are lower.

Transmyocardial revascularisation

This has been evaluated in patients who were unsuitable for either coronary artery surgery or percutaneous intervention, usually because of severe diffuse coronary artery disease.

The beating heart is exposed through a lateral thoracotomy, and a laser is used to create 10–50 small channels through the heart muscle, theoretically allowing oxygenated blood from the left ventricle to perfuse the heart. The technique is being evaluated in one major UK centre, but is not thought to offer clinical advantages over medical treatment and does not increase myocardial perfusion. It is not performed routinely in the UK.

Transmyocardial revascularisation is associated with significant risks (50% morbidity and 5% mortality). The cost is also substantial.

Other treatments that are being evaluated include neurostimulation and external balloon counter-pulsation, which are associated with a lower morbidity and mortality.

Outcome after coronary artery bypass surgery

Some grafts may thrombose and occlude shortly after the operation. Most patients are symptom-free or significantly improved for several years. The use of aggressive secondary prevention will further improve the long-term results.

Around 50% of saphenous veins occlude by 10 years due to progression of disease in native vessels, new disease distal to the graft insertion, and graft attrition (which is particularly difficult to treat with angioplasty). In contrast, over 90% of left internal mammary artery grafts are patent at 10 years. Graft patency, freedom from angina and long-term survival are better if the left internal mammary artery is used as a bypass conduit to the left anterior descending coronary artery, rather than a reversed saphenous vein. The radial artery may be used as a conduit by some surgeons, but this puts the patient at risk of hand claudication and possibly an unsightly and uncomfortable arm scar.

Comparison of percutaneous coronary intervention with coronary artery surgery

Before the widespread use of coronary artery stenting, aggressive secondary prevention and developments in coronary artery surgery, trials had shown that mortality was similar with the two methods of myocardial revascularisation. Recurrent angina, the need for anti-anginal drug treatment and repeat angiography and revascularisation in the first year were more likely in patients who had been treated with angioplasty (33% vs. 3%), but after that the incidence of angina was similar for the two methods. With the use of stenting, the incidence of death, myocardial infarction and stroke is similar and the need for repeat revascularisation is slightly greater in patients treated with angioplasty. However, in the long term angioplasty costs less than coronary artery surgery, despite the greater need for re-investigation and revascularisation during the first year. Drug-eluting stents may offer additional advantages.

Choosing the optimum treatment for each patient

Because of the similarity in outcome between the two approaches to myocardial revascularisation, a decision about the most appropriate approach is best made with the input of both an interventional cardiologist and a cardiac surgeon, together with the opinion of other specialists where necessary. The GP also has a role to play in advising the specialists about important social and general medical factors, and in providing support and advice for the patient and their family. Ultimately, the patient decides on the basis of the advice given. In many cases this is not clear-cut. If the lesions are suitable, percutaneous coronary intervention is usually the preferred initial approach.

Advice for patients before and after coronary artery surgery

- The cardiologist and cardiac surgeon have decided that you would benefit from a heart bypass operation, which is a major operation. The surgeon will explain the operation to you, and its risks and benefits.
- The operation will help your symptoms, but possibly not all of your breathlessness if this is due to damaged heart muscle or a lung problem.
- The heart artery narrowing is bypassed using one of the veins from your leg or an artery from inside the chest wall.
- You will have a scar down the breastbone. It takes 3 months to heal, but you may continue to experience odd aches and pains in the chest wall, neck and back which will probably not be due to angina. Some people develop a tender thickening of the scar called keloid, for which there is no effective cure.
- Do not drive, carry heavy objects or put any pressure on the sternum.
- You may also have a scar on your lower leg if the surgeon uses a leg vein. This may take a few weeks to heal if you are diabetic, and some patients experience pain, swelling and pins and needles for a long time. The ankle and foot may have a tendency to swell.
- You will be in hospital for around 1 week, depending on your progress, and you will be in the intensive-care unit for a night or two. Some patients do not need the intensive-care unit.
- You will have a tube in your chest for a short time, and you may experience discomfort when it is removed. You may have a sore throat for a day or so due to the breathing tube that is inserted for the operation.
- You will be able to stand and walk 2 or 3 days after the operation.
- You might find it difficult to open your bowels for a few days after the operation, but the nurses will give you medicines to help this.
- It is not uncommon for people to be depressed after the operation, but nearly everyone recovers very quickly. You are going to be tired and weak for a few weeks, so take it easy. Some people find that their memory is less sharp. If you cannot manage at home on your own, ask a friend or family member to stay with you, or move in with them. The hospital or GP may arrange for a district nurse to visit.
- Most hospitals run a cardiac rehabilitation course. Find out about your local course and see if it appeals to you.
- Get out of bed when you are ready. Have a shower and then a light breakfast. Try to walk a little further each day. Have a light lunch and then go to bed and sleep for two hours, get up, have tea and try to walk again for as long as you can. Have a light supper and go to bed early.
- You cannot drive or wear a seatbelt for 1 month. PCV and HGV drivers should not drive for 6 weeks, and must inform the DVLA. You will need to 'pass' an

exercise test before you get your licence back. Contact your insurance company to let them know that you have had a bypass operation.

- Most patients do not return to full time work before 3 months.
- Wait for 4 weeks before you have sex, but do not subject your sternum to undue pressure.
- It is very important that you do everything you can to reduce further heart problems. See your GP or practice nurse for advice and to check your tablets. These include aspirin, a statin and an angiotensin-converting-enzyme (ACE) inhibitor together with any other tablets you need. If you have had a heart attack, a β-blocker is beneficial. You will need to take these on a long-term basis under the supervision of the primary care team.
- There is no evidence that folate tablets are useful, even for patients with high levels of homocysteine.
- Stress management may be helpful.
- You should be checked every few months for blood pressure, weight, diabetes and cholesterol level, and of course you must not smoke.
- Lifestyle is important, but only you can change it. Stay optimistic and active. The more you do without straining or stressing yourself, the better.
- Look after your grafts and your grafts will look after you!

Answers to case studies

1   Check this patient's blood pressure, examine him and check his blood count, glucose, lipids and renal function. Also check his treatment. He should be on a statin and an ACE inhibitor. He should have informed the DVLA about his operation and must have an exercise test before resuming work. His cardiovascular risk factors should be monitored regularly. He should also be offered advice about his work patterns and lifestyle if this is a problem.

2   Reassure the patient that the procedure is similar to the angiogram she has already had, and go through the stages of the procedure (*see* above). She may need some help getting to and from hospital and when she arrives home. Although the risks of angioplasty and coronary artery surgery are higher in this age group, her operative risk would have been evaluated. She should understand that she may need emergency coronary artery surgery. Check, if necessary with her cardiologist, that her medication is satisfactory.

3   Assuming that this woman's husband does not mind you speaking to her (and he does not), check with the cardiothoracic registrar that all of the options have been discussed with the patient and his wife. Although angioplasty is performed in selected cases for a left main stem stenosis (e.g. patients with a protected main stem after surgery or, rarely, those who are unfit for surgery), this patient should have coronary surgery. His wife may appreciate some reassurance and optimism during this stressful period, and advice about what the patient will feel like and be able to do when he comes home.

4   This is a difficult problem. The possibilities include gastritis due to the aspirin and clopidogrel, or causes unrelated to the angioplasty. Examine the patient, check that he has no melaena, and request a blood count. If this is normal and his symptoms improve, monitor him closely. He may need a proton-pump inhibitor or an H_2-antagonist, and this should be discussed with the gastro-enterologist. Although desirable, it may not be possible to continue the antiplatelet drugs, which are particularly important for the first 4 weeks while the stent is being endothelialised. The patient should be referred back to the cardiologist and the antiplatelet medication should only be stopped if he is anaemic, in which case he may need to be referred to hospital for monitoring and possible transfusion, depending on his haemoglobin level.

5   The most likely diagnosis is a false aneurysm of the femoral artery, and this requires confirmation with a duplex ultrasound and closure. The patient will need to be referred to hospital, and you should contact the cardiologist and his team who performed the angioplasty. Obliteration of the false aneurysm is achieved either by injecting thrombin into the false aneurysm or by manual compression of the aneurysm, both procedures being performed under ultrasound guidance. Rarely, surgical closure is required. A false aneurysm with a small neck may close spontaneously, but this is unlikely to occur if it is large and the patient is on antiplatelet drugs. False aneurysms are more common in hypertensive patients.

Further reading

- Charlaon ME and Isom OW (2003) Care after coronary artery bypass surgery. *NEJM.* **348**: 1456–63.
- Diegler A, Thiele H, Falk V *et al.* (2002) Comparison of stenting with minimally invasive bypass surgery for stenosis of the left anterior descending coronary artery. *NEJM.* **347**: 551–2.
- Eagle KA, Guyton RA, Davidoff R *et al.* (1999) ACC/AHA Guidelines for Coronary Artery Bypass Graft Surgery: a report of the American College of Cardiology/American Heart Association Task Force on Practice Guidelines (Committee to Revise the 1991 Guidelines for Coronary Artery Bypass Graft Surgery). *J Am Coll Cardiol.* **34**: 1262–347.
- Schofield PM (2003) Indications for percutaneous and surgical revascularisation: how far does the evidence base guide us? *Heart.* **89**: 565–70.
- The Stent or Surgery (SoS) Trial Investigators (2002) Coronary artery bypass surgery versus percutaneous coronary intervention with stent implantation in patients with multivessel coronary artery disease (the Stent or Surgery trial): a randomised controlled trial. *Lancet.* **360**: 965–70.

CHAPTER 17

Management of valve disease

Case studies

1 An 82-year-old man complains of breathlessness and giddiness when he walks uphill. What are the possible causes and what would you do?

2 A 54-year-old man complains of breathlessness 2 weeks after a heart attack. What is the probable diagnosis and what would you do?

3 A 76-year-old man complains of fatigue, anorexia, weight loss and night sweats for the previous 4 weeks. He was seen in hospital several years ago, when he was told that he had a systolic murmur which did not need attention, and he had not thought it necessary to have this checked. What are the possible causes of his symptoms and what would you do?

4 A 35-year-old woman known to have Marfan's syndrome complains of severe back pain and sweating. What are the possible causes and what would you do?

5 A 39-year-old woman who came to the UK a year ago from the Middle East complains of recent onset of breathlessness and palpitation. What are the possible causes and what would you do?

Role of the primary care team in managing patients with valve disease

GPs and practice nurses have an important role in the diagnosis and long-term management of patients with valve disease, who may present with a variety of symptoms or problems.

'Open-access' or surgery-based electrocardiography, echocardiography and X-ray enable the GP (with, in certain areas, a visiting cardiologist) to confirm a clinical diagnosis with an anatomical and functional evaluation and a management plan. Together with surgery-based anticoagulation clinics, primary care clinicians are able to be actively involved in all aspects of management of these conditions. Close liaison with nurses working in hospitals and in community heart failure clinics adds another helpful dimension to patient care.

Patients with valve disease who deteriorate should be assessed and referred for consideration of surgery or, in the case of mitral stenosis, percutaneous balloon valvuloplasty.

Presenting symptoms in patients with valve disease

Valve disease may present in a variety of ways, including the following:

- shortness of breath, cough, tiredness, anorexia and ankle swelling due to heart failure
- palpitation and thromboembolism due to atrial fibrillation
- fever, weight loss and emboli due to infective endocarditis on either a native valve or a prosthetic valve
- haemolytic anaemia in patients with a prosthetic valve.

Management of patients with valve disease

Patients with mild valve conditions and those in whom the risks of surgery are unacceptably high are treated medically. There is increasing evidence that cardiovascular risk factor modification and medical treatment may favourably affect the natural history of certain valve conditions and their effects on the heart muscle. The need for and timing of surgery (or percutaneous mitral valvuloplasty in patients with mitral stenosis) is dictated mainly by symptoms, the clinical state of the patient (including cerebral, renal and hepatic function), the patient's wishes and supplementary test results providing information on cardiac function, size, coexistent coronary artery disease and valve conditions.

Surgery in patients with valve disease

There are several difficult aspects which need careful consideration and discussion between cardiologists, cardiac surgeons and anaesthetists. The GP's perspective of the patient's clinical state, quality-of-life aspirations and support network at home is also an important component of the decision-making process.

Surgery for valve disease is a major procedure, and it carries significant morbidity and mortality which depend on several factors (*see* Chapters 23 and 24).

Valve repair

Valve repair is recommended for most patients with mitral valve disease (both stenosis and regurgitation) because it allows retention of the native valve and avoids the risks of a prosthetic valve (e.g. lifelong anticoagulation, haemolytic anaemia, endocarditis) and the limited lifespan of a biological valve. It requires considerable surgical skills and experience.

Valve replacement

Valves may be replaced using either a prosthetic or a bioprosthetic valve.

Prosthetic mechanical valves

These have excellent durability, but because patients need lifelong anticoagulation, they are inserted in young patients (under 70 years of age) and those who require anticoagulation for other reasons. Compared with a bioprosthesis, a mechanical valve is less likely to deteriorate in patients with renal failure or hypercalcaemia. It is therefore the prosthesis of choice in patients:

- with an expected long lifespan
- with a mechanical valve in a position different from that of the valve to be replaced
- with renal failure, on haemodialysis
- who require warfarin
- aged < 65 years for aortic valve replacement
- aged < 70 years for mitral valve replacement.

Bioprosthetic valves

Anticoagulation is not necessary in patients in sinus rhythm with bioprosthetic valves, which have an average lifespan of 15 years. The recommended age for implanting a bioprosthetic valve is based on the major reduction in the rate of structural valve deterioration after the age of 65 years and the increased risk of bleeding in this age group. These valves are therefore commonly used in the following:

- elderly patients
- patients who cannot or will not take warfarin
- patients aged > 65 years who need aortic valve replacement and who do not have risk factors for thromboembolism
- patients aged > 70 years who need mitral valve replacement and who do not have risk factors for thromboembolism.

Bleeding risks of anticoagulation and antithrombotic treatment

All patients with a prosthetic heart valve and/or atrial fibrillation require warfarin. The risk of thromboembolism is higher in patients with a prosthetic valve in the mitral position than in those where it is in the aortic position.

The practical difficulties of monitoring warfarin treatment and the risks of bleeding have to be taken into account when considering valve replacement. Better anticoagulation control has reduced the incidence of major bleeding (requiring transfusion of more than 4 units of blood).

An international normalised ratio (INR) of 2.5–3.5 is recommended for patients with a prosthetic valve.

The following circumstances increase the risks of bleeding:

- elderly patients (aged > 75 years) who may be frail and forgetful, and are more likely to have other medical conditions or to be taking other medication which increases the risk of bleeding. They may have an increased sensitivity to warfarin or lower dietary vitamin K levels. The doses for warfarin loading and maintenance are lower in elderly patients
- a history of uncontrolled hypertension
- excess alcohol consumption
- peptic ulcer

- poor anticoagulation control
- certain drugs (e.g. aspirin, non-steroidal anti-inflammatory drugs).

Intracranial haemorrhage is the most serious bleeding complication. Patients who are prescribed warfarin should be warned of the risks of bruising and bleeding. INR monitoring should be performed regularly and carefully in all patients, but particularly those at high risk.

If the INR is > 5 and there is no bleeding or only minor bleeding, warfarin should be stopped or the dose reduced and the INR monitored. Oral or subcutaneous vitamin K 2–5 mg is given to patients who are bleeding, but not to patients with a prosthetic valve unless there is intracranial bleeding, because of the risk of thrombosis and obstruction of the valve. It is advisable to refer these patients to hospital, and fresh frozen plasma is given.

Management of anticoagulation in patients who require dental care

Anticoagulation should not be stopped for procedures in which bleeding is unlikely or would be unimportant if it occurred.

Aspirin should be stopped 1 week before the procedure and started as soon as it is considered safe by the surgeon or dentist.

Warfarin should be stopped before the procedure to reach an INR of < 1.5, and it should be restarted 24 hours after the procedure.

Heparin is advisable for patients:

- with a recent history of thrombosis or embolus (within 1 year)
- in whom thrombotic problems occurred previously when anticoagulation was stopped
- with three or more thrombotic risk factors (e.g. atrial fibrillation, previous thrombo-embolism, hypercoagulable state, impaired left ventricular function, mechanical prosthesis). These patients should be referred to hospital because low-molecular-weight heparin cannot be recommended at present
- metal mitral valve prosthesis.

Mitral valve stenosis

Pathology of mitral valve stenosis

Only around 50% of patients with mitral valve stenosis recall an attack of rheumatic fever in childhood. The resulting fibrosis, thickening, fusion and calcification of the valve cusps and valve apparatus lead to progressive narrowing of the mitral valve orifice. The normal mitral valve area is 4 cm^2. Moderate to severe mitral valve disease is associated with a mitral valve area of less than 1.5 cm^2, when there is restricted flow of blood from the left atrium to the left ventricle, with progressive increases in left atrial pressure, pulmonary oedema and breathlessness. Pulmonary venous pressure is increased further by atrial fibrillation, which occurs in the majority of patients.

The onset of atrial fibrillation together with increasing age and left atrial size put the patient at high risk of arterial embolism.

Symptoms usually appear between the ages of 40 and 50 years, but may appear earlier in patients from developing countries, and during pregnancy, when the plasma volume increases (*see* Chapter 20).

Signs include a loud first heart sound, an opening snap and a diastolic murmur. A systolic murmur may be heard in patients with mitral regurgitation. Other forms of rheumatic valve disease may be present. Atrial fibrillation may occur in patients with a dilated left atrium.

Investigations

ECG
This may show atrial fibrillation.

Chest X-ray
The findings depend on the severity of the stenosis and its effects on pulmonary venous pressure.

The X-ray may vary from normal in patients with mild mitral stenosis to showing pulmonary oedema. In pure mitral stenosis without right heart enlargement, the left atrial appendage may be enlarged but the heart size is normal.

Echocardiography
This essential investigation shows the extent of the pathological changes affecting the valve cusps and the whole mitral valve structure.

Measurements of the valve orifice area indicate the severity of the stenosis. Moderate stenosis is characterised by a mitral valve area of < 1.5 cm^2, and severe mitral stenosis by a mitral valve area of < 1.0 cm^2. Associated mitral regurgitation, other valve conditions and vegetations may be seen. Left and right ventricular function and dimensions are assessed and left atrial dimensions measured. This information relates clinical features to cardiac structure and function, and provides the information necessary to decide on the optimum approach to treatment, namely valve surgery or percutaneous valvuloplasty. Transoesophageal echocardiography is performed to assess possible left atrial thrombus prior to electrical cardioversion or percutaneous mitral valvuloplasty, or when a transthoracic study is unsatisfactory.

Cardiac catheterisation
This is indicated in elderly patients who may have coronary artery disease, and to obtain accurate haemodynamic data in patients who are being considered for percutaneous mitral valvuloplasty. It is not generally necessary in young patients prior to mitral valve surgery. The mitral valve gradient at rest and after exercise and the pulmonary artery pressure are high in patients with severe mitral stenosis.

Medical treatment of mitral valve stenosis

Mild symptoms may be controlled by medical treatments.

Diuretics improve breathlessness that is due to pulmonary venous hypertension and oedema.

Atrial fibrillation results from left atrial dilatation, and responds best to mechanical relief of valve stenosis. Uncontrolled atrial fibrillation should be controlled with β-blockers either alone or combined with calcium antagonists or digoxin. Other approaches to the treatment of atrial fibrillation may need to be considered (*see* section on atrial fibrillation in Chapter 18).

Anticoagulation should be considered in all patients who are in atrial fibrillation. Because emboli may occur shortly after the onset of atrial fibrillation, it is appropriate to anti-coagulate patients who are in sinus rhythm.

Prophylactic antibiotics (phenoxymethyl penicillin 250 mg twice a day by mouth) are given to patients who have had rheumatic fever until the age of 40 years, or for at least 10 years after the last attack of rheumatic fever. All patients with mitral stenosis should have prophylactic antibiotics before they undergo potentially septic procedures.

Percutaneous mitral balloon valvuloplasty for mitral stenosis

This procedure is performed in specialist units by experienced operators. Success (i.e. satisfactory dilatation) depends on the morphology of the valve and its subvalvar apparatus. Mitral regurgitation and pericardial tamponade are potential complications. Left atrial thrombus must be excluded by transoesophageal echocardiography in order to avoid the risk of arterial embolism.

The patient is sedated and the procedure is performed with local anaesthetic. It involves a right heart catheterisation and puncture of the interatrial septum to allow passage of a balloon through the mitral valve. The balloon is then inflated for a few seconds at a time (the inflated balloon obstructs the circulation) until the stenosed valve is optimally dilated. Fluoroscopy is used to visualise the balloon. Echocardiography is used during the procedure to monitor the mitral valve changes and to check for cardiac tamponade (a rare and important complication). An overnight stay is required for uncomplicated cases. There is a significant restenosis rate, which depends on the success of dilatation.

Indications for percutaneous mitral balloon valvuloplasty

- Symptomatic patients with moderate or severe mitral stenosis, favourable mitral valve morphology (pliable valve cusps with little calcification or mitral regurgitation) and absence of left atrial thrombus (risk of embolism).
- Asymptomatic patients with moderate to severe mitral valve stenosis and pulmonary hypertension.
- Symptomatic patients with moderate to severe mitral stenosis and a non-pliable valve, who are at high risk for surgery.

Indications for surgical mitral valve repair

- Symptomatic patients with moderate to severe mitral stenosis with morphology that is favourable for mitral valve repair if balloon valvuloplasty is not available, or if it is contraindicated by left atrial thrombus.
- Symptomatic patients with mitral valve stenosis with a calcified, non-pliable valve that is not suitable for valvuloplasty.

Indications for mitral valve replacement

- Symptomatic patients with moderate or severe mitral stenosis who are not candidates for either balloon valvuloplasty or valve repair.
- Patients with severe mitral stenosis but minimal symptoms who have pulmonary hypertension.

Mitral regurgitation

Pathology

Mitral regurgitation may be due to a primary valve abnormality (e.g. rheumatic valve disease, mitral valve prolapse, endocarditis) or secondary to a left ventricular problem (e.g. myocardial infarction or cardiomyopathy). Chronic progressive volume overload of the left ventricle leads to left atrial and left ventricular hypertrophy and dilatation, heart failure, pulmonary hypertension and death.

The presentation of acute mitral regurgitation is dramatic because the left heart has not had time to adapt. The acute increase in volume overload leads to sudden increases in left atrial and pulmonary venous pressure and pulmonary oedema. Surgery should be performed urgently, so these patients should ideally be referred to a surgical centre.

Mitral regurgitation is well tolerated for many years because the left ventricle is initially able to adapt to the volume overload. However, patients become symptomatic when left ventricular impairment develops. This is a sign of important mitral regurgitation indicating cardiac decompensation that is usually not reversed by mitral valve surgery, which should therefore be performed before this occurs.

Causes

Chronic mitral regurgitation
Causes include the following:

- ischaemic papillary muscle dysfunction
- cardiomyopathy
- myxomatous degeneration of the mitral valve (mitral valve prolapse).

Acute mitral regurgitation
Causes include the following:

- chordal rupture (Marfan's syndrome)
- infectious endocarditis (causes leaflet destruction, perforation and chordal rupture).

Symptoms

Symptoms depend on left ventricular function, pulmonary venous pressure and the level of activity and general medical condition of the patient. Patients with chronic, slowly progressive mitral regurgitation who take little exercise may have few or no symptoms until they are elderly, when they may develop fatigue. Patients with acute mitral regurgitation develop acute pulmonary oedema.

Signs

Patients with chronic mitral regurgitation have a pansystolic murmur and possibly a displaced apex beat. A mid-systolic click and a mid- to late systolic murmur are heard in mitral valve prolapse. Pulmonary oedema and a third heart sound may be found in patients with severe or acute mitral regurgitation.

ECG

This detects left ventricular hypertrophy with or without atrial fibrillation. It may be normal or there may be non-specific ST-segment and T-wave changes.

Chest X-ray

This depends on the severity and speed of onset of the regurgitation and left ventricular function. It may be normal, or the heart may be enlarged with signs of pulmonary oedema.

Echocardiography

This shows the morphology of the valve, the size and function of the left ventricle, left atrial size, provides a semi-quantitative assessment of the severity of mitral regurgitation, shows associated valve lesions, and gives an estimate of pulmonary artery pressure. Ruptured chordae or signs of endocarditis may be seen in patients with acute mitral regurgitation. The diagnosis of mitral valve prolapse is made clinically and confirmed by echocardiography.

Cardiac catheterisation

This is done prior to consideration of mitral valve surgery in order to:

1 investigate the possibility of coronary artery disease to determine whether this is necessary or contributing to the mitral regurgitation
2 investigate left ventricular function
3 assess the severity of mitral regurgitation
4 measure pulmonary artery pressure.

Medical treatment of mitral regurgitation

Patients with heart failure are treated medically and surgery is considered as soon as possible. Patients who pose an unacceptably high surgical risk due to their age, the presence of other medical conditions or very poor left ventricular function are treated medically.

The principles of treatment of heart failure due to mitral regurgitation are similar to those for other causes of heart failure. Diuretics for peripheral or pulmonary oedema, rhythm or rate control of atrial fibrillation, angiotensin-converting-enzyme (ACE) inhibitors and/or angiotensin II receptor antagonists, spironolactone and β-blockers may be used.

Surgical treatment of mitral regurgitation

Surgical treatment is the preferred approach.

Mitral valve repair or replacement is indicated in the following:

- symptomatic patients with a dilated heart
- as an emergency in patients with acute mitral regurgitation
- symptomatic or asymptomatic patients with impaired left ventricular function or dilatation
- asymptomatic patients with preserved left ventricular function and atrial fibrillation or pulmonary hypertension
- asymptomatic patients with signs of increasing left ventricular dilatation judged by serial echocardiography.

Surgery for associated atrial fibrillation may be performed at the same time as mitral valve repair or replacement.

Surgery for secondary mitral regurgitation should be individualised.

Mitral valve prolapse

This is a common and generally benign cardiac condition that occurs in 10% of the adult population. It is due to abnormal collagen in the mitral valve leaflets, and is a variant of normal rather than a valve abnormality. It is more common in females. It is not a cause of any cardiac symptom unless there is significant mitral regurgitation. It is diagnosed clinically by a mid-systolic click with a systolic murmur only if there is significant mitral regurgitation. The signs are variable in the same patient. Some patients are slim, have a straight back, pectus excavatum or scoliosis.

Investigations

Echocardiography shows thickening (myxomatous degeneration of the valve cusps) with varying degrees of prolapse of the valve cusps into the left atrium in systole. Serial echocardiography is indicated in patients with mitral regurgitation. The ECG is normal, and occasionally may show non-specific unimportant ST-segment and T-wave changes. Palpitation is quite common, unrelated to the valve condition, but 24-hour ECG recording may be helpful for identifying frequent arrhythmias. Cardiac catheterisation is only indicated if surgery is being considered in patients who are likely to have coronary artery disease.

Management

The prognosis is excellent, and the patient should be reassured. No medical treatment is indicated. Chordal rupture resulting in a flail leaflet and severe acute pulmonary oedema is very rare, but would necessitate urgent mitral valve repair or replacement. Cerebral embolism is rare and presents as a stroke, transient ischaemic attack or amaurosis fugax. Antibiotic prophylaxis is only necessary if there is audible mitral regurgitation.

Aortic valve stenosis

This is quite commonly seen among elderly patients in primary care. Calcific aortic stenosis is associated with atherosclerosis, so its incidence may decrease with more effective cardiovascular risk factor treatment. The diagnosis is suspected clinically and confirmed by echocardiography and Doppler examination. Coronary angiography is performed in adults who are being considered for valve replacement because of the high probability of associated coronary artery disease. The aortic valve gradient will be spuriously low in patients with significant left ventricular impairment, so the decision to replace the valve is made after considering several factors. Aortic valve replacement is effective and allows the patient to live a normal life, so it should be considered in all patients with significant stenosis.

Pathology, progression and prognosis

Aortic stenosis is caused by age-related calcification of a normal tricuspid aortic valve, which usually presents either in the elderly or as premature calcification of a congenitally bicuspid valve in middle age.

> Once symptoms develop, patients with aortic stenosis survive for only 3–5 years without aortic valve replacement. Diagnosis, monitoring of patients and specialist referral are therefore very important.

It is now recognised that aortic valve stenosis has risk factors in common with atherosclerosis. It is possible that aggressive lipid lowering may have beneficial effects in slowing down the rate of progression of valve stenosis, but statins are not yet recommended for routine secondary prevention unless other indications exist (e.g. vascular disease, hypercholesterolaemia) (see Chapter 5). Valve stenosis appears to be mediated by turbulence of blood and mechanical stresses. Rheumatic heart disease is a less common cause of aortic valve stenosis, except in immigrants. It causes mixed stenosis and regurgitation and is associated with mitral valve disease.

Symptoms

Progressive pressure overload results in left ventricular hypertrophy. The latter, even in the absence of coronary artery disease (which is present in the majority of patients), may cause angina and breathlessness due to a stiff non-compliant heart muscle. Exertional syncope or dizziness occurs due to severe obstruction of the outflow tract.

Signs

The main findings are a loud systolic ejection murmur radiating to the neck, with a slow rising or carotid artery pulse or shudder. The second heart sound, due to aortic valve closure, may be quiet in severe stenosis with calcified immobile valve cusps.

ECG

This may be normal even in severe stenosis, or it may show left ventricular hypertrophy and ST-segment and T-wave changes.

Chest X-ray

This may be normal, or it may show post-stenotic dilatation of the aorta.

Echocardiogram and Doppler examination

This is the most useful non-invasive test, showing the anatomy and function of the aortic valve, the extent of left ventricular hypertrophy, left ventricular size and function (which influences the aortic valve gradient) and other valve disease. Doppler examination will show the calculated peak gradient and thus the severity of the stenosis, which will help to decide whether aortic valve replacement is necessary.

Exercise testing

This is contraindicated in severely symptomatic patients, but is performed to assess exercise capacity and blood pressure response and signs of ischaemic heart disease which may be difficult to interpret in the presence of left ventricular hypertrophy.

Cardiac catheterisation

This is done to investigate coronary anatomy prior to aortic valve replacement. Coronary artery disease is common in patients with aortic stenosis, and coronary artery surgery is indicated for significant stenoses even in patients without symptoms, despite the associated increased perioperative risk. Cerebral emboli from the calcified valve may occur during protracted attempts to catheterise the left ventricle, so this should only be performed if it has not been possible to measure the aortic gradient by Doppler scanning.

Intervention for aortic stenosis

Balloon valvuloplasty for congenital aortic stenosis

Sudden death in the absence of symptoms is more common in infants and children than in adults. Intervention is recommended in asymptomatic patients with important stenosis (transvalvular gradient of > 50 mmHg). Prosthetic aortic valve replacement in a young patient with congenital aortic valve stenosis may necessitate a high-risk second operation if the valve fails or leaks because the patient and the aorta have grown. Therefore balloon aortic valvotomy is preferred and is performed in paediatric cardiological centres in young asymptomatic patients with non-calcified pliable significant congenital aortic stenosis. It is not performed in adults because of the risks of embolic stroke, restenosis and regurgitation.

Indications for aortic valve replacement
- Patients with severe aortic stenosis with or without symptoms.
- Patients with moderate aortic stenosis undergoing coronary artery, aortic or other valve surgery.

Medical treatment of aortic stenosis

This is necessary for patients who are not fit for or decline surgery, but it does not improve survival.

The blood count, biochemistry and thyroid function should be checked.

Diuretics are used for symptomatic pulmonary or peripheral oedema, but over-diuresis may be dangerous because it reduces the circulating plasma volume and decreases cardiac output.

Digoxin or electrical cardioversion may be necessary for atrial fibrillation.

ACE inhibitors and probably angiotensin II antagonists may be used for heart failure. These drugs increase cardiac output and improve symptoms. They should be started in hospital because of the risk of hypotension.

Aortic regurgitation

Pathology

Chronic aortic regurgitation causes volume overload of the left ventricle with compensatory hypertrophy and dilatation which are well tolerated for many years. The increased stroke volume results in hypertension, which adds a pressure overload on the heart. These changes may be reversed by timely aortic valve surgery.

Causes of aortic regurgitation

Aortic regurgitation may be due to either an abnormality of the valve cusps, resulting in mixed stenosis and regurgitation, or the aortic root.

Valve conditions that cause aortic regurgitation include the following:

- age-related degeneration of the cusps
- calcific bicuspid valve
- rheumatic heart disease
- infective endocarditis (acute aortic regurgitation).

Aortic root conditions that cause aortic regurgitation include the following:

- Marfan's syndrome
- aortic dissection
- hypertension
- ankylosing spondylitis.

Symptoms

Patients are often symptom-free until they decompensate, when they experience symptoms of heart failure.

Signs

Patients are usually in sinus rhythm, but have visible and forceful carotid artery pulsation, a wide pulse pressure with systolic hypertension and a very low diastolic pressure which results in a number of physical signs. The diastolic murmur is best heard with the patient sitting forward. A systolic murmur due to the increase in forward flow may also be heard.

ECG

This shows left ventricular hypertrophy.

Chest X-ray

This shows the following:

- increased heart size
- aortic root dilatation in aortic root conditions
- calcification of the aortic valve cusps
- signs of heart failure.

Echocardiogram

This is the most useful diagnostic test, and the findings strongly influence the timing of valve replacement. It shows left ventricular size, hypertrophy and function and any associated aortic stenosis and other valve disease which may occur in rheumatic heart disease. The proximal aortic root may be examined and measured. Doppler examination provides a guide to the severity of regurgitation.

Cardiac catheterisation

This should be performed in patients who may have coronary artery disease (those with angina or vascular disease, cardiovascular risk factors or a family history of coronary artery disease), and to define the severity of aortic regurgitation with aortography. It may not be necessary before aortic valve replacement in young patients (< 40 years of age).

Surgical management

Aortic valve replacement should be performed for severe aortic regurgitation irrespective of whether the patient has symptoms, in order to prevent left ventricular impairment becoming irreversible. Aortic valve repair is possible in certain cases.

Left ventricular impairment and dilatation may partly regress after timely aortic valve replacement.

Indications for aortic valve replacement in chronic severe aortic regurgitation

- Symptomatic patients.
- Asymptomatic patients with left ventricular dysfunction or dilatation.

Medical treatment of aortic valve regurgitation

Diuretics and vasodilators (ACE inhibitors and nifedipine) are used for symptom control in patients who are awaiting valve replacement. These drugs may also delay the time when surgery is required. They may be used in asymptomatic patients with severe chronic aortic regurgitation without left ventricular impairment or dilatation or other indications for surgery.

Acute aortic regurgitation

This condition is rare, but it requires immediate referral to a surgical centre for emergency aortic valve replacement. Causes include infective endocarditis and aortic dissection.

Tricuspid valve disease

Pathology

Isolated tricuspid valve disease is very rare in primary care. Tricuspid valve regurgitation is most commonly seen as part of severe congestive heart failure producing pulmonary hypertension. This results in right heart dilatation and stretching of the tricuspid valve ring. Rheumatic heart disease and cardiomyopathy are the commonest causes. Tricuspid regurgitation may be seen in mainlining drug addicts. Tricuspid stenosis is very rare.

Examination

Systolic 'V'-waves due to reflux of blood to the jugular veins during right ventricular contraction, signs of right heart failure (raised venous pressure, enlarged tender liver and peripheral oedema) and pulmonary hypertension (loud pulmonary component to the second heart sound) may be present.

Symptoms

Ankle swelling, breathlessness, abdominal distension due to ascites, and discomfort due to liver enlargement may be present.

Investigation

Echocardiography will provide information on both the right and left heart and valve structure and function. Cardiac catheterisation is required to assess coronary anatomy prior to revascularisation or valve replacement, and to measure the pulmonary artery pressure before cardiac transplantation.

Treatment

Peripheral oedema is treated with diuretics. Tricuspid valve replacement with or without annuloplasty is not as successful as left heart valve replacement, and patients need careful evaluation. Reducing pulmonary artery hypertension and the pressure overload on the right ventricle is difficult, and necessitates treatment of the underlying cause.

Infective endocarditis

Role of the GP

This is a dangerous condition with a high mortality and morbidity. Mortality varies according to the infective organism, ranging from 50% for fungal infections to 5% for infections with *Streptococcus viridans*. Mortality is higher with prosthetic valve endocarditis or when infection is complicated by heart failure, emboli or abscess, which are signs of aggressive, advanced, uncontrolled infection.

Infective endocarditis is treated by cardiologists in close collaboration with a microbiologist. If the diagnosis is suspected, the patient must be referred urgently to hospital for investigation and treatment.

The GP plays a crucial part in diagnosis and treatment by arranging blood tests before starting antibiotics for undiagnosed fever and non-specific illness in patients at risk (those with known heart valve disease or congenital heart disease and previous attacks of endocarditis).

Causes

Infective endocarditis may affect both normal and abnormal native valves. It presents a particularly difficult and dangerous management problem when it affects prosthetic valves.

It may arise both in the community (as a result of dental work or other procedures) and in hospital. Community-acquired infection is caused by oral viridans streptococci (now called enterococci) and *Staphylococcus aureus*, although virtually any organism may be responsible. Hospital-acquired infection may be caused by staphylococci and methicillin-resistant *Staphylococcus aureus* (MRSA). Intravenous access-site infection is a common source. Intravenous drug abuse may result in tricuspid valve endocarditis, often due to *Staphylococcus aureus*.

Clinical features

These are variable and depend on the type of infection, the valve(s) affected and the clinical state of the patient. Fever, weight loss and malaise are common, although fever may be absent in the elderly. Congestive heart failure due to valve regurgitation is the most frequent and important cardiac complication, and it is important to recognise it. Joint pain and back pain, neurological problems and headache are common, but peripheral signs due to microemboli are neither common nor diagnostic.

Prevention and management of endocarditis in primary care

Successful treatment of endocarditis depends on the following:

- the identification of patients at risk of developing endocarditis
- good oral health
- awareness of the procedures associated with bacteraemia
- antibiotic prophylaxis in appropriate cases
- prompt referral of patients with suspected infection.

Diagnosis

Infective endocarditis is often difficult to diagnose, especially in elderly patients, because the symptoms and signs in the early stages may be dismissed as part of an insignificant illness. It may be particularly difficult to distinguish infective endo-carditis from an alternative cause of fever and infection in a patient with a heart murmur.

The Duke diagnostic criteria (*see* Box 17.1) are used to confirm the diagnosis. Antibiotics may have been prescribed for a throat or chest infection and this may make subsequent microbiological diagnosis difficult. Any antibiotics that have been prescribed within the previous few weeks should be mentioned with the referral. Blood-culture-negative endocarditis occurs in 5% of cases, and may be caused by unusual or 'demanding' organisms. Serological tests and the polymerase chain reaction (PCR) are also used to investigate certain infections. The diagnosis is made on the basis of a combination of clinical features and test results (*see* Box 17.1). There is no single definitive criterion.

Box 17.1:　Criteria for diagnosis of endocarditis

Major criteria

- Persistent bacteraemia with three positive blood cultures (or both bottles of a single blood culture).

- Echocardiographic visualisation of a vegetation or abscess or dehiscence of a prosthetic heart valve.

Minor criteria

- Predisposing heart condition or intravenous drug abuse.
- Fever.
- Emboli (septic pulmonary infarcts, arterial emboli, intracranial haemorrhage).
- Immunological phenomena (glomerulonephritis with microscopic haematuria, raised C-reactive protein level and erythrocyte sedimentation rate).

Echocardiography in diagnosis and management

Transthoracic echocardiography may diagnose vegetations in only 50% of cases, and therefore failure to see a vegetation should not affect the presumptive diagnosis, which should be made using the Duke criteria.

A negative echocardiogram does not exclude infective endocarditis.

The specificity of transthoracic echocardiography is high (98%), so the absence of a vegetation in a patient in whom the diagnosis is unlikely is reassuring. Transthoracic echocardiography may be diagnostically limited in 20% of patients, and prosthetic valves are difficult to image.

Transoesophageal echocardiography should be performed in patients if:

- the transthoracic study is not of diagnostic quality
- they have a prosthetic heart valve
- the diagnosis is at least moderately likely, but the transthoracic study is normal.

Treatment

Treatment should be started immediately after sending off three sets of blood cultures. In patients who have been unwell for more than a few weeks it is reasonable to wait a day or two to confirm the microbiological diagnosis and select appropriate antibiotics before embarking on a long course of intravenous treatment. This is a combination of intravenous antibiotics for at least 2 and usually 6 weeks in hospital, but some patients with antibiotic-sensitive infection due to oral streptococci who respond within a few days may be discharged from hospital back to primary care to complete treatment on oral antibiotics. Patients who are suitable for completion of treatment at home should be haemodynamically stable, have no evidence of cardiac complications (e.g. important valve abnormality), and capable and compliant with treatment. Patients with indwelling central intravenous lines may be managed in primary care with suitable clinical support.

Cardiac surgery with valve replacement is sometimes necessary in resistant cases where there is a persistent fever, signs of heart failure or severe valvular regurgitation, abscess formation or septic emboli. Surgery carries a high risk in these patients.

Antibiotic prophylaxis

The aim is to prevent endocarditis in patients with cardiac lesions which predispose them to the condition during procedures that result in bacteraemia. Tooth brushing or flossing and chewing may be more potent causes of a bacteraemia.

The current recommendations for antibiotic prophylaxis are being reconsidered because of the risks of inducing drug-resistant organisms and the lack of scientific evidence to support the guidelines. Although infective endocarditis is seldom associated with dental procedures, currently any dental work known to induce gum bleeding and professional cleaning are included as potentially septic procedures that require antibiotic prophylaxis (*see* Box 17.2). In addition, there are patients with low-risk cardiac lesions (e.g. pulmonary valve stenosis, atrial septal defect) in whom the risk of antibiotics (allergic reactions, development of antibiotic resistance) may be greater than the risk of endocarditis. The balance of risk to benefit is particularly relevant for urological procedures, but at present it is recommended that the current guidelines published by the British Society for Antimicrobial Chemotherapy are followed (*see British National Formulary*).

Box 17.2:   Current recommendations for antibiotic prophylaxis

Procedures for which antibiotic prophylaxis is currently recommended
Dental procedures known to induce gum bleeding
Surgical operations involving the gut or respiratory mucosa
Rigid bronchoscopy
Oesophageal procedures
Cystoscopy
Gall-bladder surgery
Urological procedures
Gynaecological procedures

Procedures for which antibiotic prophylaxis is not currently recommended
Atraumatic dental procedures
Flexible bronchoscopy
Cardiac catheterisation
Gastrointestinal endoscopy
In the absence of infection:
    Insertion or removal of intrauterine contraceptive devices
    Urethral catheterisation
    Dilation and curettage, sterilisation

Answers to case studies

1   The possible causes in this patient are complete heart block, aortic valve stenosis and other medical causes, including anaemia, cerebrovascular disease with possible lung pathology or hypertensive heart disease. On examination, look for signs of aortic valve disease, hypertension, anaemia, chronic lung disease and

heart failure, and measure the heart rate. Check the patient's ECG for signs of bradycardia, heart block and left ventricular hypertrophy. Request an echocardiogram and, if this is normal, a chest X-ray and some blood tests. Prompt referral to a cardiologist is necessary if this man has significant aortic valve disease, and if he has heart block he should be sent to hospital immediately.

2   Heart failure is the likely diagnosis in this patient. Look for signs of heart failure and mitral valve regurgitation, and check his blood pressure. Ask him what drugs he was prescribed and what he is currently taking. Causes include poor drug compliance, inadequate treatment, further infarction and heart failure, mitral regurgitation or a left ventricular aneurysm. Arrange a chest X-ray to look for pulmonary oedema, and echocardiography to assess left ventricular function and size and mitral regurgitation. Check the patient's renal function and blood count. Describe to him the reasons for his breathlessness and the importance of drug treatment (which will need modification), and explain that he will need to be referred to a cardiologist for further assessment and investigation. This should include coronary angiography with a view to revascularisation.

3   The possible causes in this patient are infective endocarditis, malignancy, infection and hypothyroidism. All of these possibilities require investigation with blood tests, blood cultures (before antibiotics are started), X-rays, ECG and echocardiography. The patient will need referral to the appropriate specialist after preliminary clinical assessment. Infective endocarditis is now often community acquired and there may be no history of dental work or other septic procedures.

4   Aortic dissection is the most important cause to exclude, because of its common association with certain forms of Marfan's syndrome. If the symptoms and signs suggest this, the patient should be referred to hospital immediately. The diagnosis may be made by transoesophageal echocardiography, magnetic resonance imaging and CT scanning. If the aorta is normal, other causes of backache should be investigated. The sweating may be due to pain rather than to a fever.

5   Palpitation suggests a cardiac rather than a respiratory infective cause. Ask the patient about congenital heart disease, infections (rheumatic heart disease) and her functional capacity. Examine her heart rate and rhythm and her blood pressure, and listen to her heart. Congenital heart disease is a possibility, but she would probably know about this. Atrial fibrillation is a common consequence of mitral valve disease, and results in sudden pulmonary oedema and breathlessness. An ECG and echocardiogram should provide the diagnosis. The patient should be treated with diuretics for pulmonary oedema. If she is in atrial fibrillation, she should be given drugs to control the ventricular response (see Chapter 18) and warfarin. It may be possible to convert her medically to sinus rhythm. She should be referred to a cardiologist for assessment and further management. If she has mitral stenosis, then in view of her age it is likely that she may be suitable for percutaneous mitral valvuloplasty.

Further reading

- Bonow RO, Carabello B, de Leon AC *et al.* (2000) ACC/AHA guidelines for the management of patients with valvular heart disease: a report of the American College of Cardiology/American Heart Association task force on practice guidelines (committee on management of patients with valvular heart disease). *J Am Coll Cardiol.* **32**: 1486–588.
- Eykyn SJ (2001) Endocarditis: basics. *Heart.* **86**: 476–80.
- Working Party of the British Society for Antimicrobial Chemotherapy (1993) Recommendations for endocarditis prophylaxis. *J Antimicrob Chemother.* **31**: 437–8.

CHAPTER 18

Management of arrhythmias

Case studies

1 A 32-year-old woman complains of palpitation. She describes missed beats and extra beats when she is resting in bed and watching television. What is the probable cause and how would you manage her?
2 A 78-year-old hypertensive woman complains of short episodes of palpitation and dizzy turns but no loss of consciousness. What is the most likely diagnosis and what would you do?
3 A 38-year-old man complains of occasional palpitation without any other symptoms, which lasts for a few minutes. What would you do?
4 A 65-year-old man complains of episodes of sudden loss of consciousness. Three months ago he was treated for heart failure complicating a myocardial infarction. What is the probable cause and what would you do?
5 An 86-year-old woman becomes confused, breathless and giddy. What are the likely causes and what would you do?

Role of primary care clinicians in the management of arrhythmias

Most patients with clinically important arrhythmias are treated with drugs and monitored in primary care. Patients are referred to a cardiologist either to confirm the diagnosis or when their symptoms are unacceptable.

The roles of the primary care physician in managing patients with arrhythmias are as follows:

- to identify patients with symptoms due to arrhythmias and refer them when necessary
- to identify which patients should be managed in primary care and which should be referred to a cardiologist
- to manage commonly occurring arrhythmias
- to appreciate the value and limitations of 12-lead and 24-hour ambulatory electrocardiography and other cardiac investigations in the investigation of arrhythmias.

GPs should also be aware of the rapidly advancing non-pharmacological methods for treating arrhythmias. The indications for, availability and success of radiofrequency ablation, pacing and implantable cardiac defibrillators are increasing, and may offer a cure or relief of symptoms without drug side-effects for patients with supraventricular tachycardia, atrial fibrillation, atrial flutter, complete heart block or ventricular arrhythmias.

Clinical experience and the results of trials and observational studies are helping to define the indications for new interventional techniques and devices. The field of electrophysiology has become a major and growing cardiological specialty.

Classification of arrhythmias

Supraventricular tachycardias

These are classified as either regular or irregular according to the rhythm of the ventricular response. Most rely on a re-entry mechanism with the tachycardia initiated by an ectopic beat. The diagnosis indicates the location of the circuit.

- *Atrioventricular node re-entry tachycardia.* The re-entry circuit is in the atrioventricular node, and this is the commonest cause (90% of cases) of narrow complex regular supraventricular tachycardias. It commonly presents in early adulthood.
- *Atrioventricular re-entry tachycardia.* The re-entry circuit is an accessory pathway connecting the atrium with the ventricle (bundle of Kent in Wolff-Parkinson-White's syndrome). It may present at any age and is a regular tachycardia.
- *Atrial fibrillation.* The re-entry circuits are restricted to the atrial muscle. This is the commonest sustained arrhythmia and its prevalence is increasing. It is associated with scarring, dilatation or stretching of the atrial muscle.

The common causes of palpitation presenting in primary care include the following:

- sinus tachycardia
- atrial and ventricular ectopic beats
- atrial fibrillation
- atrial flutter
- supraventricular tachycardia.

Both ventricular tachycardia and ventricular fibrillation are rare in primary care, but they are often under-diagnosed and should be suspected as a cause of loss of consciousness or dizzy turns in patients with coronary artery disease or cardiomyopathy.

Arrhythmias and symptoms

Palpitation is a common cardiac symptom presenting in primary care.

An ECG recorded during symptoms is required to diagnose the cause of palpitation.

Symptoms are generally unreliable in diagnosing arrhythmias, and depend on the haemodynamic consequences of the arrhythmia. These relate to its cause, anatomical origin, duration, the resulting heart rate, the underlying cardiac function, coexisting valve abnormalities and the age, medical condition and level of activity of the patient.

Asking the patient to tap out the rhythm of their palpitation is usually confusing even for musically trained individuals, and provides unreliable information for making management decisions.

Patients with arrhythmias may be symptom-free. Atrial fibrillation with a ventricular rate of 100 beats/minute in an elderly patient with impaired left ventricular function or in a patient with hypertrophic cardiomyopathy may have serious haemodynamic effects resulting in heart failure or collapse, whereas it may go unnoticed by a fit person. Ventricular tachycardia related to a myocardial infarct scar may cause death or collapse. A heart rate of 30 beats/minute in a sleeping athlete is not unusual and would not be expected to result in symptoms, but if such a rate was due to complete heart block it would probably lead to syncope or heart failure.

Confusion with regard to selection of anti-arrhythmic drugs

Arrhythmias and their treatment may be confusing to primary care clinicians, and there are several reasons for this. Compared with other cardiovascular subjects, there is a relatively small evidence base on which to select anti-arrhythmic treatment which is guided by the results of observational studies, pharmacology, an understanding of the natural history of the arrhythmia and its underlying causes, and clinical experience. Drug treatment for arrhythmias should be individualised but based on the available evidence.

Electrophysiology is a complex subject compared, for example, with the simpler concept and visualisation of coronary anatomy provided by angiography and angioplasty. Arrhythmias are less frequently encountered in primary care than is the management of cardiovascular risk factors, hypertension and heart failure. The pathophysiology of some arrhythmias remains obscure, and some primary care clinicians believe that their management is a specialist subject.

Principles of prescribing anti-arrhythmic drugs

- Anti-arrhythmic drugs may result in pro-arrhythmia, particularly in patients with structural heart disease, coronary heart disease or left ventricular hypertrophy.
- Most anti-arrhythmic drugs are negatively inotropic and may precipitate heart failure in susceptible patients.
- It is essential that anti-arrhythmic drugs are only used in patients with severe symptoms or prognostically important arrhythmias.
- There is no evidence that prolonged suppression of atrial or ventricular ectopic beats with anti-arrhythmic drugs prevents sudden death in patients with structurally normal hearts. β-Blockers may increase the frequency of ectopic beats occurring in the setting of sinus bradycardia.
- Haemodynamically significant arrhythmias are difficult to treat, are associated with a high mortality and should be referred urgently to hospital.
- Anti-arrhythmic drug side-effects are more likely to occur in patients with hypokalaemia and renal and/or hepatic impairment, and in the elderly. Electrolytes and

creatinine levels should be checked as part of the clinical assessment. Drug levels only occasionally need to be checked.

- Interactions between anti-arrhythmic drugs are unpredictable. In general, only one of these drugs should be used except after specialist consultation. Significant brady-cardia may occur with the combination of a β-blocker with any anti-arrhythmic drug, particularly verapamil or digoxin, although these combinations are occasionally prescribed for patients with uncontrolled atrial fibrillation.
- Anti-arrhythmic drugs may occasionally cause ventricular tachycardia, ventricular fibrillation or, rarely, torsades de pointes, which are usually associated with widening of the QRS complex and prolongation of the QT interval. Anti-arrhythmic drugs should be stopped if significant ECG changes occur.
- Patients with symptomatic regular narrow complex supraventricular tachycardia and intolerable atrial fibrillation should be referred to a cardiologist.
- The data sheet and the *British National Formulary* should be consulted before prescribing these drugs.

Torsades de pointes

This is an uncommon and dangerous form of ventricular tachycardia that is diagnosed on an ECG if the QRS complex appears to be twisting around a baseline. It usually degener-ates to ventricular fibrillation and cardiac arrest. It results from prolongation of the QT interval. There is a genetic predisposition in some cases. There are several causes, including any anti-arrhythmic drug which prolongs the QT interval, and interactions between anti-arrhythmic drugs and other drugs, including antidepressants, anti-histamines and antibiotics (e.g. intravenous erythromycin). Hypokalaemia, hypo-magnesaemia, hypocalcaemia and bradycardia are predisposing factors.

Treatment of torsades de pointes involves admitting the patient to hospital as an emergency to deal with the possibility of cardiac arrest, stopping the offending drug(s) and correction of predisposing biochemical abnormalities. Bradycardia is corrected by tem-porary cardiac pacing.

Anti-arrhythmic drugs should only be prescribed after a precise diagnosis of the arrhythmia and any underlying heart disease has been made. The benefits, risks and duration of treatment should be carefully considered and explained to the patient.

Box 18.1:   Vaughan Williams classification of anti-arrhythmic drugs commonly used in the UK

This classifies anti-arrhythmic drugs into four categories according to their main pharmacological action. Members of each drug class (particularly β-blockers) may have different pharmacological properties which are used in marketing the drug, but that do not often translate into significant clinical differences.

Class IA

Disopyramide
Indications
- Maintenance of sinus rhythm after electrical cardioversion.
- Suppression of atrial or ventricular arrhythmias after surgery.
- Prevention of paroxysmal supraventricular tachycardia or atrial fibrillation.

Dose
300–800 mg per day orally. The intravenous preparation should only be given if there are facilities for cardiac monitoring or defibrillation.

Contraindications
- Sinus node disease.
- Unpaced heart block or bundle branch block.
- Severe heart failure.
- Long QT syndrome.
- The sustained-release preparation is contraindicated in patients with renal or hepatic impairment.
- Atropine-like side-effects (ocular hypotension in patients with narrow-angle glaucoma), acute urinary retention in patients with prostatism, aggravation of myasthenia gravis, dry mouth, impotence.

Class IB

Lignocaine
This is used intravenously in hospital to treat significant ventricular arrhythmias.

Class IC

Flecainide
This is a sodium-channel blocker that can be administered both orally and intravenously. Tablets may be used to treat acute non-life-threatening arrhythmias.
   It is useful for treating supraventricular tachycardias.

Indications
- Atrioventricular-node-reciprocating tachycardia.
- Wolff-Parkinson-White's syndrome.
- To convert paroxysmal atrial fibrillation to sinus rhythm.
- Sustained ventricular tachycardia.
- Symptomatic ventricular ectopic beats.

Dose
50–300 mg per day in two divided doses.

Contraindications
- Heart failure.
- Unpaced heart block, bundle branch block, sinus node disease and bradycardia.

One study showed a doubling of mortality or non-fatal cardiac arrest when flecainide was used to treat asymptomatic ventricular ectopic beats after myocardial infarction. Therefore it should not be used in patients with prior myocardial infarction or those with known coronary artery disease, and it should be used with caution in elderly patients. There is no evidence that it increases the risk of sudden death in patients with supraventricular tachycardia.

Side-effects
- Ventricular tachycardia.
- Congestive heart failure.
- Conversion to atrial flutter.

Propafenone
Indications, contraindications and side-effects
Similar to those for flecainide.

Dose
150–300 mg three times a day.

Class II

β-Blockers
Several β-blockers are available, and there is little significant clinical difference between them. They improve the prognosis in patients when given early after myocardial infarction and with controlled heart failure. They are effective in hypertension and angina, and are particularly useful in patients with both conditions. They may be considered the drug of first choice for patients with paroxysmal atrial fibrillation and normal left ventricular and sinus node function. Patients with sinus node disease are susceptible to both tachycardia and bradycardia, and β-blockers may precipitate severe symptomatic bradycardia. They are also used to prevent migraine and to blunt the sympathetic effects of acute hyperthyroidism.

Contraindications
Even though some β-blockers are 'cardioselective', they should not be used in patients with airways disease. They may be used with caution in patients with diabetes and claudication. They are contraindicated in patients with bradycardia, heart block or uncontrolled heart failure.

They should be started at a low dose, which may be increased according to the clinical and heart rate response.

Side-effects
A significant proportion of patients find the common side-effects of physical and mental fatigue, cold hands and feet and impotence unacceptable. Sudden withdrawal of treatment may lead to myocardial ischaemia in patients with significant coronary heart disease.

β-Blockers may be prescribed inappropriately to treat palpitations which may be due to benign ectopic beats occurring in the setting of bradycardia and sinus node disease. Under these circumstances, β-blockers may increase the frequency of arrhythmia.

Class III

Amiodarone
This is a useful and effective anti-arrhythmic drug. It is more effective than propafenone and sotalol in maintaining sinus rhythm in patients with paroxysmal or persistent atrial fibrillation. It is generally used as a second-line drug because it has significant side-effects in 20% of patients and complex pharmacokinetics resulting in a long half-life (around 2 months). It has comparatively little negative inotropic activity, so is used as a first-line drug in patients with impaired left ventricular function and significant arrhythmias.

Indications
- All tachyarrhythmias of any origin.
- Ventricular arrhythmias in patients with structural heart disease (e.g. hypertrophic cardiomyopathy).
- Prior to elective electrical cardioversion, and afterwards to maintain sinus rhythm.

Contraindications
- Thyroid abnormalities.
- Unpaced severe conduction abnormalities.

Interactions
Amiodarone is strongly protein bound, and it raises the plasma concentration of warfarin, digoxin and phenytoin. The doses of these drugs should therefore be reduced in order to avoid side-effects, and the INR/prothrombin time should be checked more frequently.

Amiodarone prolongs the QT interval. Although rarely causing torsades de pointes, it should not be prescribed with class IA and III anti-arrhythmic drugs, antipsychotics, tricyclic antidepressants, antihistamines, antimalarials or bradycardic agents.

Dose
200 mg three times a day for 1 week, 200 mg twice a day for the second week and then 200 mg per day. The dose may need to be reduced in elderly or small patients. The minimum effective dose should be used in order to avoid side-effects, and a weekly dose of 300 mg (100 mg on alternate days) may be sufficient.

Side-effects
- Sensitivity to sunlight resulting in erythema and burning is not a major problem for patients living in the UK, but patients should be warned to cover up and use a high-protection sunscreen cream in sunny weather, and they should be advised not to sunbathe.

- Amiodarone contains iodine, and both hypothyroidism and hyperthyroidism may occur after prolonged use. Interpretation of thyroid function tests is difficult because they may be abnormal even if the patient is euthyroid. Thyroid function tests should be checked before starting treatment, 6-monthly thereafter and also after stopping treatment. Regular clinical assessments are recommended. Amiodarone-induced thyroid abnormalities usually resolve within 3 months of drug withdrawal.
- Pulmonary fibrosis, which may be fatal even if recognised early, is diagnosed with a chest X-ray and usually resolves within a few months after drug withdrawal. Amiodarone should be used very cautiously in patients with lung disease.
- Impaired liver function tests may resolve spontaneously, but the drug should be stopped if they do not.
- Microdeposits in the eyes are benign, rarely affect vision and do not necessitate drug withdrawal.
- Peripheral neuropathy and myopathy are rare and may not be reversible. Impotence may also occur.

Sotalol
This has both class II and III actions, and it shares the indications and contraindications of other β-blockers and class III drugs.

Indications
- Supraventricular and ventricular arrhythmias.
- As for other β-blockers.

Dose
40 mg twice a day increased gradually if necessary to 160 mg twice a day. The dose should be reduced in patients with renal impairment.

Side-effects
Torsades de pointes is the most important side-effect, and caution should be used when prescribing sotalol for patients with predisposing factors, congestive heart failure or exacerbation of chronic obstructive airways disease.

Class IV

Verapamil
This is a calcium antagonist which blocks the inward flow of calcium into heart muscle, coronary arteries and conduction tissue. It lowers peripheral vascular resistance, slows electrical conduction through the atrioventricular node, slows the heart rate and lowers myocardial oxygen consumption.

Indications
- Hypertension.
- Angina.
- Controlling the ventricular response in atrial fibrillation.
- Paroxysmal supraventricular tachycardia.

Contraindications
- Atrial fibrillation/flutter complicating Wolff-Parkinson-White's syndrome. This is because it may lead to atrioventricular block and increased conduction down the accessory pathway leading to ventricular tachycardia.
- Hypotension/cardiogenic shock.
- Bradycardia.
- Second- or third-degree heart block.
- Patients taking digoxin or β-blockers (bradycardia).

Side-effects
- Constipation and flushing.
- Caution should be used in patients with liver disease.

Dose
120 mg twice a day orally increasing to 160 mg twice a day or 240 mg every morning in slow-release formulation.

The intravenous formulation has been replaced by adenosine for treating supraventricular tachycardia, mainly because of associated hypotension.

Diltiazem

This has similar pharmacology, indications and contraindications to verapamil. It is useful for treating angina. It can be used in combination with β-blockers, but should be used with caution in patients who have or are predisposed to bradycardia. It is generally well tolerated.

Digoxin

This drug does not fit into a single Vaughan-Williams class and it has multiple actions. It slows the ventricular response to atrial fibrillation in patients at rest, but is not as effective as verapamil or β-blockers in controlling the ventricular rate response in exercising patients. Compared with class I anti-arrhythmic drugs or amiodarone, it has relatively little effect in converting patients to sinus rhythm. It has a weak positive inotropic action.

Dose
A loading dose should be used. The maintenance dose is judged according to the age, weight and renal function of the patient. A loading dose of 0.5 mg followed by 0.25 mg 6 hours later and a maintenance dose of 0.25 mg every morning is usually

adequate in most adults. Lower doses are used in elderly patients with hypokalaemia and renal impairment. A dose of 0.0625 mg (after loading with 0.375 mg in divided doses) is usually sufficient in small elderly patients.

Side-effects
- Bradycardia and heart block.

Contraindications
- Atrial fibrillation/flutter complicating Wolff-Parkinson-White's syndrome (*see* verapamil above).
- Its positive inotropic action may increase the outflow tract gradient in hypertrophic obstructive cardiomyopathy.

Serum levels
Some physicians prefer to check the serum drug level, but overdose is rare in patients treated with the doses suggested above. Serum levels are useful in patients with suspected non-compliance. Toxic side-effects include nausea, vomiting, visual disturbance and arrhythmias.

Indications
- Atrial fibrillation/flutter with or without heart failure.
- Sinus rhythm and heart failure.

Selecting anti-arrhythmic drugs

Although some anti-arrhythmics are contraindicated in certain situations, no anti-arrhythmic drug is clearly superior for treating specific arrhythmias. There may be a preference for one drug for other reasons.

Patients should be told that it may be necessary to try a number of drugs in order to find the one that is most effective for them.

Pro-arrhythmic action of anti-arrhythmic drugs

Pro-arrhythmias are tachyarrhythmias and bradyarrhythmias, and they represent the most serious and unpredictable side-effect of anti-arrhythmic drugs. Predisposing conditions include hypokalaemia, left ventricular hypertrophy, bradycardia and potassium-channel blockers.

The ablation procedure

The investigation and treatment are performed at the same time. The procedure involves inserting small electrodes intravenously into the right heart (and occasionally the left heart via the interatrial septum), under local anaesthesia, sedation and analgesia if required. X-ray guidance or, more recently, non-fluoroscopic, computer-generated, electro-anatomical maps are used to guide electrode positioning. Radiofrequency energy is used to ablate tissue, leaving it electrically inert, and during ablation some patients experience warmth or chest pain. Depending on the problem, the procedure lasts around an hour, requiring an overnight stay at most.

Results of ablation for supraventricular tachycardia

Ablation (destruction) of part of the re-entry circuit that facilitates tachycardia is associated with high cure rates (over 98% for supraventricular tachycardia and atrial flutter) and a complication rate of 1%.

The procedure is less successful in treating atrial fibrillation, with cure rates of around 50%. There is a higher procedural complication rate because a trans-septal puncture is required to ablate and 'isolate' the cuff of pulmonary vein from which the atrial fibrillation originates. Ablation is offered to patients with intolerable atrial fibrillation despite medical treatment.

Non-pharmacological management of ventricular arrhythmias

These conditions are rarely encountered in primary care. Ventricular tachycardia and fibrillation may present as 'failed sudden death', brief changes in conscious level or palpitation. Most commonly they result from an arrhythmia focus in a scarred and weak left ventricle due to myocardial infarction or a cardiomyopathy. Occasionally, ventricular tachycardia may be benign when it originates from the right ventricular outflow tract. It is important to optimise the medical treatment of patients with impaired cardiac function.

The implantation of a cardioverter-defibrillator reduces the risk of sudden cardiac death in patients at high risk. Indications include the following:

- patients who have survived an attack of sudden death due to ventricular tachycardia or fibrillation that did not have a reversible cause
- symptomatic patients with ventricular tachycardia associated with impaired cardiac function (most often due to infarction or cardiomyopathy)
- patients with spontaneous sustained ventricular tachycardia that is not amenable to other forms of treatment and who do not have structural heart disease
- structural heart disease and non-sustained ventricular tachycardia that are not controlled by drugs
- cardioverter-defibrillators are also implanted in patients with severe left ventricular function.

These devices provide bradycardia support like a normal pacemaker, but they also recognise important ventricular arrhythmias and deliver a shock until normal rhythm is restored.

The first device was implanted in 1980, and at that time they were cumbersome, requiring a thoracotomy. They are now similar in size to a pacemaker, with a single electrode that is positioned in the right ventricle. They are implanted under local anaesthesia and tested with the patient fully anaesthetised. The batteries last for 3 to 6 years depending on the number of shocks delivered. The complications include infection, pneumothorax, inappropriate shocks which may result in major psychological disability, and lead failure. Although the modern devices are simpler to implant, device checks, follow-up and problem solving require highly skilled and experienced technical support.

Cardiac resynchronisation

Ventricular tachycardia leading to ventricular fibrillation is often the cause of death in patients with heart failure. Pacemakers with facilities for cardioversion/defibrillation/bradycardia support and resynchronisation may be used (*see* Chapter 13).

Ablation treatment for ventricular arrhythmias

Ventricular arrhythmias originating from the right ventricular outflow tract and a focal point in the left ventricle may be treated with radiofrequency ablation. Patients with myocardial scarring who remain symptomatic despite having an implantable cardioverter-defibrillator may benefit from ablation of foci of arrhythmias in the ventricle.

Adjunctive anti-arrhythmic drug treatment

This may be necessary in order to reduce arrhythmia and symptoms in patients who have an implantable cardioverter-defibrillator or who have had ablation.

Management of sinus tachycardia

This is common, particularly in younger patients and during pregnancy. It is generally benign, and is often related to anxiety and less commonly associated with anaemia or thyrotoxicosis. It must be distinguished from other causes of a fast heart rate. It may be related to drug therapy, particularly inhaled β-agonists that are used to treat airways obstruction and over-the-counter cold cures containing sympathomimetic agents, and illicit recreational drugs. Treatment involves excluding these causes and explaining the condition to the patient with the aid of an ECG recorded during an attack. Drugs are not indicated.

Management of atrial and ventricular ectopic beats

Patients may describe 'missed and extra beats' or a temporary difficulty in catching their breath. When benign, ectopic beats occur with a slow resting heart rate and disappear as the heart rate increases with exercise, and patients find this reassuring and therapeutic. Ectopic beats are more common in patients with left ventricular hypertrophy due to hypertension, resting bradycardia due to regular exercise, or hypertrophic heart muscle disease.

Twenty-four-hour ambulatory electrocardiography will show the frequency and number of ectopic beats, and is useful for establishing the diagnosis. The recording shows the patient that their symptoms are real but benign, and have been taken seriously. Echocardiography may be used to measure left ventricular wall thickness and function. Ectopic beats are benign and do not require treatment or investigation unless they are associated with underlying structural heart disease. The use of β-blockers is not advised because, by slowing the heart rate, they may increase the number of bradycardia-related ectopic beats as well as having other side-effects.

Management of atrial fibrillation

This is the commonest significant arrhythmia seen in primary care. Its prevalence increases with age, and it is becoming more common. It is due to electrical re-entry circuits in the atrial muscle or the muscle of the pulmonary veins. Most patients are treated with drugs. The treatment for persistent atrial fibrillation remains controversial.

Risks of atrial fibrillation

Patients with atrial fibrillation have a sixfold increased risk of stroke and a twofold increased risk of death.

Atrial fibrillation is a major cause of the following:

- palpitation
- heart failure due to cardiac dilatation, tachycardia and loss of atrial contraction
- thromboembolism due to thrombus formation in the left atrial appendage. Embolic strokes resulting from non-valvular atrial fibrillation are more severe than ischaemic strokes, and are associated with a higher mortality. It is important that anti-coagulation is considered in all patients (*see* below).

Clinical evaluation of atrial fibrillation (from the Joint American College of Cardiology, American Heart Association and European Society of Cardiology guidelines)

The following points should be ascertained and determine management:

- symptoms
- clinical type of atrial fibrillation
- date of onset (patients may be symptom-free)
- frequency, duration, precipitating factors and modes of termination
- response to anti-arrhythmic drugs
- presence of underlying cardiac or reversible medical conditions.

The following investigations confirm the diagnosis and also assess associated cardiac conditions and the likely response to different forms of treatment, including cardioversion.

Clinical features of atrial fibrillation

The average age of patients with atrial fibrillation is 75 years, with the majority older than 65 years. Around 10% of people aged over 75 years are in atrial fibrillation.

Most patients have symptoms, but these are very variable and depend on the type and duration of atrial fibrillation, the ventricular response rate, and the age and clinical status of the patient. For example, in a patient who has a stiff left ventricle due to hypertrophic cardiomyopathy and whose cardiac output depends on left atrial contraction, acute atrial fibrillation may cause collapse. Elderly sedentary patients may be symptom-free and the arrhythmia may be detected by chance. It may present with palpitation, breathlessness due to congestive heart failure, syncope due to either a fast or slow heart rate or, alarmingly, with emboli.

The heart and pulse rate are completely irregular, and this results in a discrepancy between the apex and radial heart rate. Low-volume cardiac contractions may not be palpable at the wrist. Examination may show hypertension, signs of heart failure, alcoholism, a pericardial rub, mitral valve disease, recent cardiac surgery or congenital heart disease.

Classification of atrial fibrillation

Atrial fibrillation may be classified according to the duration of attacks, and this is helpful in management.

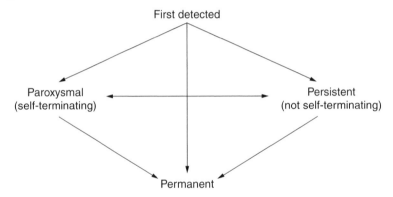

Figure 18.1: Clinical classification of atrial fibrillation.

- *Paroxysmal* attacks usually last less than 1 day and are self-terminating.
- *Persistent* attacks last more than 7 days, but may be terminated with cardioversion by drugs.
- Atrial fibrillation is classified as *permanent* if it has been present for more than 1 year, or cannot be terminated with drugs or electrical cardioversion, or if electrical cardioversion is not indicated.
- Both paroxysmal and persistent attacks may be recurrent (defined as two or more attacks).

Box 18.2: Medical conditions associated with atrial fibrillation that are commonly seen in primary care

Hypertension
Coronary heart disease and myocardial infarction
Infection in patients who are predisposed to atrial fibrillation
Cardiomyopathy

Mitral valve disease
Thyrotoxicosis
Sinus node disease
Alcohol (either an acute binge or chronic heavy consumption)
'Lone' atrial fibrillation (patients with a structurally normal heart)

Prognosis of atrial fibrillation

The prognosis of atrial fibrillation depends on its cause and the patient's age, underlying cardiovascular status and other medical conditions.

It has a good prognosis in young fit individuals with no cardiovascular disease ('lone atrial fibrillation'). Similarly, atrial fibrillation usually resolves without consequences within a few days after an alcohol binge, acute pericarditis or cardiac surgery. It is usually persistent and associated with haemodynamic impairment and thromboembolism in patients with a dilated cardiomyopathy due to chronic alcohol consumption, viral myocarditis, mitral valve disease or coronary heart disease.

Permanent atrial fibrillation in the elderly is associated with a poor prognosis due to the risk of stroke (which is largely preventable with warfarin) and heart failure.

Investigations in patients with atrial fibrillation

ECG
This identifies the following:

- rhythm and ventricular rate
- left ventricular hypertrophy
- pre-excitation
- bundle branch block
- prior myocardial infarction.

Chest X-ray
This should be undertaken if pulmonary oedema or a lung lesion is suspected.

Blood tests
These should include the following:

- thyroid function tests
- electrolytes and urea
- blood count.

Echocardiography
This identifies the following:

- valvular heart disease
- left and right atrial size
- left ventricular size and function
- left atrial thrombus (transoesophageal echocardiography is more sensitive than transthoracic echocardiography, and guides cardioversion)
- pericardial disease.

Supplementary tests

Exercise testing
This is used:

- to assess the heart rate response to exercise (rate control) and to assess the need for pacemaker implantation in patients with atrial fibrillation and bradycardia as part of sinus node disease
- to provoke atrial fibrillation in patients with suspected exercise-induced arrhythmia
- to assess underlying ischaemia in order to guide drug treatment and the need for angiography.

Twenty-four-hour Holter monitoring
This is used:

- to assess the duration and frequency of attacks and to confirm the diagnosis if this is in doubt
- to evaluate the heart rate in relation to symptoms.

Electrophysiology
This is performed as a prelude to catheter ablation.

Anticoagulation in atrial fibrillation

Anticoagulation should be considered in all patients with atrial fibrillation, and the decision as to whether to use it will depend on the risk of stroke and thromboembolism. This varies by a factor of 20 according to the patient's age and clinical and cardiovascular factors (*see* Box 18.3). Elderly patients have most to gain from anticoagulation because they are at greatest risk.

Box 18.3:   Factors which increase the risk of thromboembolism in patients with atrial fibrillation of any type

Atrial fibrillation for more than 7 days
Dilated impaired heart
Prosthetic heart valve
Left atrial thrombus
History of thromboembolism
History of transient ischaemic attack
Family history of thromboembolism
Mitral valve disease
Any cardiovascular risk factor
Age > 75 years
Haematological disease predisposing to thrombosis
Malignancy

For example, the risk of stroke is small (< 2% per year) in young patients (< 75 years) with lone atrial fibrillation who may be treated with aspirin.

For patients at high risk (*see* Box 18.3), adequate doses of warfarin should be prescribed and monitored to achieve an INR of > 2.0 and < 3.5. In this range, the risk of severe disability and death due to stroke is reduced compared with that associated with 'low-dose' warfarin and INR levels of < 2.0. The risk of intracranial haemorrhage is not significantly increased at INR levels of < 3.9.

Patients with a history of previous stroke are at particularly high risk (12% per year). The number of patients with atrial fibrillation who need treatment with warfarin in order to prevent one stroke is therefore about three times higher in primary prevention (*n* = 37) than in secondary prevention (*n* = 12).

Doctors seem to be reluctant to advise patients to start warfarin, possibly because of the fear of haemorrhage, although this risk is only slightly increased if the INR is closely controlled.

Antithrombotic and anticoagulant treatment guidelines for patients with permanent atrial fibrillation

- For patients under 60 years of age without cardiovascular risk factors, aspirin 300 mg every morning is currently recommended.
- For patients aged over 60 years, warfarin with an INR of 2–3 is recommended at present, or with an INR of 2.5–3.5 in patients with rheumatic heart valve disease, prosthetic valve(s) or a history of previous thromboembolism.

Testing the INR in primary care
Responsibility for management of anticoagulation is increasingly being devolved to primary care, and this has great advantages for patients. There are a number of instruments available for testing the INR, and they have been shown to be as reliable as laboratory measurements. Self-measurement and control of anticoagulation is safe and may become common practice in the same way that diabetics measure and control their blood sugar levels.

Antithrombotic treatment (aspirin or clopidogrel) should be used in patients at low risk of stroke, in those who do not wish to take warfarin, in cases where it is logistically difficult to monitor the INR and in patients in whom warfarin is contraindicated. Clopidogrel is a platelet inhibitor with similar risks of bleeding to aspirin (2%). It is used in patients who cannot tolerate aspirin, and has a half-life of several days.

Treatment of paroxysmal self-terminating atrial fibrillation in symptom-free patients

Attacks usually last less than 24 hours, but it is difficult to know how long a first attack will last when the patient is first seen.

If the patient is symptom-free or only mildly symptomatic, prescribe aspirin 75 mg every morning and review them within a few days.

No anti-arrhythmic treatment is necessary for attacks that last less than 24 hours.

Treatment of symptomatic patients with paroxysmal or persistent atrial fibrillation

The aim is to try to convert the patient to sinus rhythm as soon as possible in order to reduce the risk of embolism. Symptoms usually improve with ventricular rate control. Pharmacological cardioversion is less likely to be successful in patients who have been fibrillating for more than 7 days (persistent atrial fibrillation).

Antithrombotic or anticoagulation treatment

- Treat with aspirin 300 mg immediately and then 75 mg every morning or clopidogrel 75 mg once a day.
- Use warfarin instead of antithrombotic drugs if the patient has severe cardiac dilatation, rheumatic mitral valve disease, a history of previous thromboembolism or left atrial thrombus on echocardiography. For elective cardioversion of atrial fibrillation of more than 48 hours' duration, start warfarin and keep the INR in the range 2–3 for 3 weeks before and continue for 4 weeks after cardioversion.
- Continue warfarin (and do not start aspirin) if the patient is already on long-term warfarin for any reason (e.g. prosthetic heart valve, pulmonary embolus). Continue warfarin in patients with multiple risk factors or those at risk of recurrent thromboembolism.

No anticoagulation is required for patients with supraventricular tachycardia or atrial fibrillation of less than 48 hours' duration.

Anti-arrhythmic treatment options

These are as follows:

- flecainide 200–300 mg orally or 150 mg slowly intravenously. This is successful in around 95% of patients if given within 24 hours of the start of the attack, *or*
- dofetilide (dose depends on the patient's renal function, age and weight), *or*
- propafenone (450–600 mg orally), *or*
- amiodarone (for dose, *see* above), *or*
- digoxin (second-line drug or for hypotensive patients).

If the patient reverts to sinus rhythm, the decision to continue warfarin will depend on the risk of the patient reverting to atrial fibrillation and other risk factors for thromboembolism weighed against the risks of bleeding.

Catheter ablation may be used in patients with unacceptable symptoms despite anti-arrhythmic drug therapy.

Pacing for atrial fibrillation

Dual-chamber pacing with pacemaker software designed to recognise and pace the heart at specified rates to terminate atrial fibrillation reduces the frequency and duration of attacks of palpitation in symptomatic patients with bradycardia-dependent atrial fibrillation. 'Prevent AF' pacing is appropriate in these patients, who may develop symptomatic bradycardia at a later stage. Patients need aspirin and may require anti-arrhythmic drugs. They should be referred to a specialist with expertise in this developing field.

Rhythm vs. rate control in patients with persistent atrial fibrillation

The decision either to try to convert the patient back to sinus rhythm (*rhythm control*) or to accept permanent atrial fibrillation and aim for satisfactory ventricular *rate control* should be individualised. This is because the probability of maintaining sinus rhythm after electrical cardioversion is influenced by the age of the patient, the characteristics of their arrhythmia and the underlying heart condition. The decision is also influenced by the need for anticoagulation and its potential risks and practicalities in patients considered for rate control. Aspirin may be used in low-risk patients or in cases where warfarin is contraindicated.

Which approach is better?

In patients aged over 75 years with risk factors for stroke or death, neither approach is clearly superior with regard to mortality, quality of life, exercise capacity or risk of stroke. However, the risk of warfarin-associated bleeding is lower in the 40% of patients who remain in sinus rhythm after successful cardioversion, and this is clinically important in this age group.

Cardioversion and other non-pharmacological approaches should be considered in younger patients with lone atrial fibrillation, symptomatic patients of any age and those with structural heart disease. These patients should be referred to an electrophysiologist.

Rhythm control reduces (but does not completely abolish) the risk of thromboembolism and heart failure, palpitation resolves and warfarin treatment (with its complications) is generally avoided. Mortality is lower in patients who remain in sinus rhythm after cardioversion.

Cardioversion is mainly effective in patients with structurally normal hearts and paroxysmal or persistent atrial fibrillation.

This approach should be considered in patients who have a physically active lifestyle, in whom warfarin treatment is dangerous or unacceptable, and in whom cardioversion is likely to be successful in the long term.

Restoration of sinus rhythm may be achieved with electrical cardioversion, drugs, ablation or surgery (which is associated with a higher morbidity and mortality than other approaches). However, only 60% of patients remain in sinus rhythm after electrical cardioversion, even with additional anti-arrhythmic drug treatment.

Rate control is used in patients with a low probability of successful cardioversion, namely the elderly, those who have been in atrial fibrillation for more than a year, those with a dilated heart and those who require anticoagulation for other reasons (e.g. thrombotic disease, prosthetic heart valve). One of the potential complications of permanent atrial fibrillation is cardiac dilatation and impairment, termed 'atrial fibrillation-related cardiomyopathy'. This is one of the mechanisms of thromboembolism and it leads to heart failure.

Rate control is achieved with anti-arrhythmic drugs (digoxin, β-blockers, diltiazem, verapamil or various combinations of these), but necessitates the use of warfarin.

In patients whose ventricular rate remains fast despite drug treatment, atrio-ventricular node ablation may occasionally be necessary. This isolates the atria (which continue to fibrillate) electrically from the ventricles (which contract at their intrinsic rate of around 30 beats/minute). The atrioventricular block created is irreversible, and a permanent pacemaker is virtually always necessary and is implanted as part of the procedure.

Electrical cardioversion

This should be considered in all patients with persistent atrial fibrillation. It involves the patient being anticoagulated for 4 weeks prior to the procedure to reduce the likelihood of embolism and for at least 4 weeks after the cardioversion because the patient may revert back to atrial fibrillation shortly after cardioversion. Cardioversion may be performed without anticoagulation if atrial fibrillation started within 48 hours, because the risk of left atrial thrombus formation in that time and consequent thromboembolism is small. The absence of left atrial thrombus on transoesophageal echocardiography provides further reassurance that the risk of thromboembolism is negligible.

Cardioversion has a lower long-term success rate in elderly patients, who may be more appropriately managed with rate control and anticoagulation.

Indications for electrical cardioversion

- After failed anti-arrhythmic drug treatment in patients with paroxysmal atrial fibrillation and a fast ventricular rate complicated by heart failure, angina, hypotension or unacceptable symptoms, particularly in individuals with acute myocardial infarction or diastolic dysfunction (e.g. hypertrophic cardiomyopathy), and during pregnancy.
- To prevent ventricular fibrillation in patients with Wolff-Parkinson-White's syndrome in whom atrial fibrillation occurs with a rapid ventricular response and haemodynamic instability.
- In patients with persistent atrial fibrillation when early recurrence after cardioversion is unlikely.
- To restore sinus rhythm in patients having their first attack of atrial fibrillation.
- For repeated cardioversion with prophylactic drug therapy in patients who revert back to atrial fibrillation after successful cardioversion without drug therapy.

The procedure

Most cardiologists recommend an anti-arrhythmic drug to be taken both before cardioversion, to improve the likelihood of success, and for several weeks at least after the procedure to decrease the likelihood of reversion back to atrial fibrillation. Outpatients are admitted to hospital starved. The heart rhythm is monitored with an ECG, the patient is given a short general anaesthetic and cardioversion is performed. The patient is generally able to leave hospital after a few hours, but should not drive home, and should not go to work until the following day. They may experience skin burn or discomfort over the chest which resolves after a few days in response to application of a steroid cream.

Management after cardioversion

The patient should be reviewed after 1 week. If they are in sinus rhythm, their anti-arrhythmic drug(s) and anticoagulation should be continued because of the ongoing likelihood of recurrent atrial fibrillation. They should be reviewed again 1 month later to assess their need for long-term anticoagulation or antithrombotic and anti-arrhythmic drugs, which may be stopped in patients at low risk of recurrence. These drugs may need to be continued in individuals with risk factors for recurrent atrial fibrillation.

Patients may continue to experience mild palpitation and have 24-hour ECG evidence of recurrent paroxysmal atrial fibrillation which does not result in haemodynamic upset. This may be viewed as an incomplete but satisfactory result. These patients can be reassured, and will require intermittent review to assess whether the attacks become troublesome and require different treatment.

For patients who have reverted back to atrial fibrillation at any stage it may be appropriate to try cardioversion again, possibly using a different anti-arrhythmic drug but continuing anticoagulation. Alternatively, if the chances of long-term successful cardioversion are small, the patient should be treated with rate control and anti-coagulation. Occasionally, non-pharmacological treatments for atrial fibrillation are used for symptomatic patients, and these individuals should be referred to a cardiologist.

Anti-arrhythmic drugs for maintaining sinus rhythm in patients with recurrent paroxysmal or persistent atrial fibrillation

First-line drugs: oral daily doses
These include the following:

- flecainide 200–300 mg every morning (if there is no significant coronary artery disease)
- sotalol 240–320 mg every morning
- propafenone 450–900 mg.

Second-line drugs
These include the following:

- amiodarone (first-line drug in patients with heart failure) 100–400 mg every morning
- disopyramide 400–750 mg every morning.

Atrial flutter

This often occurs with atrial fibrillation, and is associated with similar conditions in elderly patients.

Treatment of atrial flutter

Drug treatment using amiodarone or flecainide may reduce recurrence rates but permit fast ventricular rates and heart failure. It is often better to use digoxin combined with β-blockers to slow the ventricular rate, and this encourages atrial fibrillation to develop.

Catheter ablation of atrial flutter is more successful than drug treatment, can be performed quickly with a low risk of complications, and in many patients is probably the treatment of first choice.

Management of bradycardia in primary care

Bradycardia may be defined as a heart rate slower than 50 beats/minute while the patient is awake. The heart rate may fall to rates of 40 beats/minute during sleep, particularly in young people and atheletes. Bradycardia is mainly due to degenerative disease affecting the sinus node and atrioventricular node.

Sinus node disease

This is common in primary care, and is associated with coronary heart disease, hypertension, cardiomyopathy, anti-arrhythmic drugs, hypothyroidism, and infection in patients with predisposing conditions. In contrast to sinus bradycardia related to exercise, the heart rate in patients with sinus node disease does not increase with exercise (chronotropic incompetence).

This may present as 'tachybrady' (or 'sick sinus') syndrome, which is the presence of intermittent sinus bradycardia and paroxysmal atrial fibrillation. It is a common cause of syncope and palpitation.

The diagnosis is made with a combination of ECG and 24-hour ambulatory ECG recording. For patients with occasional episodes, loop recorders may be used. The patient places the device over their heart during an attack and transmits the recording to hospital over the telephone. Implantable event recorders are occasionally used, and are utilised for patients with undiagnosed syncope thought to be due to a cardiac arrhythmia.

Assessment of the heart rate response to exercise provides useful information in patients with exercise-related symptoms or those who feel that their heart rate is too slow. An appropriate increase in heart rate during exercise differentiates physiological sinus bradycardia (e.g. in athletes whose heart rate increases with exercise) from sinus node disease and chronotropic incompetence. This assessment can be made in the GP surgery by recording the ECG with the patient at rest and then asking them to perform fast straight leg raising and recording an ECG after exercise. An inadequate heart rate response (chronotropic incompetence) may be due to inadequate exercise, drugs (β-blockers) or sinus node disease.

Management of sinus node disease

No treatment is necessary in symptom-free patients without atrial fibrillation, because their prognosis is good.

Pacing for sinus node disease

Sinus node disease is the commonest indication for pacing in the UK. It is important to have evidence that the symptoms relate to bradycardia before implanting a pacemaker. Atrial rather than single-chamber ventricular pacing is recommended because it reduces the incidence of permanent atrial fibrillation and thromboembolism. Dual-chamber pacing (with the electrodes positioned in both the right atrium and the right ventricle) is only indicated in patients who have or are likely to develop atrioventricular node disease.

Patients should be referred for implantation of a pacemaker if they have any of the following:

- symptomatic bradycardia
- paroxysmal atrial fibrillation that requires anti-arrhythmic drugs because of resulting symptomatic bradycardia
- symptomatic chronotropic incompetence.

Rate-responsive pacing, where a sensor in the pacemaker determines the heart rate depending on the activity of the patient, improves the physiological response to exercise.

Management of atrioventricular node disease

Stokes–Adams attacks, defined as syncope due to bradycardia diagnosed by examination of the jugular venous pulse, were first described nearly 200 years ago.

There are three degrees of heart block.

First-degree heart block

The PR interval is > 0.2 seconds, and there is a delay in conduction within the atrioventricular node.

First-degree heart block does not result in symptoms, is benign, and no treatment is necessary.

Second-degree heart block

There are two types, which have different implications and management. The block is in the atrioventricular node.

Type I (Wenckebach) second-degree atrioventricular block

Typically, the ECG shows progressive lengthening of the PR interval until a P-wave is not conducted to the ventricles and the sequence starts again. There are other atypical patterns.

This type of heart block is benign if there is no other conduction disorder. These patients are usually symptom-free and pacing is not indicated.

However, if it is associated with bifascicular block, there is a significant chance that it will progress to complete heart block. These patients should be kept under review because they may need pacing if they become symptomatic or develop more severe heart block.

Type II (Mobitz) second-degree atrioventricular block

The PR interval is constant, but P-waves are intermittently not conducted to the ventricles, resulting in pauses equal to two P–P intervals. This type of heart block is usually associated with bundle branch block. Pacing is indicated even in symptom-free patients because the majority of patients progress to complete heart block.

Third-degree (complete) atrioventricular block
The P-waves are dissociated from the QRS complexes because they reflect independent electrical activity. Congenital complete heart block is seen with narrow QRS complexes at a rate of 50 beats/minute which increases with exercise, because the block is in the atrioventricular node. Acquired complete heart block affects the His-Purkinje tissue below the atrioventricular node, and this results in a wide QRS complex with a rate of 30 beats/minute. It is important to exclude drugs (most commonly digoxin and β-blockers) as the cause of the problem, as this would avoid pacemaker implantation which is otherwise necessary and urgent.

Bundle branch block
The QRS complex exceeds 120 milliseconds (3 little squares) on the ECG.
   Pacing is indicated if bundle branch block occurs with atrioventricular block.

- Right bundle branch block is usually benign. No treatment is required.
- Left bundle branch block is usually associated with heart disease (cardiomyopathy, coronary heart disease), and 5% of patients may progress to complete heart block. The prognosis depends on the underlying cardiac condition.

Who should be referred to a cardiologist?

Patients with any of the following should be referred:

- unpleasant palpitation, loss of consciousness or dizzy turns
- symptomatic regular supraventricular tachycardia
- atrial flutter
- poorly controlled atrial fibrillation
- unpleasant symptomatic ventricular ectopic beats
- ventricular tachycardia
- palpitation and impaired cardiac function
- bradycardia.

Answers to case studies

1   The most likely cause is atrial and/or ventricular ectopic beats. It is important to try to capture the arrhythmia on an ECG or 24-hour ECG recorder to prove the diagnosis. Assuming that the patient has no cardiac history, no other cardiac symptoms and no abnormality on examination, no other investigations are necessary. It is helpful to explain the mechanism of the ectopic beats and their relationship to a slow heart rate. Echocardiography should be performed if there is any suggestion of structural heart disease, and a normal echocardiogram dispels concerns and indicates that any ectopic beats recorded are very unlikely to be of prognostic importance. Anxious patients find this very reassuring, and this reduces the likelihood of further consultations for the same symptoms.

2   The most likely diagnosis is paroxysmal atrial fibrillation. This patient needs the assessment described above and should be referred to a cardiologist.

3   This patient should be assessed clinically, and if this shows no abnormality, he should have an ECG. A normal ECG does not exclude the possibility of supraventricular tachycardia due to atrioventricular node re-entry or a bypass tract, although the latter is less likely. The patient should be referred to a cardiologist for a 24-hour ECG in an attempt to capture the arrhythmia because he may have silent short attacks, and echocardiography should also be performed.

4   The most likely cause is ventricular tachycardia related to a possible left ventricular scar or aneurysm resulting in 'failed sudden death'. Check the patient's medical treatment. If possible he should be on aspirin, an ACE inhibitor or angiotensin II blocker, spironolactone, a β-blocker and a diuretic. Check his electrolytes and ECG. A 24-hour ECG recording will be taken in hospital. He should be referred urgently to a cardiologist, preferably in a specialist centre that provides electrophysiology facilities. He will need coronary angiography, possible revascularisation, and should be considered for an implantable cardioverter-defibrillator combined with biventricular pacing.

5   Examination is important, and if this shows bradycardia the most likely explanation is heart block, which is easily diagnosed by ECG. This patient should then be referred urgently for pacemaker implantation. Other possible causes include anaemia, hypothyroidism, cerebrovascular disease, infection and malignancy, and these should be excluded if no cardiac cause is found.

Further reading

- Fuster V, Ryden LE, Asinger RW *et al.* (2002) ACC/AHA guidelines for the management of patients with atrial fibrillation – executive report. *J Am Coll Cardiol.* **38**: 1231–65.
- Hylek E, Go AS, Chang Y *et al.* (2003) Effect of intensity of oral anticoagulation on stroke severity and mortality in atrial fibrillation. *NEJM.* **349**: 1019–26.
- Markides V and Schilling RJ (2003) Atrial fibrillation: classification, pathophysiology, mechanisms and drug treatment. *Heart.* **89**: 939–43.
- Pedersen OD, Bagger H, Keller N *et al.* (2001) Efficacy of dofetilide in the treatment of atrial fibrillation–flutter in patients with reduced left ventricular function: a Danish investigation of arrhythmia and mortality on dofetilide (Diamond) study. *Circulation.* **104**: 292–6.
- Wyse DG, Waldo AL, DiMarco JP *et al.* (2002) A comparison of rate control and rhythm control in patients with atrial fibrillation. *NEJM.* **347**: 1825–33.

CHAPTER 19

Coronary heart disease in women

Case studies

1 A 68-year-old obese woman complains of breathlessness when shopping and doing housework. She has well-controlled type 2 diabetes and smokes 15 cigarettes per day. What would you do?

2 An 86-year-old woman with previously well-controlled angina returns from holiday and tells you that she can now walk only 20 yards before experiencing chest pain, which she also experiences at night when lying in bed, and after tea. What would you do?

3 A 28-year-old woman comes to see you complaining of stress-induced chest pain. Her mother died at the age of 49 years, apparently from a heart attack. What would you do?

Problems in managing coronary heart disease in women

For many years, doctors were taught that women were at lower risk of coronary heart disease compared with men, and that coronary heart disease was a 'male disease'. Epidemiological studies focused on men. There was a higher threshold for investigating women with ischaemic symptoms, particularly with coronary angiography. This would result in an under-diagnosis of coronary artery disease in women. Even now, women may erroneously believe that they are at greater risk from breast cancer than from coronary heart disease, and so may not adopt a 'healthy heart lifestyle'.

Gender differences in coronary heart disease

However, coronary heart disease affects men and women equally. Although mortality from vascular and coronary heart disease appears to be decreasing in men, it is increasing in women and this presents a major challenge to primary care clinicians. The prevalence of hypertension, smoking and obesity is higher in men, but these risk factors are becoming more common in women. In Europe, smoking is more common in young women than in young men.

The prevalence, presentation and management of coronary heart disease and certain risk factors differ in women. Diabetes and LDL- and HDL-cholesterol levels exert a relatively greater atherogenic effect, and the menopause is a cardiovascular risk factor. Coronary heart disease develops approximately 10 years later in women.

One in three women die from coronary heart disease, which is the commonest cause of death in women.
The risk of coronary heart disease rises in women after the age of 45 years.
Two-thirds of women never fully recover after myocardial infarction.

Gender differences in myocardial infarction

Women appear to be at higher risk of stroke and reinfarctions but not of death.

Gender differences in lipids

Total cholesterol and LDL-cholesterol
The levels of total cholesterol and LDL-cholesterol are lower in premenopausal women than in men, and these levels increase after the menopause, peaking between the ages of 55 and 65 years, approximately 10 years later than in men. HDL-cholesterol levels are higher in postmenopausal women than in men.

Age and hypercholesterolaemia
The impact of hypercholesterolaemia as a cardiovascular risk factor varies with a woman's age. A cholesterol level of > 6.1 mmol/l confers a relative risk of coronary heart disease of 2.4 in a woman under 65 years of age, but of only 1.1 in a woman aged over 65 years. However, there are no significant gender differences relating to homozygous familial hyperlipidaemia. The myocardial infarction rate is lower in women with the heterozygous form.

HDL-cholesterol
Levels of HDL-cholesterol are higher in women both before and after the menopause, and appear to exert greater protection against coronary heart disease risk than in men.
   A low level of HDL-cholesterol is an independent predictor of coronary heart disease in both men and women.

LDL-cholesterol levels
LDL-cholesterol levels increase slightly with age, and raised levels increase the risk of coronary heart disease by threefold in young women (under 65 years of age), but not in older women.

Triglycerides
High triglyceride levels are an independent risk factor for both men and women, but high levels appear to exert a comparatively greater atherogenic effect in women, although the reasons for this are unclear.

Combined dyslipidaemias

The risks of coronary heart disease and its consequences are synergistic, and in both men and women are greater where the usual combination and interactions of lipid abnormalities exist.

Hypertension

Hypertension is unusual in young women, and usually coexists with other cardiovascular risk factors. The diagnosis must be confirmed with 24-hour ambulatory recordings where necessary after comprehensive general medical management, before a diagnosis is made and medication is prescribed (*see* Chapter 12).

The prevalence of hypertension increases after the menopause. Compared with normotensive women, hypertensive women have a 3.5-fold higher risk of developing coronary heart disease, although this risk is lower than in hypertensive men.

Smoking

Smoking increases the risk of peripheral vascular disease by sevenfold and the risk of coronary artery disease and myocardial infarction by fivefold. Although the proportion of male and female adult smokers has decreased over the last three decades, the incidence of smoking has increased among female teenagers. Women who smoked more than 15 cigarettes per day and used 'high-dose' oestrogen oral contraceptives (now rarely prescribed) were found to have a 20-fold increase in coronary heart disease risk. Passive smoking increases coronary risk in men and women by 30%.

Diabetes

Type 2 diabetes is associated with a higher atherogenic risk in women than in men, but the reasons for this are unclear. Type 2 diabetes increases coronary risk by threefold in women and by twofold in men compared with non-diabetic subjects. Diabetes reduces the protective effect of the premenopausal state.

Obesity

This is a major and increasing health problem in both young people and adults, and is associated with other cardiovascular risk factors, including hypertension, insulin resistance, diabetes, hyperlipidaemia and physical inactivity. Slight obesity increases coronary risk by sixfold.

Physical inactivity

Physical inactivity is associated with other cardiovascular risk factors, and regular physical activity reduces cardiovascular risk by at least 50%. The reduction in coronary risk is related to the intensity, duration and frequency of physical exercise, which reduces stress and anxiety and gives a greater sense of well-being. People who exercise regularly tend to have a healthy lifestyle and are less likely to have associated risk factors.

Inflammatory markers

C-reactive protein is an acute-phase protein, and its levels increase with age and are higher in smokers. They may be predictive of coronary events, and are implicated in acute ischaemic syndromes, although their role has not been defined. C-reactive protein levels are high in postmenopausal women with cardiovascular events, but this may reflect the ischaemic inflammatory process rather than the genesis of the event.

Menopause

Coronary heart disease risk increases after the menopause regardless of whether this is a natural 'early' menopause or medically induced. The increased risk is attributed to lower oestrogen levels in these women. The menopause is associated with various unfavourable changes in lipids, glucose levels and thrombotic tendency. Total cholesterol, LDL-cholesterol and triglyceride levels increase, glucose levels increase and insulin sensitivity decreases, fibrinogen levels increase and vascular endothelial dysfunction may occur.

Hormone replacement therapy, cardiovascular disease and general health

Experimentally, oestrogen improves lipid profiles by reducing LDL-cholesterol and increasing HDL-cholesterol levels. Observational studies have suggested that post-menopausal hormone replacement therapy reduces the risk of coronary heart disease, but this has not been confirmed in randomised trials.

Recently, postmenopausal hormone replacement therapy has been shown to cause small increases in coronary events, stroke, pulmonary embolism and breast cancer. Two of each of these events result from treating 1000 women for 1 year. One serious event occurs per 100 women treated for 5 years. In addition, although hormone replacement therapy improves the severity and frequency of flushing by 80%, it does not improve quality of life (e.g. depression, insomnia, sexual function, cognition) in asymptomatic patients. Women with flushing are generally young and usually require treatment for only a year. The absolute risk of hormone replacement therapy will therefore be much lower when it is used in these patients, and is estimated at one serious adverse event per 1000 women treated for 1 year.

Hormone replacement therapy should be started at a low dose and increased gradually until symptoms resolve and then reduced every 6 months to assess whether it needs to be continued. It is not recommended for asymptomatic postmenopausal women.

Oral contraceptives and heart disease

Oral contraceptives should not be prescribed to women over 35 years of age if they have cardiovascular risk factors.

Approach to diagnosis of women with suspected coronary heart disease

Women with suspected coronary heart disease should be managed in the same way as men. They should be given similar advice on primary and secondary cardiovascular prevention. Women with diabetes are at particularly high risk, and should be managed accordingly.

Diagnostic tests

Exercise testing may give rise to a 20% false-positive rate in women, but the reasons for this are unclear. This may dissuade a physician from investigating a woman for possible coronary heart disease, although this principle may not deter him or her from requesting a mammogram which may have a similar false-positive rate in fibrocystic breast disease.

Despite its reduced accuracy in women, exercise testing should be used as the preferred stress test to investigate ischaemia in patients at intermediate coronary risk, as well as for the other indications discussed in Chapters 14 and 25.

Stress echocardiography may be useful in patients who cannot exercise, and when interpretation of the ECG is complicated by left bundle branch block and other re-polarisation changes.

Nuclear imaging is complicated in women because breast tissue often obscures the inferior surfaces of the heart, and this reduces the accuracy of the technique. The inherent concerns of injecting radioactive pharmaceuticals and the long duration and expense of the tests need to be weighed against, at best, a marginal benefit in women with resting electrocardiographic abnormalities.

At present there are insufficient data comparing the diagnostic and prognostic value of electron beam computed tomography in men and women. The technique is experimental, expensive, not available on the NHS, and it adds no useful or incremental information over conventional clinical risk estimations. It is discussed in Chapter 6.

Coronary angiography remains the only investigation that provides accurate ana-tomical information on coronary artery anatomy and atherosclerotic disease. It is indicated in patients who cannot exercise, when the results of stress testing suggest the presence of coronary artery disease or when obstructive coronary artery disease needs to be excluded in order to define management. Complications are generally no more frequent in women than in men.

Cardiovascular medical therapy

Apart from pregnancy and breastfeeding, there are no major differences between the sexes when considering cardiovascular medication.

When starting treatment in women with a low body mass index, the lowest recommended drug doses should be prescribed, and these may be increased gradually if necessary.

Dihydropyridine calcium antagonists used to treat hypertension may be unacceptable in women who develop significant peripheral oedema.

Cardiac surgery and myocardial revascularisation

Although there was formerly concern that the short- and long-term results of coronary artery and valve surgery and coronary angioplasty were poorer in women, this is no longer thought to be the case. The original findings may have been due to a variety of other patient characteristics, including age, severity of disease at presentation, body size and coexisting disease.

In summary, gender is not a factor when considering cardiac surgical or percutaneous interventions.

Answers to case studies

1 Asthma, chronic bronchitis, anaemia, hypothyroidism and obesity need to be considered, and should be assessed clinically and investigated. This patient may have angina, and if she can exercise you should arrange for her to have an exercise test. If not, a stress echocardiogram might be helpful. If coronary artery disease is suspected, then if the symptoms are not severe the patient should be prescribed aspirin and GTN, which she should take prophylactically as well as to abort spontaneous attacks of angina. She may need to be referred to a cardiologist if she does respond or if there is evidence of important ischaemia, as both suggest significant coronary artery disease. She should be advised and helped to stop smoking and to lose weight, and her other cardiovascular risk factors should be reviewed.

2 Unstable angina is the most likely diagnosis, and this patient should be referred urgently to hospital for a specialist opinion. Her anti-anginal medication should be reviewed and increased if possible. Exercise testing will add little diagnostic or prognostic information. Coronary angiography with a view (preferably because of her age) to coronary angioplasty is indicated if the patient's symptoms do not respond to medical treatment, although the possibility that she may need coronary artery surgery should be discussed with her and her family.

3 Despite this patient's family history of premature coronary heart disease, it is unlikely that she has coronary heart disease. However, if she has symptoms which suggest angina she should have an exercise test, and if this shows ischaemia she should be referred for a specialist opinion. If she has a low absolute coronary risk and her symptoms do not suggest angina, other causes of chest pain should be considered and investigated.

Further reading

Hormone replacement treatment

- Grady D, Herrington D, Bittner V *et al.* (2002) Cardiovascular disease outcomes during 6.8 years of hormone therapy: Heart and Estrogen/Progestin Replacement Study follow-up (HERS II). *JAMA.* **288**: 49–57.
- Hays J, Ockerne JK, Brunner RL *et al.* (2003) Effects of estrogen plus progestin on health-related quality of life. *NEJM.* **348**: 1839–54.
- Herrington DM, Reboussin DM, Brosnihan B *et al.* (2000) Effects of estrogen replacement on the progression of coronary artery atherosclerosis. *NEJM.* **343**: 522–9.
- Hlatky MA, Boothroyd D, Vittinghoff E *et al.* (2002) Quality-of-life and depressive symptoms in post-menopausal women after receiving hormone therapy: results from the Heart and Estrogen/Progestin Replacement Study (HERS) trial. *JAMA.* **287**: 591–7.
- Preventive Services Task Force (2002) Post-menopausal hormone replacement therapy for primary prevention of chronic conditions: recommendations and rationale. *Ann Intern Med.* **137**: 834–9.

CHAPTER 20

Management of heart disease in pregnancy

Case studies

1 You hear a new systolic murmur in a 20-year-old, symptom-free, pregnant woman at a routine antenatal check (16 weeks). What would you do?

2 A 33-year-old woman who had successful corrective heart surgery for tetralogy of Fallot in early childhood comes to see you because she is pregnant. She is generally fit. She wants to know the risk of her baby having heart disease and whether she will be well enough to go through the pregnancy. What advice would you give her?

3 A 28-year-old woman with Marfan's syndrome and normal blood pressure wants to have 'natural childbirth'. What would you advise her to do?

4 A 33-year-old woman who is taking warfarin for an aortic valve replacement inserted 8 years previously is 12 weeks pregnant and wants reassurance from you that all is well and will continue to be so. What would you advise?

The role of primary care clinicians in the management of pregnant women with heart disease

Maternal heart disease may be first diagnosed during pregnancy by the GP. The majority of patients with significant heart conditions will be managed jointly by the primary care team, obstetrician, cardiologist and the midwives.

Healthy pregnant women commonly have symptoms consistent with cardiac disease, and it is important to distinguish them from those with cardiac disease. Patients who are identified as being at low risk can be managed in a similar way to pregnant women without cardiac disease, and the risks of pregnancy to mother and fetus are not significantly higher than for healthy women. Patients with high-risk cardiac conditions pose difficult management problems and have to be carefully assessed and closely monitored by both the primary care team and specialists.

The pregnant patient with a cardiac condition often consults the GP for advice and guidance. It is therefore important that primary care clinicians have an understanding of the differential risks that pregnancy poses in specific cardiovascular conditions. After delivery, patients with significant heart disease may require advice and support with baby care.

Management of pregnant women with cardiac disease is individualised because there are few randomised trials on the basis of which to form evidence-based practice guidelines.

Physiological and haemodynamic changes during pregnancy

Cardiac output increases by about 50% during pregnancy due to increases in blood volume, red cell mass and heart rate, and this accounts for the common finding of a benign systolic murmur. Systemic vascular resistance decreases. Blood pressure falls due to a reduction in peripheral vascular resistance resulting from gestational hormones and prostaglandins. Blood pressure and cardiac output increase during delivery, and these increases are influenced by the mode of delivery, which is important in women with hypertension and those at risk of heart failure. Blood reaching the circulation from the uterus increases the cardiac output early postpartum, so pulmonary oedema may occur only after delivery. The haemodynamic changes that occur during delivery and in the postpartum period usually resolve within 1 week of delivery.

Haemodynamic effects of pregnancy in cardiac conditions

The haemodynamic effects of pregnancy on the mother depend on the underlying anatomical and physiological abnormality, and vary during pregnancy, at delivery and postpartum.

Pulmonary artery pressure increases during the period just before and after delivery, so patients with pulmonary arterial hypertension are at highest risk at this time. Patients with Eisenmenger's syndrome may deteriorate and become more cyanosed and breathless during pregnancy because of increased right to left shunting resulting from systemic vasodilatation and right ventricular overload.

The increase in cardiac output, particularly during and after delivery, puts a strain on both ventricles. Heart failure may occur in patients with right or left ventricular outflow tract obstruction (aortic or pulmonary valve stenosis) or a weak heart muscle (cardiomyopathy, or after corrective surgery for congenital heart disease).

The increase in blood pressure during delivery poses a risk of aortic dissection, aortic aneurysm, rupture and dissection in patients with a weak aortic wall due to Marfan's syndrome.

The increase in heart rate and blood volume increases the transmitral gradient in mitral valve stenosis.

Clinical evaluation of pregnant women

Shortness of breath, tiredness and ankle swelling are common during pregnancy, and are partly due to increasing abdominal girth, generalised weight gain and restricted chest expansion. Palpitation is usually benign and due to ectopic beats.

Hypertension is the commonest cardiovascular problem during pregnancy. It is discussed in Chapter 12.

> The majority of previously well pregnant women who present with cardiac-sounding symptoms or a systolic murmur do not have underlying cardiac disease. However, it is important that cardiac disease is considered and investigated where appropriate, but that the patient is not made unduly anxious until a diagnosis has been made.

Investigating possible cardiac symptoms during pregnancy

- An ECG and rhythm strip recorded during palpitation is helpful, and if normal it is reassuring and indicates that there is no arrhythmia to account for the symptoms. Possible anxiety with a sinus tachycardia may account for the palpitation.
- A 24-hour ambulatory ECG recording may be helpful for patients with intermittent palpitation.
- Echocardiography is indicated to evaluate patients with murmurs or heart failure and those with known structural heart disease.
- Chest X-ray examination with abdominal shielding is more accurate than clinical assessment in diagnosing pulmonary oedema, and is occasionally necessary.

Management and risk stratification of pregnant women with cardiovascular disease

- Assess the patient's clinical and functional status and general medical health (blood pressure, anaemia, thyroid status, smoking, alcohol consumption and diet).
- Characterise the lesion, anatomy and haemodynamics (pulmonary artery pressure, valve area and gradient, intracardiac shunts, cardiac function).
- Determine the risk of pregnancy to the mother and the fetus.
- Discuss management strategies for high-risk cases.
- Discuss termination when appropriate.
- Reassure the patient when appropriate.
- Avoid teratogenic drugs.
- Liaise with specialists (cardiologist and obstetrician).
- Assess the need for antibiotic prophylaxis.
- Assess the need for genetic counselling.

Risk stratification

Before conception
Women with congenital heart disease, acquired heart valve disease or cardiovascular disease are usually diagnosed before conception, and should be advised of the potential

risks of pregnancy and the risk of congenital heart disease in any offspring. Possible options for corrective surgery, medical treatment and genetic counselling should be explored and explained.

After conception
Diagnosis of maternal heart disease after conception is less usual, but it is important that this is done as soon as possible so that management can be planned. Women with congenital heart disease constitute a larger population than those with rheumatic heart disease in pregnancy.

Close collaboration and clear communication between primary care and hospital specialists is important, and reduces both patient anxieties and complications.

Pregnancy is not recommended for patients with high-risk conditions, and termination of pregnancy should be considered and discussed in these cases.

Specific high-risk conditions
Structural and haemodynamic conditions that put the mother and fetus at high risk include the following:

- cyanotic heart disease of any cause (e.g. uncorrected tetralogy of Fallot)
- significant right to left shunt without cyanosis
- exercise-induced hypoxaemia (< 85%)
- pulmonary arterial hypertension (> 35 mmHg)
- weak aortic wall (Marfan's syndrome)
- breathlessness of any cause (New York Heart Association classes III and IV)
- severe aortic or mitral valve stenosis
- severe left ventricular impairment.

Pregnancy is generally not advised for patients with these high-risk conditions, although women with these conditions who have become pregnant have been known to have a successful pregnancy. An individual evaluation and risk assessment is necessary.

Pulmonary arterial hypertension

The maternal mortality rate is around 50% due to the increase in pulmonary artery pressure during the peripartum period. In patients with Eisenmenger's syndrome (right to left shunt through a septal defect), the fall in systemic vascular resistance and increased right ventricular overload increases the right to left shunt, and this results in reduced pulmonary artery blood flow and increased cyanosis.

Acquired heart valve disease

Management before conception
Referral to both cardiac and obstetric specialists is recommended if pregnancy is contemplated, so that those at high risk can be identified, their medical management reviewed and any intervention necessary performed if appropriate before conception.

Patients with significant mitral valve stenosis should be considered for mitral valvuloplasty before conception and during pregnancy if they remain symptomatic despite treatment with diuretics and vasodilators. Similarly, aortic valve surgery should be considered for patients with severe aortic stenosis. Percutaneous valvuloplasty should be considered for patients with severe pulmonary valve stenosis before conception, although it may be necessary during pregnancy.

Patients with valvular disease who may be relatively symptom-free before or during early pregnancy may deteriorate suddenly and unpredictably during pregnancy or delivery.

Management after conception

Serial echocardiographic studies are often necessary in patients with stenotic valvular heart disease, as the effective gradient increases during pregnancy due to the increased blood volume and cardiac output and reduced systemic vascular resistance. However, it is difficult to predict the haemodynamic effects of pregnancy in individual cases.

Aortic and mitral regurgitation are generally well tolerated in patients without symptoms, because the degree of valve regurgitation decreases during pregnancy as the systemic vascular resistance falls.

Severe mitral stenosis

This is the commonest form of acquired valve disease in pregnant women, and it is more common in patients born outside the UK.

The transmitral valve gradient increases during the second and third trimester, with a consequent increase in left atrial pressure and risk of pulmonary oedema. The prognosis of patients with rheumatic mitral valve stenosis is determined mainly by the degree of stenosis which, if severe (< 1.5 cm^2), may result in sudden pulmonary oedema and maternal and fetal distress. The left atrial pressure increases with tachycardia. Patients should be reviewed monthly from 20 weeks' gestation. Diuretics and β-blockers may be necessary to treat pulmonary oedema. Percutaneous mitral valvuloplasty should be considered in suitable patients with significant mitral valve stenosis if they develop pulmonary oedema or are likely to do so at any stage during or after pregnancy.

Severe aortic stenosis

This is usually well tolerated during pregnancy unless the patient is symptomatic at rest or on minimal exertion. Aortic valvuloplasty is occasionally necessary.

Cyanotic heart disease

These patients are at high risk. The maternal mortality rate is 2%. The risk of complications (which include infective endocarditis, heart failure and arrhythmias) is around 30%. The fetal prognosis is poor, with a 50% risk of spontaneous abortion, 40% risk of premature delivery and a high risk of small-for-dates babies.

Management of high-risk patients

Most cardiologists and obstetricians recommend termination of pregnancy in women with a high-risk cardiac condition. The risks of early termination are lower than the risk of continuing the pregnancy.

For women who decide to continue with their pregnancy, rest, prompt treatment of heart failure, and frequent, vigilant clinical monitoring are necessary. Hospital admission, often at 20 weeks, may be necessary if the patient deteriorates, becomes hypoxic or develops arrhythmias.

Patients with hypertension and/or pre-eclampsia should be admitted to hospital for bed rest, antihypertensive treatment and consideration of early delivery. Precautions should be taken against thromboembolism, particularly before and after Caesarean section or in patients who are resting in bed.

Marfan's syndrome

Women with a dilated aortic root (> 4.8 cm) who are contemplating pregnancy should be assessed by a vascular surgeon experienced in the management of this condition. Aortic stenting or grafting should be considered because the risk of aortic dissection or rupture of an aortic aneurysm during pregnancy, particularly delivery with associated hypertension, is around 10%. Segments of the aorta that are not treated may also dilate or dissect. Pregnant patients with Marfan's syndrome should be monitored with echocardiography to measure the aortic diameter throughout pregnancy and for several months after delivery. β-Blockers should be continued during and after pregnancy.

Mitral valve repair may be necessary if the patient is symptomatic, has had heart failure or has a dilated left ventricle.

Indications for cardiology referral during pregnancy

Patients with the following conditions should be referred:

- high-risk cardiovascular conditions
- unexplained, new or troublesome cardiac symptoms or signs
- heart failure
- hypertension
- structural heart disease or previous cardiac surgery
- Marfan's syndrome
- previous thrombotic disease
- anxious patients who want reassurance from a cardiologist.

Fetal assessment

There is a risk of congenital heart disease in the fetus of an affected mother of around 10%. If the mother has a congenital bicuspid aortic valve, the fetal risk of this abnormality is nearly 20%.

The possibility of fetal heart disease should be investigated in pregnant women. Termination of pregnancy or early delivery should be considered in women at high risk. The survival rate of babies delivered at 32 weeks is high (> 95%), but it is relatively low (< 75%) in babies delivered before 28 weeks.

Low-risk cardiac conditions

In the absence of symptoms, cyanosis, pulmonary hypertension, significant cardiac impairment or arrhythmias, pregnancy is usually safe. The frequency of clinical assessments and the need for cardiac investigations are determined individually.

Pregnancy is usually well tolerated in patients with low-risk cardiac conditions, although arrhythmias, deterioration of left ventricular function and progression of pulmonary hypertension may occur. Patients who have had cardiac surgery without prosthetic valves generally do well.

Normal spontaneous vaginal delivery is usually possible in patients with low-risk conditions such as the following:

- small left to right shunts (atrial and ventricular septal defects, patent ductus arteriosus)
- insignificant left ventricular outflow tract obstruction (mild aortic valve stenosis, hypertrophic obstructive cardiomyopathy)
- pulmonary valve stenosis
- surgically corrected structural disease without important residual heart defects
- Marfan's syndrome without cardiovascular involvement – this affects 1 in 5000 members of the population and is a comparatively common and important condition. There is often a family history. It is due to a defect in collagen synthesis, and affects the skeleton, eyes and cardiovascular system in 80% of patients.

  The commonest cardiac abnormality is mitral valve prolapse. Most patients with only insignificant mitral valve prolapse have an uncomplicated pregnancy and less than a 1% risk of heart failure, infective endocarditis or aortic dissection. β-Blockers are used to lower and blunt the systolic pressure surges, and should be continued during pregnancy
- patients who have had valve replacements with non-prosthetic valves
- acquired valve disease.

Management of arrhythmias during pregnancy

Arrhythmias, most commonly atrial and ventricular ectopic beats, are common in healthy individuals and are usually only of importance if they increase during exercise. They may be more frequent during pregnancy due to haemodynamic, hormonal and emotional factors, particularly in patients with structural heart disease.

Specialist referral and 24-hour ECG recordings may be necessary for patients with unpleasant symptoms, or when the diagnosis is in doubt.

Atrioventricular node ablation for frequent haemodynamically significant supraventricular tachycardia due to an accessory pathway or atrioventricular node re-entry tachycardia may be necessary during pregnancy. The patient should be referred to an electrophysiology centre.

Permanent pacemaker implantation for serious symptomatic bradycardia is occasionally necessary. Both procedures may be performed with lead shielding of the uterus and restricted use of X-ray screening.

Drug treatment of pregnant patients with arrhythmias

Because of the risk of teratogenicity associated with the use of any drug during pregnancy, particularly in the first trimester, anti-arrhythmic drugs should be avoided unless the patient has severe symptoms or the arrhythmia has haemodynamic consequences. Most anti-arrhythmic drugs are negatively inotropic and must be used with caution in patients with impaired cardiac function.

Digoxin may be used to slow the ventricular rate in atrial fibrillation. β-Blockers and verapamil may be used to treat supraventricular arrhythmias. Amiodarone should only be used for important arrhythmias, and after other drugs have been tried but have failed. Long-term use may result in neonatal thyroid abnormalities.

Infective endocarditis

This is rare during pregnancy, but should be considered in women with predisposing cardiac conditions who develop fever, anaemia, heart failure or new murmurs with signs of emboli. Check the C-reactive protein and the erythrocyte sedimentation rate. Prompt specialist referral and high-quality echocardiography are essential, and the patient should be treated with appropriate antibiotics after consultation with a bacteriologist.

Antibiotic prophylaxis during pregnancy

These are the same as for non-pregnant patients undergoing dental or other potentially septic procedures that are likely to cause a Gram-positive bacteraemia.

Antibiotic prophylaxis is indicated before surgical delivery and cardiac surgery in all women with valve disease, intracardiac shunts, prosthetic valves and previous endocarditis.

Even though the risk of endocarditis during normal delivery is very low, antibiotic prophylaxis is indicated in women with prosthetic heart valves and shunts and previous endocarditis. It is discretionary for normal delivery in women with rheumatic heart disease and those with mitral regurgitation due to mitral valve prolapse. Gentamicin levels must be checked because of the risks of fetal deafness.

Peripartum cardiomyopathy

This is an uncommon form of dilated cardiomyopathy that is diagnosed by the presence of new heart failure or, less commonly, emboli or arrhythmias occurring in previously healthy women. Patients with pre-existing dilated cardiomyopathy usually deteriorate and present before the last month of pregnancy. Echocardiography shows a dilated, poorly contracting heart. Most cases resolve with medical treatment, but severe cases may require intensive-care support, inotropes, oxygen treatment and ventricular assist devices. Cardiac transplantation is reserved for the very worst refractory cases.

Patients with persistent symptoms and signs of heart failure and echocardiographic evidence of an established dilated heart have a poor prognosis, and further pregnancies are not recommended. There are no guidelines about further pregnancies in patients who make a complete recovery, in whom repeat episodes are possible but unlikely.

Dilated cardiomyopathy

Pregnancy is not recommended in patients with dilated cardiomyopathy because of the high risk to both the mother and the fetus. Termination of pregnancy is advised if the left ventricular ejection fraction is < 50% and the heart is dilated, because of the possibility of further deterioration. If termination is refused, admission to hospital is recommended for symptomatic patients, and frequent clinical and echocardiographic monitoring and avoidance of exertion are advisable.

Hypertrophic cardiomyopathy

The systolic murmur of hypertrophic cardiomyopathy may be first diagnosed during pregnancy and attributed to the pregnancy. The condition is diagnosed by echo-cardiography and ECG. Patients without a family history will need reassurance that they are at low risk of sudden death. Patients with diastolic impairment are at risk of haemodynamic deterioration if they develop atrial fibrillation, and DC conversion and anticoagulation with heparin are required. Digoxin to control the ventricular response to atrial fibrillation is only contraindicated if there is a significant left ventricular outflow tract gradient. Transoesophageal echocardiography is used to identify patients with left atrial thrombus before cardioversion. Symptomatic patients may be treated with rest, β-blockers and diuretics.

Answers to case studies

1   The murmur is probably benign and associated with the physiological changes of pregnancy. You should explain this to the patient and discuss the merits of echocardiography, which if normal would be reassuring and would provide useful information for her future management.

2   The maternal and fetal prognosis will depend on the presence of residual shunt, right ventricular outflow tract obstruction, right and left ventricular function and pulmonary hypertension. The patient will probably already be under the care of a cardiologist, but if not, she should be referred. Assessment should include her functional class, the precise anatomical and haemodynamic status and presence of hypoxaemia. The risk associated with pregnancy is low after successful correction of tetralogy of Fallot. The risk of fetal congenital heart disease is 2–16%, and the mother should be assessed in a suitable unit. Termination of pregnancy for an affected fetus may be necessary and depends on maternal functional class and the presence of cyanosis. It is likely that this mother will have a successful pregnancy and be able to have a normal delivery.

---

3   This patient should be referred to a centre with the necessary expertise and experience for aortic imaging and blood pressure assessment. Patients with a normal aortic root and no significant cardiac involvement tolerate pregnancy well and are at low risk. In the presence of aortic root dilatation, there is an increase of approximately 1% in maternal mortality and 20% in fetal mortality. Patients with a significantly dilated root should be advised of the 10% risk of death and offered termination. It is possible that stenting for disease affecting the thoracic aorta may allow pregnancy to continue. β-Blockers and rest are advised for all such patients.

4   The risks associated with pregnancy are small in this patient. The problems relate to anticoagulation. Warfarin carries a 5% risk of teratogenicity if used in the first trimester, but is the most effective and most convenient form of anticoagulation. Unfractionated heparin does not cross the placenta, and osteoporosis and thrombocytopenia are rare side-effects. Warfarin is recommended during the second and third trimesters and should be replaced by heparin at week 36 to avoid the risk of neonatal intracranial haemorrhage during delivery. At present low-molecular-weight heparin is not recommended as anticoagulation for pregnant patients with prosthetic valves. The risks of each approach should be explained to the patient.

Further reading

- Siu SC and Colman JM (2001) Heart disease and pregnancy. *Heart.* **85**: 710–15.
- Task Force on the Management of Cardiovascular Diseases During Pregnancy of the European Society of Cardiology (2003) Expert consensus document on management of cardiovascular diseases during pregnancy. *Eur Heart J.* **24**: 761–81.

CHAPTER 21

Management of sexual problems in male patients with cardiac conditions

---

Case studies

1 A 55-year-old man who sustained a myocardial infarction 6 months ago is depressed and having marital problems. What would you do?
2 A recently married couple in their seventies come to see you together because the wife is worried about starting a sexual relationship with her husband, as her previous husband died of a heart attack. What would you do?
3 A 74-year-old man develops symptoms of prostatism and impotence and is worried that the two conditions are related. What would you do?

Erectile dysfunction

This is defined as the inability to achieve and maintain an erection sufficient to permit satisfactory intercourse.

Prevalence

Some degree of erectile dysfunction is thought to affect around 50% of all men over the age of 40 years. However, this may be an underestimate because men may be embarrassed to discuss what they consider to be a personal and private matter unrelated to their heart problem.

Role of the GP in management

The willingness of men to discuss their sexual problems depends on their age, culture, religion, upbringing, marital status and the impact that the problem has on their life, as well as their understanding of the problem and its causes. To some men it may be an occasional irrelevant inconvenience, but to others it can be a major concern and source of misery. Some young men may view it as a natural part of life, like balding. Older men, who may be embarking on a new relationship, may find it a major impediment to an enjoyable and fulfilling life.

It is important that GPs offer patients (particularly those with risk factors for erectile dysfunction) and their partners the opportunity to discuss erectile dysfunction in the same way as one might ask routinely about angina or breathlessness. The GP plays an important role in educating patients about the condition and reassuring them about the increasing success of treatment. These consultations demand skill and sensitivity, but are rewarded with immense gratitude from patients.

The GP's unique insight into the patient's medical and social history and domestic situation enables him or her to provide helpful individualised advice on the management of this common condition.

Over the last few years men have become less reticent about discussing this problem with their GP. The social stigma of erectile dysfunction is gradually being replaced by an understanding of the unfortunate impact it has on quality of life for the patient and his partner. This has been brought about by the efficacy and popularity of Viagra and newer related preparations, and the endorsement by the NHS of their use in certain conditions, together with greater public awareness and discussion of the condition both in the media and in GP surgeries.

Risk factors for erectile dysfunction

These are similar to those for cardiovascular disease. Erectile dysfunction is more common in individuals who smoke or have hypertension, diabetes or hyperlipidaemia. Urological, neurological, hormonal and other medical causes, including diabetes and adverse drug effects, should be investigated and excluded.

Depression, anxiety, psychological disorders, marital conflict and work-related problems are other common causes and also consequences of erectile dysfunction. Patients should be referred to the relevant specialist. Cardiovascular causes should be considered after other causes have been excluded.

The association of sexual dysfunction with cardiovascular disease

A primary objective in the treatment of cardiac conditions is to allow patients of all ages to live a fulfilled and active life. Sexual activity is considered by many patients to be an important part of their life and something they wish to continue. Primary care clinicians should question patients with cardiovascular disease about sexual activity in the same way that they might enquire about exercise, diet and other components of lifestyle. They should also appreciate that some patients are unwilling to discuss these matters or feel uncomfortable talking about them.

Erectile dysfunction is common in men over 60 years of age, particularly after myocardial infarction and cardiac surgery. It adversely affects their quality of life and self-esteem, and may be an important cause of marital conflict and depression, which are improved after successful treatment.

Sexual dysfunction and cardiovascular disease are commonly associated with each other. Erectile dysfunction is also understandably common in men during and after any illness or hospitalisation.

Most men with erectile dysfunction have one or more cardiovascular risk factors, especially diabetes, hypertension or hyperlipidaemia. It is possible that cardiovascular risk factors are as relevant in patients with erectile dysfunction as they are in the development of coronary artery disease, although a causal relationship is not as firmly established. Sexual dysfunction may be a marker of subclinical cardiovascular disease. The vigorous treatment of cardiovascular risk factors is thus fundamental to the management of both conditions.

Sexual activity as a trigger for acute cardiac conditions

Sexual activity is generally safe and is encouraged as part of a normal healthy lifestyle in male and female patients with heart disease. Cardiac symptoms including breathlessness and angina, acute decompensation of heart failure, acute coronary syndromes and acute myocardial infarction (and, more tragically, sudden death) may be experienced for the first time during sexual activity. Increases in heart rate and systolic blood pressure during intercourse lead to a sudden increase in myocardial oxygen demand, and theoretically can trigger atheromatous plaque rupture and infarction. Sudden decreases in heart rate and blood pressure result in sudden reductions in coronary blood flow and myocardial oxygen supply and can trigger angina.

Left ventricular work and myocardial oxygen consumption are determined by the product of heart rate and systolic blood pressure during peak exertion. This can be reduced by modifying the mechanics and dynamics of sexual activity.

Is sexual activity dangerous in cardiac patients?

Sexual activity is safe in the majority of cardiac patients. It is only contraindicated in high-risk patients, who can usually be identified clinically without the need for cardiac investigations.

Cardiac risk associated with sexual activity and medication for erectile dysfunction

The annual risk of myocardial infarction in a healthy man is 1%, which increases to 1.01% as a result of sexual activity, and this risk increases tenfold to 1.1% in a man with coronary heart disease, which is equivalent to a chance of 20 in a million.

Patients at low cardiac risk

These include individuals with controlled hypertension, mild angina, full recovery and no or minimal symptoms after myocardial revascularisation, full recovery 2 weeks after myocardial infarction and insignificant valvular disease. Patients at low risk (i.e. able to run up two flights of stairs or able to complete 12 minutes of the Bruce treadmill protocol or the WHO cycle protocol without ischaemia and who have a normal haemodynamic response) can be safely encouraged to resume or continue full unrestricted sexual activity.

Most patients with erectile dysfunction and cardiovascular disease are in the low-risk group.

Patients at high cardiac risk

These include individuals recovering from recent (less than 1 week previously) myocardial infarction, severe heart failure or recent (less than 2 months previously) sternotomy for cardiac surgery (in order to avoid compression or rotation strain to the sternum and costochondral joints), and patients with cardiac conditions resulting in severe breathlessness and/or angina during intercourse (e.g. unstable angina, decompensated heart failure, obstructive cardiomyopathy, severe aortic stenosis), uncontrolled hypertension or significant arrhythmias (including bradycardia, which can be induced during a Valsalva manoeuvre, or atrial fibrillation due to sudden increases in blood pressure).

These patients require cardiac review, particularly of their cardiovascular risk factors and medication, and they may require specialist referral and further investigations (*see* Chapters 5, 7–10, 12–17).

Giving advice about sexual activity in primary care

It is helpful if someone in the practice is interested in and able to discuss these matters with patients and their partners, who are often too embarrassed to initiate the discussion directly.

There are few hospital-based specialists, particularly with an understanding of the cardiac aspects of the problem, in the UK. There remains a need for trained personnel to provide an integrated service in this field. Sexual matters for patients, particularly those with cardiac conditions, are as important as other lifestyle issues and should be given equal consideration and care.

Their treatment and cardiovascular risk factors should be reviewed, and patients with angina and/or heart failure may need specialist review. Both the patient and his partner may feel understandably anxious about the possible dangers of sexual intercourse, and may ask for advice directly or hint at it during the consultation. Primary care clinicians should be willing to discuss this openly, sympathetically and constructively as they would discuss any clinical problem. It is important that after the cause of erectile dysfunction has been identified, primary care staff try to enhance and restore the emotional well-being and quality of life of the patient. Coexisting depression should be managed appropriately. These matters may also be discussed in conjunction with secondary prevention and lifestyle factors in a cardiac rehabilitation clinic.

Patients and their partners often want to know when it is safe to resume a sexual relationship after a heart attack, angioplasty or heart surgery. It is difficult to generalise, and it depends on a number of factors, including the age of the patient and his partner, the haemodynamic status and the presence or absence of ischaemia. Patients at low risk are generally young, with normal or near normal left ventricular function and no reversible ischaemia more than 2 weeks after an uncomplicated infarct. Patients with significant left ventricular impairment and/or known coronary artery disease should be referred to a cardiologist for assessment, including an exercise test. The GP should be prepared to discuss sexual practices with those patients who want further detailed advice.

Drug-induced erectile dysfunction

Drug-induced erectile dysfunction is common and well recognised with regard to β-blockers and thiazide diuretics, and is less commonly associated with statins. Patients may feel convinced that they only became impotent after they started a certain drug. The side-effects of the drug should be researched. If there are no reports that impotence is a recognised adverse effect, it may be necessary to withdraw the incriminated drug and ask the patient whether their symptoms have improved after a week or so. If their sexual function has improved and they are willing, they should be rechallenged with the drug. Recurrent symptoms suggest a drug side-effect which is generally related to the class of drug.

Drug withdrawal and rechallenge are probably not necessary if the problem started after taking β-blockers because impotence is a well-recognised side effect. Drug withdrawal may be necessary if patients with heart failure or hypertension are on angiotensin-converting-enzyme (ACE) inhibitors (which are recognised as causing erectile dysfunction) or angiotensin II antagonists, which are an important component of their treatment and for which there are no other classes of drug with similar benefits.

Phosphodiesterase type 5 (PDE5) inhibitors in erectile dysfunction

These drugs inhibit the breakdown of cyclic GMP and improve the rigidity and duration of erections. As long as they are prescribed and used according to the manufacturer's recommendations, they are safe in patients with stable coronary artery disease. Treatment with these drugs is successful in over 80% of cases.

PDE5 inhibitors are contraindicated in patients who are taking nitrates or nicorandil because of the risk of potentiating important hypotension, and in those in whom sexual activity is inadvisable. They should be used with caution in patients who are taking doxazocin. Around 80% of patients with cardiovascular disease who are taking PDE5 inhibitors are at low cardiac risk and are therefore unlikely to be taking long-acting nitrates.

PDE5 inhibitors may be given together with β-blockers and ACE inhibitors.

Sildenafil (Viagra)

A full review of the cause of the patient's erectile dysfunction and their medication is required before starting sildenafil. This drug is otherwise safe for the vast majority of patients with cardiovascular disease. It is not indicated for use in women.

Sildenafil has had a major impact in the treatment of erectile dysfunction, and is generally safe in most cardiac and hypertensive patients. It is a vasodilator and results in a reduction in blood pressure. There are no other important interactions, and it is not contraindicated with antihypertensive drugs. The commonest side-effects are headache and facial flushing, which occur in around 10% of patients.

The recommended dose is 50 mg (25 mg in the elderly) to be taken 1 hour before sexual activity. The drug is effective 30 minutes after taking it, and the effects last for 4–6 hours. The recommended maximum dose is 100 mg. It is contraindicated in patients taking nitrates. Further information is provided on the data sheet.

Other newer compounds

Tadalafil and vardenafil are similar in structure to sildefanil, and the trial data have shown them to be as safe as placebo, with no excess cardiovascular mortality compared with age-matched controls or placebo.

The duration of onset, action and efficacy of vardenafil are similar to those of sildenafil. Tadalafil has a longer half-life, and its effects may last for over 36 hours.

Answers to case studies

1   It is important to be sure of this patient's precise symptoms. If he is impotent, there are several possible causes. He might require more than one consultation, but will need time, sympathy and understanding, and possibly psychological and marital counselling. It is important to exclude angina and heart failure, possibly with further cardiac tests, and to review his cardiovascular risk factors and medication and optimise his secondary prevention. If he is taking β-blockers, these may need to be stopped or the dose reduced.

2   If the husband has no erectile dysfunction and no cardiac problem, he is at low risk of a cardiac problem during sexual activity. If necessary he could be prescribed Viagra.

3   This patient will need a full medical assessment and should be referred to a urologist to exclude a primary urological problem.

Further reading

- Carrier S, Brock G, Kour NW *et al.* (1993) Pathophysiology of erectile dysfunction. *Urology.* **42**: 468–81.
- DeBusk R, Drory Y, Goldstein I *et al.* (2000) Management of sexual dysfunction in patients with cardiovascular disease: recommendations of the Princeton Consensus Panel. *Am J Cardiol.* **86**: 175–81.
- Lue TF (2000) Erectile dysfunction. *NEJM.* **342**: 1802–13.

CHAPTER 22

Congenital heart disease

Case studies

1 You hear a systolic murmur in a previously fit teenage boy with a chest infection. What would you do?
2 A 38-year-old woman who is pregnant for the first time comes to see you for a routine prenatal check at 16 weeks. She is concerned that her sister gave birth to a baby with congenital heart disease, and she wants reassurance. What would you do?
3 A 47-year-old woman who had successful repair of an atrial septal defect 10 years ago forgot to ask her gynaecologist if she needed antibiotics before a D & C (dilatation and curettage). What would you advise her to do?
4 A 53-year-old woman comes to see you complaining of chest pain which you feel is not related to her heart, but you hear a loud systolic murmur. She was told that she was born with a hole in the heart, but did not have an operation. What would you do?

Prevalence and diagnosis of congenital heart disease

The overall prevalence of congenital heart disease is 8 per 1000 live births. Ventricular septal defects account for 30% of all cases, atrial septal defects account for 10% and patent ductus arteriosus accounts for 10%. Other cardiac malformations occur infrequently and will be seen only rarely in primary care. Mitral valve prolapse is considered to be a variant of normal mitral valve anatomy and, together with congenital bicuspid valve, is discussed in Chapter 17. Not all affected babies survive to infancy, so there would be less than 80 patients with congenital heart disease in a general practice with 8000 patients.

Fetal echocardiography, magnetic resonance imaging and computerised tomography are used alone or in combination to diagnose affected babies in mothers at risk during pregnancy. Mothers with babies at risk from Down's syndrome should be investigated with amniocentesis. Some congenital heart defects may be corrected *in utero*, while others are corrected during the neonatal period.

Role of primary care in the management of patients with congenital heart disease

Optimal long-term survival and quality of life are achieved by early diagnosis and intervention for patients with simple shunt lesions or single obstructive valvular lesions. The management and follow-up of patients with complex congenital heart disease demand the skills and experience of regional paediatric cardiological centres and adult congenital heart disease units. Patients with known congenital heart disease should, depending on their age, be referred to the relevant centre for long-term monitoring. Similarly, patients with suspected undiagnosed congenital heart disease should be referred for evaluation.

Primary care physicians should educate and remind patients with congenital heart disease about the importance of excellent dental and oral hygiene, regular visits to a dentist, and antibiotic prophylaxis before potentially septic procedures (*see* Chapter 17). Antibiotic prophylaxis is recommended for all patients with congenital heart disease except isolated secundum atrial septal defect and successful repaired atrial and ventricular septal defects and patent ductus arteriosus.

Risk factors for congenital heart disease

The causes of congenital heart disease are unclear, but are thought to involve genetic and environmental factors during formation of the heart, including the following:

- maternal rubella
- alcohol abuse
- lithium
- certain drugs
- radiation
- congenital heart disease in the mother
- congenital heart disease in a previous pregnancy or in a first-degree relative.

Congenital heart disease in infancy

Causes

The principal causes of heart failure in infancy are age related:

- newborn small preterm – persistent patent ductus arteriosus
- full-term newborn – hypoplastic left heart, coarctation of the aorta
- over 2 weeks – ventricular and atrial septal defects.

Presentation

Feeding difficulties, failure to put on weight, a fast pulse rate and a fast respiratory rate are serious signs, and the infant should be referred urgently to hospital.

Ventricular septal defect

This is the commonest congenital cardiac abnormality in infants and children, account-ing for 30% of all cases of congenital heart disease and occurring equally frequently in boys and girls. A large proportion of defects close spontaneously, completely or partially, within the first year of life leaving the patient symptom-free but with a loud systolic murmur and a risk of endocarditis, for which they should receive prophylactic antibiotics.

Closure of the defect in patients with an insignificant shunt is not necessary, and their prognosis is good because there is a minimal increase in pulmonary blood flow. Follow-up is advisable.

Patients with a persistent significant ventricular septal defect present in the first year of life with congestive heart failure and a harsh systolic murmur, which necessitates recognition and urgent referral to a specialist centre where echocardiography will provide the diagnosis. Closure of the defect by either surgical repair or a double umbrella device is necessary to avoid the risk of pulmonary hypertension, which reverses the shunt (Eisenmenger's syndrome).

Atrial septal defect

Atrial septal defect accounts for one-third of cases of congenital heart disease in adults, and is three times more common in females. It may occur with other cardiac abnormal-ities, particularly mitral valve prolapse and mitral regurgitation. It may present in childhood or in adults, and is commonly associated with Down's syndrome.

The symptoms depend on the size of the defect and its haemodynamic consequences. The left-to-right shunt across the inter-atrial septum results in increased pulmonary blood flow with gradually progressive pulmonary hypertension, dilatation of the atria, right ventricle and pulmonary arteries, and right heart failure and atrial fibrillation. It is an uncommon cause of palpitation, breathlessness or unexplained stroke in young adults.

The diagnosis may not be made until adulthood because most patients remain symptom-free until their thirties. These patients are vulnerable to heart failure and stroke by their fifties. Atrial septal defect is diagnosed by clinical findings of fixed splitting of the second heart sound, chest X-ray showing large pulmonary vessels, ECG and echocardiography.

Uncomplicated atrial septal defects should ideally be diagnosed and closed in child-hood, or before adulthood if possible, percutaneously with an umbrella device in a specialist centre. Surgical closure is otherwise effective and carries a low risk of around 1%. Successful closure before the development of pulmonary hypertension results in a normal life expectancy. Surgical closure of atrial septal defects in symptomatic adults over the age of 40 years with significant left-to-right shunts results in a better survival and exercise tolerance compared with medical treatment, but does not reduce the risk of stroke or the risk of development or persistence of atrial fibrillation. Patients with symptomatic atrial flutter or fibrillation should be managed as discussed in Chapter 18. Closure is too late once pulmonary hypertension has occurred. The decision to close atrial septal defects in a symptom-free adult is controversial, but with advances in low-risk, percutaneous umbrella-device closure many specialist units believe that this will prevent symptomatic deterioration in the long term. Long-term cardiological follow-up is recommended for patients with unclosed atrial septal defects, and for those in whom closure was performed in adulthood. Antibiotic prophylaxis against infective endocarditis is not recommended for patients with atrial septal defect (repaired or unrepaired) unless there is an associated valve abnormality.

Patent foramen ovale

This is found in 25% of the normal population. Approximately 10–40% of strokes have no obvious cause, and 50% of these are thought to be due to a patent foramen ovale. The latter is diagnosed by transoesophageal echocardiography. Although it is not yet clear whether all of these lesions should be closed, the safety and ease of percutaneous closure provide an attractive method of reducing the risk of stroke. In the UK this procedure is mainly performed by paediatric interventional cardiologists.

Patent ductus arteriosus

The ductus arteriosus connects the descending aorta (distal to the origin of the left subclavian artery) to the main pulmonary artery trunk at the origin of the left pulmonary artery. In the fetus, it allows arterial blood to bypass the unexpanded lungs and enter the descending aorta for oxygenation in the placenta.

Normally it closes spontaneously shortly after birth. Non-closure (a patent ductus) accounts for 10% of cases of congenital heart disease. The persistent left-to-right shunt leads to pulmonary hypertension, right heart failure and a high mortality rate in the first year of life.

Most patients should be diagnosed shortly after birth with echocardiography and have a machinery murmur. The duct is closed using percutaneous catheter techniques or ligated in infancy, which results in a normal prognosis. Rarely, a patent ductus is diagnosed in adults. Closure is recommended in adults with a murmur because of the risks of endarteritis and heart failure. Closure is not recommended in patients without a murmur because they may have already developed Eisenmenger's syndrome, or the shunt may be too small and pose a negligible risk of endarteritis and heart failure.

Life expectancy is normal with a small patent ductus, but carries a risk of endocarditis. Large shunts may lead to left ventricular failure and flow reversal. Survival is possible without closure, but the patient will experience breathlessness and palpitation in adulthood, and is at risk from infective endarteritis and endocarditis and heart failure in adulthood. Death occurs in one-third of patients with a persistent ductus by the age of 40 years, and in two-thirds by the age of 60 years. Therefore closure or ligation is recommended for even a small patent ductus.

Coarctation of the aorta

This is a fibromuscular narrowing of the descending aorta in the region of the ductus distal to the left subclavian artery. It occurs in 0.4 per 1000 live births, and is much more common in males. It is associated with a bicuspid aortic valve, patent ductus arteriosus, ventricular septal defect, Turner's syndrome and aneurysms of the circle of Willis.

The presentation and prognosis vary according to age. Neonates, even after repair, have a poorer prognosis than children and adults. Coarctation of the aorta may be detected during the first week of life in a breathless, pale neonate with a history of poor feeding and absent foot pulses due to reduced or absent blood flow through the coarct. Urgent referral is necessary because the coarct restricts blood flow down the aorta, leading to increased left ventricular afterload and heart failure. Prostaglandin infusion to re-establish patency of the ductus may be life-saving. Even with prompt intervention and repair of the coarct using either angioplasty or surgical intervention, patients remain at risk of premature atherosclerosis, hypertension and premature death.

The older child or adult may be symptom-free with upper limb hypertension and leg claudication with absent or diminished foot pulses. The 25-year survival rate is 80% if the coarct is repaired in childhood.

In adults, coarctation may present as hypertension, aortic dissection, heart failure, aortic stenosis, infective endocarditis, premature coronary artery disease and cerebrovascular disease. Pregnant women with aortic coarctation are at high risk of aortic dissection.

The ECG may be normal and the chest X-ray may be abnormal in severe cases. Doppler echocardiography, CT scanning and magnetic resonance imaging of the aorta provide information on its location and severity. Long-term survival is optimised by repair performed in childhood. Hypertension persists in 50% of patients if repair is performed after the age of 40 years, when the 15-year survival rate is only 50%.

Surgical repair is performed if the transcoarct gradient exceeds 30 mmHg, but restenosis occurs in 30% of adults after surgical resection. Restenosis and aortic aneurysm repair are more frequent after angioplasty, which is currently used mainly for restenosis occurring after surgery.

After repair of the coarct, the patient remains at risk of complications of hypertension, which may be difficult to control, and they need long-term follow-up to monitor blood pressure and signs of heart failure. Two-thirds of patients over the age of 40 years with uncorrected coarctation have heart failure. Around 75% die by the age of 50 years, and 90% by the age of 60 years.

Answers to case studies

1 The murmur may be innocent and/or related to the chest infection. Other possibilities include congenital aortic stenosis, ventricular septal defect, mitral valve prolapse and other structural congenital heart disease. The patient and his parents should be advised that an echocardiogram may be necessary if the murmur is still present when he is re-examined after the chest infection has resolved.

2 This patient is at risk and should be referred to a paediatric cardiac unit for assessment, including fetal echocardiography.

3 Antibiotic prophylaxis is not necessary after successful closure of an atrial septal defect.

4 It would be helpful to have all of this patient's previous notes. If she has been generally fit and well, the murmur is most probably due to a small, restrictive, residual and harmless ventricular septal defect, and she has a good prognosis.

She should be given antibiotic prophylaxis. An echocardiogram should be performed if this has not been done within a year, to confirm the diagnosis and exclude associated valve abnormalities.

Further reading

- Freedom RM, Nykanen DG (1998) Congenital heart disease. In: EJ Topol (ed.) *Comprehensive Cardiovascular Medicine*. Lippincot-Raven, Philadelphia.
- Marelli AJ, Moodie DS (1998) Adult congenital heart disease. In: EJ Topol (ed.) *Comprehensive Cardiovascular Medicine*. Lippincot-Raven, Philadelphia.

CHAPTER 23

Heart disease in the elderly

What is old age?

With an increasing proportion of the population living and working for longer and hoping and expecting that their retirement years will be enjoyable and active, primary care clinicians need to understand how increasing age affects the cardiovascular system and how medical advances can be applied safely, sensibly and intelligently to benefit this growing population of patients.

> Old age should not be defined simply by a number, but by the individual's biological and psychological state, which determine their prognosis, lifestyle and view of their future.

There is no general agreement on an age watershed that identifies an elderly patient. Current medical literature includes people aged 80 years or over as elderly. The proportion of the population aged over 80 years is increasing rapidly. It constitutes the fastest growing segment of the population and accounts for 11% of those over 60 years of age worldwide. An 80-year-old has a life expectancy of approximately 8 years.

The patient's perspective in clinical management decisions

Each elderly patient will have a different and personal perspective of what they expect and hope to achieve from the remainder of their life, and what they are willing to tolerate with regard to disability and symptoms and the impact that these have on their lifestyle. If they are ill and in need of an operation or merely a tablet, they will have to decide whether their symptoms and the impact that the condition has on their lifestyle merit the risks and side-effects of the proposed intervention. Explaining these matters simply, directly and in a way that the patient understands is not always easy, and demands communication skills and empathy from the clinician, who must be able to understand and respect the patient's aspirations and wishes and, importantly, their whole clinical state and social and personal circumstances.

Giving advice on the pros and cons of aortic valve replacement in a 90-year-old who is keen to pursue an active life is not easy. The more common situation of deciding whether to recommend angiotensin-converting-enzyme (ACE) inhibitors, statins, aspirin and β-blockers to an elderly patient after myocardial infarction is equally difficult.

Giving elderly patients advice based on clinical trials

Although observational clinical studies have reported on the outcome of certain interventions (cardiac surgery, valve replacement and coronary angioplasty) in elderly patients, randomised clinical trials evaluating medical treatments have not included patients over 80 years of age, usually because they may be on other medication which cannot be stopped or they have comorbidity which would exclude them from the trial. It is therefore difficult to provide elderly patients with quantitative information concerning outcome and risk in certain areas of cardiology. However, outcome data gleaned from personal, prospective databases, including prognostically useful clinical information, can provide the clinical team with relevant information to guide decision making.

Advice to elderly patients must be individualised.

Age-related medical changes

The following conditions become increasingly common with advancing age and complicate the management of elderly patients.

General medical conditions
- Renal impairment with increases in serum creatinine levels.
- A decrease in bone density, leading to a loss of mechanical strength and increased vulnerability to fracture.
- Cerebrovascular disease.
- Impaired mental state due to dementia.
- Neurological and musculoskeletal conditions.
- Thyroid disorders.
- Renal impairment.
- Liver impairment.
- Diabetes.

Cardiac conditions
- Coronary artery disease and acute myocardial infarction.
- Hypertension.
- Heart failure.
- Aortic valve disease.
- Atrial fibrillation.
- Heart block.
- Infective endocarditis.

Because elderly people have a reduced physiological and anatomical resistance, they are vulnerable to a 'domino effect' of illnesses once a clinical problem occurs. For example, an elderly patient with visual impairment may trip and fall. Her osteoporosis predisposes her to a fractured hip, which requires surgery, but this puts her at high perioperative risk of myocardial infarction due to underlying coronary heart disease and heart failure due to diastolic left ventricular dysfunction. Her poor mobility puts her at risk of deep vein thrombosis and pulmonary embolism. Involvement of all the relevant medical and surgical specialties is likely to improve management, and enables the team to predict and possibly prevent potential complications.

> A full general medical assessment should be made and coexisting conditions corrected wherever possible.

Risk–benefit analysis in cardiological treatments

Risk–benefit analysis is particularly important in these high-risk patients. Advice should be individualised based on a detailed and comprehensive knowledge of the patient's clinical, social and psychological circumstances, considered in the context of patients with a similar risk profile who have undergone a similar intervention.

This is a particularly difficult aspect of clinical care in elderly patients. The prevalence of nearly every cardiac condition increases with advancing age. In the absence of guidelines specifically written for elderly patients, clinicians are forced to rely on their clinical judgement and experience when deciding on certain interventions that have a finely balanced risk–benefit ratio. Warfarin treatment is a common and important example.

Certain interventions (e.g thrombolysis or primary coronary angioplasty for acute myocardial infarction) carry greater risks in elderly patients, but are also associated with a correspondingly greater potential benefit.

Elderly people may be less motivated to exercise, mix socially or take on new psychological or intellectual challenges. Their social networks and personal circumstances may have changed and their horizons may have altered. They are more likely to have comorbidities (e.g. arthritis, neurological conditions, hypertension, diabetes and gastrointestinal conditions). These conditions alter their resilience with regard to physical and psychological challenges, operations and interventions, and they are usually more sensitive to medication and more likely to develop side-effects.

Cost implications of treating the elderly

The cost implications of certain expensive interventions, such as cardiac surgery, must also be borne in mind, although this is a secondary consideration when deciding to offer a patient treatment.

Changes in the ageing cardiovascular system

The following changes occur.

- Hypertension.
- The left ventricular wall becomes thicker and amyloid is deposited independent of blood pressure.
- Diastolic dysfunction may lead to heart failure.
- The heart valves become fibrosed and calcified, and in particular this affects the mitral valve annulus and the aortic valve cusps. Aortic valve sclerosis may not result in outflow obstruction, but confers significant morbidity and mortality.
- Sinus node and conducting tissue disease.
- Arterial thickness, tortuosity and calcification.
- Coronary artery structural changes resulting in reduced laminar flow and lipid deposits.

Clinical features in the elderly

Isolated systolic hypertension with visible carotid artery and brachial artery pulsation, systolic heart murmurs, added heart sounds and difficulty in measuring the jugular venous pulse due to local skin and fascial anatomical changes in the neck are clinical findings which require elucidation.

Most elderly people have systolic heart murmurs due to mitral valve regurgitation and/or aortic valve sclerosis or stenosis.

Prescribing principles in the elderly

Elderly patients are likely to have other treated conditions, and therefore the prescribing of cardiovascular medications may result in drug interactions and confusion about which drugs to take at recommended times. This may reduce compliance.

Only essential drugs should be prescribed. Compliance is likely to be better if a simple, once daily, 'all-at-once' regime is devised, which may need to be supervised by the person living with or caring for the patient.

Elderly patients have reduced muscle mass and reduced liver and renal function, and these factors mean that drug frequency and dosages may need to be decreased. In addition, age-related changes in pharmacokinetics mean that smaller doses of nearly all cardiovascular drugs should be used and the doses increased gradually with careful monitoring of biochemistry.

Hypertension

Isolated systolic hypertension is the commonest form of hypertension and is discussed in Chapter 12. A diuretic and dihydropyridine calcium-channel blocker combination has been used in placebo-controlled trials, but a third or fourth drug may need to be used to achieve a target blood pressure of < 140/90 mmHg. Lowering the diastolic blood pressure to < 55 mmHg may compromise coronary blood flow and increase the risk of angina or myocardial infarction. Maintenance of a normal serum potassium concentration is important.

Healthy lifestyle measures should be encouraged by advising patients to reduce their salt intake by avoiding consumption of too many ready-to-cook meals, snacks, crisps, nuts and convenience foods. Obesity should be treated and an individualised exercise programme advised, although it may be very difficult to implement all of these lifestyle measures.

Diabetes

The prevalence of type 2 diabetes is increasing in both the young and the elderly. Apart from the well-recognised diabetic microvascular complications (including retinopathy, nephropathy and neuropathy) and macrovascular complications (including coronary heart disease, stroke and peripheral artery disease), there are other less well-known complications which have similarly devastating effects in the elderly. These include cognitive disorders and physical disability (either causing or resulting from falls or fractures). These conditions have a major impact on the lifestyle of these patients, with loss of independence, increased demands on carers and family, and loss of independence, and they represent a major drain on social, human and financial resources.

The primary care team will be central to the multi-disciplinary approach to the management of these patients.

Hyperlipidaemia

Statins reduce the risk of secondary coronary events in people over 60 years of age, as well as the risk of stroke and transient ischaemic attacks.

Heart failure in the elderly

Diastolic rather than systolic heart failure is the commonest haemodynamic abnormality in the elderly. Around 70% of elderly patients with heart failure have preserved left ventricular systolic function. In contrast, only 10% of patients under 60 years of age have preserved left ventricular systolic function. Infection, uncontrolled blood pressure and myocardial infarction (which may be silent) may each present as heart failure.

The prognosis of elderly patients with heart failure remains poorer than for many forms of cancer, and the management of patients with end-stage disease requires highly developed clinical and organisational skills in co-ordinating input from specialists, geriatricians, general physicians and experts in palliative care.

Clinical features

The presenting symptom may be breathlessness, but in common with other conditions, including infections, heart disease may present as a non-specific illness, confusion, depression, falls, anorexia and weight loss or immobility.

The physical signs may be difficult to elicit. A raised venous pressure may be obscured by fascia in the neck, which may be affected by cervical spine arthritis. The presence of added heart sounds due to ventricular stiffness may make auscultation difficult. In some patients who have very thin arms and ankylosis of the elbow, it may be difficult to record the blood pressure.

Investigations

An ECG will show the heart rhythm and signs of myocardial infarction. Echocardiography is a very helpful investigation for assessing and characterising left ventricular function, valve structure and competence, and for assessing aortic valve stenosis.

Thyrotoxicosis should be excluded as a possible cause of atrial fibrillation which may not result in symptoms. Occasionally, anaemia may contribute to symptoms of breathlessness and tiredness. The possibility of coexisting diabetes and renal impairment should be investigated.

Management

Ill patients and those who cannot cope at home may need to be admitted to hospital. Bed rest should be avoided unless the patient is unable to sit in a chair, because of the risks of venous thrombosis and embolism, chest infection and limb weakness.

Subcutaneous fractionated heparin, compression stockings and timely physiotherapy to facilitate early mobilisation are important.

Fluid restriction is no longer advised, as it makes the patient very uncomfortable and can aggravate malnutrition. A low-salt diet is advised, but prepared ready-to-cook meals and salty convenience foods may be a major component of the patient's usual diet.

Atrial fibrillation with an uncontrolled ventricular rate should be treated with digoxin, which acts as a weak inotrope in patients with heart failure and is beneficial even in individuals who are in sinus rhythm. The decision to anticoagulate must be made with due attention to all of the risks and benefits.

Diuretics are used to treat pulmonary and peripheral oedema. Resistant oedema may require intravenous loop diuretics (frusemide). All diuretics may cause incontinence and urinary retention. A thiazide diuretic can be added to a loop diuretic in patients with severe peripheral oedema, but is less likely to be effective if the glomerular filtration rate is less than 40 ml/minute, and gout is a possible side-effect.

Hyperkalaemia may result from the use of potassium-sparing diuretics or supplemental potassium, particularly when combined with ACE inhibitors. Renal function should be monitored in all patients.

ACE inhibitors may, particularly in fluid-depleted patients, result in hypotension and an intolerable cough, so the dose increases should be slow. The patient may need to be switched to angiotensin II blockers. Both classes of drug may unmask renal artery stenosis.

Adverse effects of β-blockers, including tiredness, fatigue, bradycardia, hypotension and exacerbation of airflow obstruction are common in the elderly, and may necessitate stopping these drugs. It is important that medication used to treat heart failure is started at the lowest possible dose, which should only be increased very slowly and gradually. Drugs may need to be started and increased one at a time in order to avoid adverse haemodynamic effects.

A combination of hydralazine and isosorbide may be used in patients who cannot tolerate ACE inhibitors or angiotensin II blockers.

Isolated systolic hypertension may cause heart failure, and should be treated.

The patient's social circumstances and support require frequent review in order to reduce the need for hospital readmissions. Domiciliary visits by heart failure nurses may be very useful for monitoring the clinical, biochemical and social status of the patient and, importantly, ensuring compliance with medication.

Coronary artery disease and angina

Angina is a clinical diagnosis (*see* Chapter 2), but other causes of chest pain need to be excluded.

It may be argued that the lifestyle of patients who have survival past the age of 80 years must be satisfactory, but conventional risk factors should still be reviewed and treated when appropriate, even where there are areas of doubt or lack of evidence that intervention improves survival. These aspects are difficult to prove in this population of patients.

Isolated systolic hypertension may result in angina, and should be controlled. Obesity in the elderly is uncommon, possibly because the obese are selected out of the old-age population. Diabetes, smoking and hyperlipidaemia should be treated in the same way as in younger patients. A low-fat diet is recommended, although elderly patients may find it even more difficult to change their diet than younger patients.

Medical treatment is the preferred option, and this should be pursued with anti-anginal drugs added one at a time and with gradual dose increases. If it is tolerated, aspirin should be given to all patients. β-Blockers, short- and long-acting nitrates (which may be given both orally and transdermally), calcium-channel blockers and potassium-channel-opening agents should be used, adding one class of drug at a time and starting with low doses.

Intolerable angina despite optimal medical treatment

Non-invasive angina or ischaemia provocation tests may be impractical and do not generally provide further diagnostic information. Exercise testing provides an indication of exercise capacity, and this is clinically useful. Stress echocardiography and nuclear tests are both open to observer bias and may confirm myocardial ischaemia. However, they add little to clinical management decisions in the elderly patient with clear-cut angina, whose pre-test likelihood of having coronary artery disease is over 95%.

Myocardial revascularisation

Patients with angina that is refractory to maximum tolerated or recommended doses and who have had a full review and treatment of cardiovascular risk factors should be considered for revascularisation, preferably with coronary angioplasty (which has a lower perioperative risk than coronary artery bypass grafting). There are no reliable data from randomised trials including patients over 80 years of age, so these procedures are performed primarily for relief of symptoms. Intuitively, however, it is difficult to imagine that the survival benefit applicable to a 60-year-old patient with a critical stenosis of the left main coronary artery or three-vessel coronary artery disease would not be extended to an 80-year-old patient with similar coronary artery anatomy.

If the patient agrees, the management should be discussed with their family and the risks of treatment explained and put in context, as far as possible, with a non-interventional conservative strategy.

Coronary angiography should preferably be performed in a cardiothoracic centre, which would allow the possibility of immediately proceeding to coronary angioplasty, obviating the need to readmit the patient for another procedure and arterial cannulation. However, a staged procedure may be desirable both for clinical reasons and to reduce the dose of radiographic contrast medium and potential serious renal impairment.

Patients who are scheduled for coronary angioplasty should also consent to emergency coronary artery bypass grafting, which may be necessary in approximately 2% of cases due to abrupt vessel closure, which is more common in an elderly and often calcified coronary artery. Peripheral vascular complications are also more common in the elderly.

Treatment of myocardial infarction in the elderly

Patients over 75 years of age represent around 30% of those with acute myocardial infarction and 50% of those who die acutely from their infarct. The 30-day mortality rate in elderly patients treated with thrombolysis for acute ST-elevation myocardial infarction is around 20%, compared with 11% for patients under 80 years of age. This indicates that, whenever possible, mechanical thrombolysis should be attempted for elderly patients with acute myocardial infarction. In order to salvage jeopardised myocardium as soon as possible by reperfusing it with blood, the 'door to balloon time' should be less than 60 minutes, and this service is only available in a few centres at present in the UK. For suitable elderly patients who are treated in major centres with experienced operators, primary coronary angioplasty is superior to thrombolysis in reducing mortality. In the elderly, streptokinase is associated with a lower risk of intracerebral bleeding and death compared with tissue plasminogen activator.

Valve disease

Mitral valve regurgitation

This can be due to mitral annulus calcification (which is more common in women), papillary muscle dysfunction due to ischaemia or degeneration, or mitral valve leaflet prolapse. All of these conditions are common in people over 70 years of age.

ACE inhibitors can be used for their vasodilatory action in patients with coexisting hypertension and coronary heart disease.

Aortic stenosis and sclerosis

Senile calcific aortic stenosis develops in relation to the same risk factors that are associated with cardiovascular disease. It may progress rapidly, so prompt diagnosis and quantification of its severity using echocardiography and Doppler examination is important.

Infective endocarditis

This condition is uncommon, and is often difficult to diagnose due to its insidious nature and atypical presentation. Elderly patients may not have the classic features of fever, changing heart murmurs and signs of emboli, and may present with weight loss, anorexia and fatigue with no fever. This leads to delayed diagnosis and often a worse outcome in a patient with other medical problems and a reduced resistance to infection. At 25%, the in-hospital mortality rate is twice that of patients aged 50–70 years. The aortic and mitral valves are most commonly affected.

The digestive tract is the most frequent portal of entry, due to the higher incidence of colonic lesions. *Streptococcus bovis* is the predominant organism. In men, prostatic lesions are common. Whereas intravenous drug abuse is a common cause in younger patients, this is not the case in the elderly. This highlights the importance of prophylactic antibiotics for gastroenterological and urological procedures in high-risk patients. Pace-maker endocarditis is also more common in the elderly.

It is important to suspect infective endocarditis in elderly patients, and to take blood cultures and check the C-reactive protein level (the erythrocyte sedimentation rate is diagnostically less helpful in the elderly because it is generally higher than in younger patients), as well as other haematological and biochemical tests.

Transoesophageal echocardiography is more sensitive than a transthoracic study for detecting vegetations and abscesses, and it is usually well tolerated.

If the diagnosis is suspected, treatment with appropriate antibiotics should be started as soon as possible after consultation with a microbiologist and when blood cultures and other investigations have been undertaken. Attention to the patient's general medical and haemodynamic state is important.

Surgery carries higher risks in the elderly, but should be performed if patients develop heart failure, an aortic abscess or other infective embolic complications. However, patients should be carefully selected.

Cardiac surgery

Elderly patients are now being referred for cardiac surgery more frequently. In-hospital complications and mortality rates are higher and hospital stays are longer due to coexisting cerebrovascular and peripheral artery disease, diabetes, pulmonary disease and renal impairment.

Difficult and common questions include the following.

1 Should surgery be performed at all or is there an alternative strategy?
2 How and when should surgery be performed?

3   In a patient with both valve and coronary artery disease, should coronary artery bypass surgery be performed at the same time as valve replacement or can coronary angioplasty be used to revascularise the patient?

There are also cost–benefit considerations.

Table 23.1:   Outcomes of cardiac surgery in people over 80 years of age

	Coronary artery surgery (CABG)	Aortic valve replacement (AVR)	CABG+AVR	Mitral valve replacement (MVR)
Death (%)	10	9	27	25
Stroke (%)	3	3	4	8
Five-year survival rate (%)	66	63	62	57

Cardiac surgery in patients over 80 years of age

- The overall operative mortality for these different and combined elective and routine operations is 13%.
- Post-operative complications included one or more of the following: chest infections, pulmonary oedema, pulmonary embolism, arrhythmias (most commonly atrial fibrillation), stroke, renal failure requiring dialysis, myocardial infarction. The incidence of one or more of these complications is approximately 60%.
- The 5-year survival rate is 63%, but this depends largely on the age of the patient at the time of surgery.
- Most patients (87%) believed that they made the right decision, but many factors influence this type of retrospective quality-of-life assessment.

Predictors of death include New York Heart Association functional class and procedure time. Atheromatous aortic disease increases the risk of stroke. Pre-operative myocardial infarction increases the risk of late out-of-hospital death. Cardiac surgery can be performed with an 'acceptable' risk in patients with near-normal left ventricular function.

Atrial fibrillation

This is discussed in Chapter 18. It is a common arrhythmia in the elderly, with a prevalence of around 10% in those over 75 years of age and 15% in those over 80 years.

Both chronic and intermittent paroxysmal atrial fibrillation are often detected during routine examination or on a 24-hour ECG performed during the investigation of dizzy turns. Most patients can be managed in primary care and then discussed with a cardiologist. Patients with disabling symptoms or in whom further investigation or intervention are being considered should be referred to a cardiologist.

Clinical features

Atrial fibrillation usually results in no palpitation and may be discovered coincidentally. Symptoms depend on the ventricular response and rate, the underlying state of the coronary arteries and left ventricular function. For example, the loss of atrial contraction in a patient with diastolic dysfunction results in a low cardiac output, leading to heart failure, dizziness and (rarely, with very fast ventricular rates) loss of consciousness. Compared with young patients, elderly individuals are more likely to experience transient ischaemic episodes, stroke, and peripheral arterial or mesenteric emboli, because they are more likely to have coexisting vascular risk factors.

Management

Confirmation of the diagnosis and, in the case of paroxysmal atrial fibrillation, quantification of the frequency and duration of attacks with ambulatory electrocardiography is important and guides treatment. It is important to exclude hyperthyroidism, overuse of or sensitivity to β-agonists, alcohol, hypokalaemia (due to diuretics) and chronic obstructive lung disease as causes or contributory factors.

Warfarin

The risk–benefit ratio must be judged carefully for each patient, taking into account the risk factors for left atrial thrombosis and embolisation. Patients with a structurally normal heart and no vascular risk factors are at low risk, whereas those with a dilated heart, mitral regurgitation, hypertension and diabetes are at high risk.

There are no guidelines regarding the upper age limit at which warfarin is contraindicated because of gastrointestinal bleeding or stroke, and the decision to anticoagulate should be made after evaluating the patient's risk. Most clinicians would be very cautious about recommending warfarin for or continuing its use in patients over 90 years of age. Similarly, warfarin is contraindicated in patients who fall repeatedly, those with dementia or with a history of recent gastrointestinal bleeding, patients taking non-steroidal anti-inflammatory drugs, and those with anaemia, liver disease, excess alcohol consumption or underlying carcinoma.

If there are no major indications and the patient is willing and able to have blood tests to monitor the international normalised ratio (INR), which should be tightly controlled at between 2 and 3, then warfarin is advised for elderly patients who:

- have had transient ischaemic attacks, *or*
- have had stroke (to be started not less than 2 weeks after the stroke and only if the blood pressure is controlled), *or*
- have risk factors which further predispose them to stroke or emboli.

Aspirin

Compared with warfarin, this is less effective in preventing emboli but also less liable to result in major bleeding complications. Concomitant use of a proton-pump inhibitor to reduce the risk of gastrointestinal bleeding is advisable.

Heart rate control

It is important to control the ventricular rate in all patients, and digoxin, diltiazem, verapamil and β-blockers may be used, depending on the clinical state of the patient and coexisting conditions.

Atrial fibrillation may be part of sinus node disease, and because of the risk of inducing bradycardia, these drugs are contraindicated unless the patient has a pacemaker.

Cardioversion

This may have no advantage over rate control and anticoagulation in the elderly, unless the patient has a history of recent atrial fibrillation and haemodynamic compromise due to diastolic dysfunction. Sinus rhythm is maintained in 30–60% of patients, but this can be very advantageous by making anticoagulation unnecessary, although aspirin may be recommended for patients with long episodes of paroxysmal atrial fibrillation.

The use of anti-arrhythmic drugs, including flecainide, amiodarone and sotalol, may help to maintain sinus rhythm.

Pulmonary vein isolation using radiofrequency ablation

Evolving and more sophisticated approaches, including pulmonary vein isolation using radiofrequency ablation, are not a preferred option in the elderly.

Atrioventricular node ablation and pacemaker implantation

This should be considered for patients with resistant and haemodynamically compromising atrial fibrillation when associated with bradycardia as part of sinus node disease and conduction tissue disease.

Pacing for bradycardia

Pacemakers are indicated for patients with symptomatic bradycardia and heart block, which become increasingly common with advancing age due to degeneration of the sinus node and cardiac conducting tissue in the His-Purkinje system. This leads to sinus bradycardia, sinus pauses, atrial fibrillation, bundle branch block and complete heart block.

Pacing is a cost-effective procedure because it corrects bradycardia which otherwise results in falls and possible fractures.

Pacing (*see* Chapter 18) is performed under local anaesthesia, usually with mild sedation, and the procedure takes approximately an hour and involves an overnight stay in hospital.

Ventricular tachycardia

This is under-diagnosed, and should be suspected in patients with hypertensive heart disease and previous myocardial infarction where a thickened or scarred heart muscle acts as the substrate. It may present as dizzy turns, syncope and breathlessness.

It may be diagnosed with a fortuitous ECG or (more commonly) by ambulatory electrocardiography showing a broad complex tachycardia with independent atrial and ventricular activity, and it can be difficult to distinguish from a supraventricular tachycardia with bundle branch block. It can be treated satisfactorily with amiodarone, although other anti-arrhythmic drugs may be used after discussion with a cardiologist. Referral is appropriate, and occasionally an automatic implantable cardiac defibrillator may be indicated for patients with resistant arrhythmia.

Further reading

Hypertension

- SHEP Co-operative Research Group (1991) Prevention of stroke by antihypertensive drug treatment in older persons with isolated systolic hypertension. *JAMA*. **265**: 3255–64.
- Staessen JA, Fagard R, Thijs L *et al.* (1997) Morbidity and mortality in the placebo-controlled European trial on isolated systolic hypertension (Syst-Eur) in the elderly. *Lancet*. **350**: 757–64.

Heart failure

- Murray SA, Boyd K, Kendall M *et al.* (2002) Dying of lung cancer or cardiac failure: prospective qualitative interview study of patients and their carers in the community. *BMJ*. **325**: 929–32.

Cardiac surgery

- Glower DD, Christopher TD, Milano CA *et al.* (1992) Performance status and outcome after coronary artery bypass grafting in persons aged 80 to 93 years. *Am J Cardiol*. **70**: 567–71.
- Kohl P, Kerzmann A, Lahaye L *et al.* (2001) Cardiac surgery in octogenarians: perioperative outcome and long-term results. *Eur Heart J*. **22**: 1235–43.

Infective endocarditis in the elderly

- Di Salvo G, Thuny F, Rosenberg V *et al.* (2003) Endocarditis in the elderly: clinical, echo-cardiographic and prognostic features. *Eur Heart J*. **24**: 1576–83.
- Hoen B, Alla F, Selton-Suty CH *et al.* (2002) Changing profile of infective endocarditis. Results of a 1-year follow-up in France. *JAMA*. **288**: 75–81.

CHAPTER 24

Perioperative risk assessment in cardiac patients

Case studies

1 An 80-year-old man presents with an acute ascending aortic dissection. He has a chest infection and is hypertensive. What would you do?
2 A fit 68-year-old man who had coronary artery surgery 4 years ago and has no cardiac symptoms is scheduled for a total hip replacement. What pre-operative assessment does he need?
3 A 75-year-old hypertensive man, who is unable to walk more than 100 yards on the flat due to breathlessness, has diabetes and mild angina and needs a prostatectomy. What pre-operative assessment should he have?
4 An 84-year-old woman is admitted to hospital for a gastroscopy and is found to be diabetic and in atrial fibrillation. What would you do?
5 A 68-year-old woman with a previous myocardial infarction and decompensated heart failure is admitted for peripheral arterial surgery. She has moderate renal impairment. What would you do?

Role of the primary care team in explaining risks of surgery in patients with heart disease

The primary care team has an integral role in the risk assessment of patients undergoing non-cardiac surgery. They are part of a multi-disciplinary team that includes the surgeon, anaesthetist, cardiologist, intensivist, nurses, physiotherapists, technicians and other specialists.

The risks of non-cardiac surgery are most frequently due to coronary artery disease and impaired cardiac function as well as other medical conditions. Perioperative risks can be prevented or reduced if they are predicted pre-operatively and appropriate measures taken. This necessitates a comprehensive and detailed knowledge of the patient's clinical risk profile.

Good communication between all members of the team and documentation of relevant previous medical conditions are important. Because the GP is very often the clinician responsible for making the diagnosis and recommending referral for a surgical opinion, the patient may want to consult their GP after their specialist consultation to seek further advice and reassurance that the proposed operation is really necessary, is safe and will improve their quality of life (questions that some patients may be reticent about asking the surgeon).

Explaining the risks of non-cardiac surgery to patients with heart disease is difficult and requires an understanding of the patient's clinical profile and how this affects their risk from the proposed operation. This aspect of the work for primary care clinicians will probably increase, as the likelihood of comorbidity and the likelihood of patients needing surgery both increase as people live longer.

Aims of risk assessment and its effect on clinical management

The aim is to prevent or reduce perioperative risk. Some risk factors may be correctable. For example, myocardial ischaemia may be corrected by revascularisation and anaemia may be corrected by blood transfusion. Hypertension and diabetes can be controlled. Age is a major predictor of risk but is not correctable. The problems posed by other conditions, such as recent (less than 4 weeks old) myocardial infarction, can be reduced by delaying the operation and assessing cardiac function and residual ischaemia, improving cardiovascular risk factors and starting appropriate treatment for left ventricular impairment. Temporary cardiac pacing may be necessary for patients with symptomatic bradycardia and for those at risk of heart block.

Identification of patients at high risk who need further investigation is a skill that is gained from experience. The surgeon and the relevant specialists have to weigh up the risks of surgery against the risks of not operating, and the views of the patient must be taken into consideration.

Perioperative risk depends on the following:

- the type of procedure to be performed
- the patient's risk profile
- the experience and quality of the medical team and hospital facilities (which will not be discussed here).

Classification of risk according to the operation

High risk (risk of death and non-fatal infarction > 5%)
- Urgent major operations in the elderly.
- Aortic and other major vascular surgery.
- Peripheral vascular surgery.
- Prolonged abdominal operations.

Intermediate risk (risk of death and non-fatal infarction < 5%)
- Intraperitoneal and intrathoracic surgery.
- Carotid endarterectomy.
- Head and neck surgery.

- Orthopaedic surgery.
- Prostate surgery.

Low risk (cardiac risk < 1%)
- Endoscopic procedure.
- Superficial procedures.
- Cataract surgery.
- Breast surgery.

Assessing the patient's risk

A thorough clinical history and examination are important and useful, and provide a fairly accurate estimation of perioperative risk.

Clinical evaluation

All patients with known or suspected heart disease should be evaluated for the presence of heart failure, coronary artery disease, arrhythmia and previous myocardial infarction.

The following factors help to determine risk.

- Age.
- Functional capacity. This is an important predictor of risk, and patients with a very restricted functional capacity and who are breathless at rest may have underlying heart failure with significant cardiac impairment and structural heart disease, myocardial ischaemia, lung disease and/or other medical conditions. They are at high risk and require a comprehensive pre-operative evaluation. Patients who can walk up two flights of stairs quickly without breathlessness or angina would generally have an acceptable functional capacity and be at low perioperative risk.
- Comorbid conditions (diabetes, peripheral vascular disease, renal impairment, chronic lung disease).
- Type of surgery to be performed.

The following features provide useful information for risk assessment.

Major clinical predictors of increased perioperative risk
- Heart failure with breathlessness at rest.
- Unstable coronary syndromes (myocardial infarction within 4 weeks, unstable angina, new or severe angina).
- Ischaemia induced within 3 minutes of the Bruce treadmill protocol.
- Heart block.
- Significant ventricular arrhythmias.
- Uncontrolled supraventricular arrhythmias.
- Severe valvular disease.

Pre-operative evaluation of high-risk patients
- Specialist cardiology assessment.
- ECG.

- Chest X-ray.
- Blood tests (renal function, blood count, glucose levels).
- Echocardiography.
- Test(s) for ischaemia.
- Coronary angiography for patients with symptomatic or objective features of significant ischaemia if not done within the last year.

Intermediate and low predictors of increased perioperative risk
Most cardiac patients will be in this category.

- Advanced age (> 80 years).
- Inability to climb one flight of stairs without symptoms.
- Mild angina.
- Comorbid conditions (diabetes, peripheral vascular disease, renal impairment, chronic lung disease).
- History of myocardial infarction.
- Compensated heart failure.
- Controlled atrial fibrillation.
- Left bundle branch block.
- History of stroke.
- Uncontrolled hypertension.
- Renal impairment.
- Poor functional capacity (restricted to light gardening or housework, and only able to walk slowly on the flat).

Note: No ischaemia and an exercise tolerance of 12 minutes on the Bruce treadmill protocol predicts low risk.

Pre-operative evaluation of patients at intermediate risk
- Specialist cardiology referral.
- ECG.
- Chest X-ray for patients with breathlessness while walking on the flat.
- Echocardiography.
- Exercise testing (or other test for ischaemia) for patients with breathlessness when walking on the flat and those who are to undergo a high-risk procedure.
- Patients who can walk up two flights of stairs quickly with no symptoms and who are to undergo a low-risk procedure do not need exercise testing or echocardiography.
- Hypertension should be controlled.

Quantification of the risk

The doctor's perspective
This remains difficult, and only approximate percentage risks can be given. A number of risk indices have been formulated for weighting and scoring risk factors, but these are not widely used. Better pre-operative assessments, anaesthesia and an improved understanding and treatment of risk factors have reduced the perioperative risks. Quantification of perioperative risk has to be individualised, and may be obtained from the surgeon's

personal results for the procedure performed in patients with a similar risk profile to the patient under consideration.

The patient's perspective

In general, patients understand the implications of the terms 'high' and 'low' risk, but assume that surgery would only be performed if necessary and with an acceptable risk. Trying to quantify risk is an inaccurate business because there are many variables which interact in a complex and inconsistent way in different patients. Ultimately it is the decision of the surgeon to explain the operative risks to the patient. A risk prediction of 20% is very high, but only if the patient is one of the 20%!

When is urgent or emergency surgery necessary?

In certain circumstances surgery has to be performed as an emergency, so only a post-operative evaluation can be undertaken.

Who should be referred to a cardiologist?

The aim is to identify patients at high and intermediate risk of cardiac problems.

Patients with known heart failure, angina and coronary artery disease, previous infarction, myocardial revascularisation, valvular disease or significant conduction tissue disease, and those with a poor functional capacity or major clinical markers of risk should be referred to a cardiologist for assessment. Specialist referral is advisable for those with other medical conditions which increase the perioperative risk.

Patients with major predictors of risk and those at intermediate risk who are to have high-risk surgery should be referred and investigated. Patients with a poor functional capacity and more than one minor predictor of risk may also be considered for further testing prior to arterial surgery.

Cardiac investigations

The indications for invasive and non-invasive testing are similar to those in the non-operative setting. Patients with coronary artery disease, renal impairment or diabetes, a poor functional capacity and those who are to have a high-risk surgical procedure should undergo cardiac testing.

When is cardiac testing not necessary?

- In patients who have a high functional capacity, no evidence of heart or vascular disease or those who have had a full cardiac and medical assessment within the last year.
- In patients with known coronary artery disease but who are symptom-free and have no evidence of ischaemia on an exercise test performed within the last year.

When should surgery be delayed or cancelled?

- If one or more *major* predictors of risk are present.
- If the patient or their family do not wish to proceed, or if they want a second opinion.

Evaluation of cardiac function

Echocardiography

This is a useful, widely available method for evaluating left and right ventricular function and valve structure. Patients with a resting left ventricular ejection fraction of < 35%, those with severe diastolic dysfunction, those with uncompensated heart failure and those with significant valve disease are at high risk.

12-Lead ECG

This is recommended for patients with a history of coronary artery disease, and for those who are to undergo a high- or intermediate-risk procedure, patients with diabetes and those aged > 50 years who have more than one cardiovascular risk factor.

Reversible myocardial ischaemia

The main indications for tests to assess myocardial ischaemia are as follows.

- In patients with an intermediate pre-test probability of coronary artery disease.
- Prognostic assessment of patients with known or suspected coronary artery disease or a significant change in their clinical status.
- Documentation of reversible myocardial ischaemia.
- Assessment of patients after an acute coronary syndrome.
- Evaluation of exercise performance when subjective assessment is unreliable.

Exercise testing

Treadmill or cycle exercise testing is widely available, and is useful for quantifying exercise tolerance and haemodynamic responses and diagnosing ischaemia. These variables can accurately identify patients at low risk of cardiac events, who probably do not require coronary angiography. Patients with ischaemia should have coronary angiography. Failure to exercise to 85% of the age-predicted heart rate confers a high risk of perioperative cardiac events (around 25%). In patients with previous myocardial infarction or angina, exercise testing provides no additional diagnostic information, and coronary angiography should be performed.

Alternative tests to assess myocardial ischaemia

If exercise testing cannot be performed because the patient cannot walk or cycle due to arthritis, claudication or lung disease, or if the patient has other conditions which make interpretation of the exercise test result difficult, stress echocardiography and nuclear perfusion imaging may be used to identify patients at high and low perioperative risk.

Pharmacological stress testing

This is useful for patients who are unable or unwilling to perform an exercise test. Dobutamine echocardiography performed by an experienced operator provides useful diagnostic and prognostic information, is safe, and allows the examination of resting right and left ventricular function, valve structure and function, and the effects of dobutamine on regional and global left ventricular function.

Nuclear perfusion imaging

This may be used instead of exercise testing in patients with bundle branch block, but it does not offer any significant advantages over exercise testing in predicting peri-operative complications or long-term outcomes. It is significantly more expensive than exercise testing, and because of its limitations is only performed in a few centres in the UK. The dose of radioactivity is not inconsiderable, although it is probably not clinically significant for a single isolated test.

On the basis of currently available information, there is no justification for the use of either dobutamine echocardiography or nuclear perfusion imaging as a screening test in low-risk populations.

Medical management of angina

Patients may need to stop aspirin and other antithrombotic treatment before certain types of operations.

Patients with angina, hypertension, asymptomatic coronary artery disease or major cardiovascular risk factors should take β-blockers, which have been shown to reduce perioperative ischaemia and cardiac events in high-risk patients.

Coronary angiography

This provides anatomical rather than physiological information, as well as the opportunity to improve myocardial blood supply with angioplasty performed at the same time.

Coronary angiography may be appropriate for the following patients:

- those at high risk
- patients at intermediate risk prior to a high-risk procedure (e.g. vascular reconstruction), without preliminary non-invasive testing
- those with angina at rest or on minimal exertion

- those with equivocal non-invasive test results
- those with recent myocardial infarction who need urgent surgery.

Myocardial revascularisation prior to non-cardiac surgery

Coronary artery surgery and/or angioplasty may need to be performed in patients with angina and those with prognostically significant coronary artery disease (left main stem, proximal three-vessel coronary artery disease and severe left ventricular impairment).

Surgery should be delayed for 1 week after plain angioplasty and for 4 weeks after coronary stent implantation to allow for endothelialisation of the stent. Clopidogrel is recommended as long-term antithrombotic treatment in patients with coated stents, and the decision to stop this must be individualised.

Management of hypertension prior to surgery

This is a common clinical management problem. Patients may have well-controlled hypertension during normal activities, but their blood pressure may rise to a high level when they are admitted to hospital. These patients should be referred to a cardiologist, and their blood pressure must be controlled prior to surgery. Surgery should only be undertaken in patients with uncontrolled hypertension if it has to be performed as an emergency, in which case the blood pressure can be controlled with intravenous agents including nitrates, labetalol and nitroprusside (*see* Chapter 12). Sometimes the high blood pressure may be due to anxiety and a pronounced 'white-coat syndrome,' and anxiolytics and sedation may be effective in the short term. Patients should be restarted on oral antihypertensive treatment as soon as possible after surgery.

Valvular heart disease

Dental care and antibiotic prophylaxis

Depending on the procedure to be performed, all patients should be considered for appropriate antibiotic prophylaxis, and some patients may require a dental assessment and treatment before surgery. Pulmonary valve lesions are rare and do not usually require antibiotic prophylaxis.

Stenotic valvular lesions

Patients with these lesions should be referred to a cardiologist before surgery. Surgery in patients with symptomatic aortic and mitral valve stenosis may precipitate heart failure and pulmonary oedema. A comprehensive physical examination, echocardiography and (where appropriate) cardiac catheterisation and angiography should be performed.

Patients in whom valvuloplasty or valve replacement is required will need to be transferred to a cardiac surgical centre, and non-cardiac surgery will have to be delayed.

Regurgitant valvular lesions

Aortic and mitral regurgitation is usually well tolerated, but patients should be referred to a cardiologist for a full assessment and appropriate investigations.

Cardiomyopathy

Patients with both dilated and hypertrophic cardiomyopathy should be referred to a cardiologist for assessment of functional capacity and cardiac function and, in patients with symptomatic arrhythmias, vulnerability to serious arrhythmia (Holter monitoring).

Management when the patient returns home

When they return home, patients should be reviewed from both surgical and cardiovascular viewpoints. Risk factors and all treatments for cardiovascular disease and heart failure should be reviewed. In particular, treatment of smoking, hypertension, diabetes and lipid status should be optimised. Symptoms of heart failure, angina and breathlessness may be more noticeable to patients after orthopaedic and peripheral vascular surgery because of an improvement in their mobility. Despite careful pre-operative risk assessment, some patients may develop perioperative cardiovascular problems, and these individuals will need further cardiac review and investigation.

Answers to case studies

1 Repair of the aortic dissection is an emergency and should be performed without delay. All of the relevant specialists should be advised about the procedure and consulted.

2 This patient needs only a pre-operative assessment by the anaesthetist and an ECG, and can then proceed to surgery without any further cardiac investigations because he is at low risk and is to undergo an intermediate-risk procedure.

3 This patient has a poor functional capacity and a number of intermediate predictors of perioperative risk, and he needs a cardiological opinion and further cardiac testing before surgery. If he can exercise, he should have an exercise test to assess his exercise capacity and the severity of reversible myocardial ischaemia. If he cannot exercise sufficiently to 85% of his age-predicted maximal heart rate, dobutamine stress echocardiography should be performed to look at his cardiac structure and function at rest and under pharmacological stress. If there are signs of significant reversible ischaemia or underlying left ventricular dysfunction at rest or during stress, then the patient should have a coronary angiogram and revascularisation if necessary.

4 This patient should be referred to a cardiologist and assessed prior to gastroscopy, which is a low-risk procedure that is performed under light sedation.

Her atrial fibrillation will need to be controlled, and her diabetes may need review by a diabetologist both perioperatively and in the long term. If she is generally fit and active, she will not need further cardiac tests other than an ECG. After her gastroscopy, she should be reviewed and, depending on the result and her other risk factors for embolisation (*see* Chapter 18), she should be considered for rate control and anticoagulation.

5   This patient has major predictors of risk, and is scheduled to have a high-risk operation which should be postponed until she has been fully assessed by a cardiologist and other relevant specialists. Before surgery is performed she will need investigation with ECG, chest X-ray, echocardiography and, if there is evidence of residual ischaemia, coronary angiography in view of her previous myocardial infarction. She will need treatment for her heart failure, and her renal function and blood count will require review. If there is a compelling need to operate as an emergency, she must be treated urgently and the perioperative risks minimised as much as possible.

Further reading

- Eagle KA, Berger PB, Calkins H *et al.* (2002) ACC/AHA guideline update for perioperative cardiovascular evaluation for non-cardiac surgery – executive summary: a report of the American College of Cardiology/American Heart Association Task Force on Practice Guidelines (committee to update the 1996 guidelines on perioperative cardiovascular evaluation for noncardiac surgery). *J Am Coll Cardiol.* **39**: 542–53.

CHAPTER 25

Cardiac tests and procedures

Case studies

1 A 55-year-old hypertensive man, who smoked cigarettes until a year ago, complains of intermittent chest pain related to exercise. What would you do?

2 An 82-year-old woman who had aortic valve disease diagnosed 15 years ago, but who has not been back to hospital since, feels unwell, has lost her appetite and has lost 7 pounds in weight over the last 3 months. What are the likely causes and what would you do?

3 A 78-year-old woman has had one or two dizzy turns without loss of consciousness. What would you do?

Using cardiac tests in primary care

Cardiac tests are increasingly being performed in primary care because a larger proportion of patients with cardiovascular disorders are being diagnosed, treated and monitored by primary care clinicians. Patients may often prefer to ask their GP about a cardiac test rather than the hospital specialist. They will want to know why the test is being performed, what it entails, what the risks are, what the result means and how it might affect their treatment. Several new imaging and physiological tests are now being used in patients with cardiovascular disorders, and it is important that GPs understand what the tests are for, what they involve for the patient and how the results influence management.

Open-access investigations

ECGs have been performed by GPs for many years, and primary care clinicians now have open access at their local hospital for exercise testing, echocardiography, chest radiography and blood tests. The rationale is that open-access investigations reduce the length of time for which patients need to wait to be investigated. This may paradoxically increase waiting times to see a specialist, because the test requested may reveal unexpected or irrelevant findings which the GP feels obliged to refer for clarification and reassurance. Inappropriate investigations may lead to further inappropriate and expensive tests, patient and doctor anxiety, and inappropriate, expensive and potentially dangerous treatment. An example is atherosclerosis imaging and screening with Electron Beam Computed Axial Tomography (EBCAT) scanning in low-risk individuals.

It is therefore essential that all tests are requested and performed with a knowledge of the value and limitations of the test in the patient's individual clinical situation, and with an understanding of the possible implications of the result and how that result will influence clinical management.

It is helpful to discuss the clinical case with the consultant cardiologist or a senior medical member of the team if there is doubt about any aspect of a patient's investigations.

The quality of the test report will depend on the information that is provided on the request form.

An abnormal test result does not necessarily indicate that the patient's diagnosis is only due to the reported abnormality. For example, breathlessness may be due to both heart failure and lung disease, and this highlights the importance of the clinical examination and a questioning mind.

The cost implications of an investigation and the effects that both the test and the result may have on the general well-being and psychological state of the patient should also be considered before requesting the test.

Test interpretation and blind management advice

An intrinsic limitation of most open-access investigations is that the result may be interpreted by the reporting physician in the absence of a detailed knowledge of the patient's clinical background. In some cases it is unlikely that management advice included in the report will be relevant to the patient. For example, a specialist consultation would not be necessary in the management of a young woman whose echocardiogram report confirms a clinical diagnosis of a mitral valve prolapse. However, a specialist referral would be required for an elderly man with echocardiographic evidence of significant aortic stenosis. In addition, the test may be interpreted in the absence of detailed clinical information, and the reporting physician may not have had the opportunity to interpret the test result with a knowledge of the patient's clinical background. An exercise test showing ST-segment depression in a patient with a low probability of having coronary artery disease will probably be a false-positive result, and this may lead to confusion and anxiety (and often to further inappropriate testing).

GPs therefore need to understand the value and limitations of the more commonly used cardiac tests so that these are used appropriately and efficiently. Primary care clinicians need to be able to explain to patients why the test has been requested, how the test helps in their management, what it involves, and the implications of the results.

The reader is referred to detailed texts for information about the diagnostic criteria and examples of pathology.

Test result quality

The diagnostic quality of a test and the information obtained from it depend on factors relating to the equipment, the patient and the reporting physician. For example, a high-quality ECG recording depends on a properly maintained and calibrated ECG machine, good-quality electrodes and paper, correct skin preparation to obtain a satisfactory electrical signal, and a relaxed patient. Physicians who report tests will need to be provided with adequate clinical information.

Variability in the interpretation of test results

All cardiac tests involve interpretation, and are not purely objective measurements like a blood test. There is a well-recognised inter- and intra-observer variability in test result interpretation. There is also a patient component in the variability of exercise test results, but this is not clinically significant.

Questions to ask before requesting or performing a test

The value of any test result depends on a number of factors, and the following points should be considered before requesting cardiac tests.

- What is the most likely clinical diagnosis?
- Do I need to perform an investigation at all to confirm the diagnosis, to obtain prognostic information or to help me to decide on the best management option for the patient, or can I rely solely on my clinical assessment?
- Will the test result influence clinical management and in what way will it do so?
- What is the most appropriate and efficient way to investigate the problem?
- Is the patient willing and able to be subjected to the test?
- What do I need to tell the patient about the test and what it involves?
- What will I need to do if the test result is unhelpful or does not explain the clinical problem?

Chest X-ray

This is invaluable in the assessment of patients who present with breathlessness due to either cardiac or lung disease. Despite having been in use for over a century as the oldest method of imaging the heart, it remains a useful investigation, although other imaging techniques provide more detailed and accurate anatomical and physiological information about the heart.

Value and limitations

A plain chest X-ray will show pulmonary oedema but not necessarily the cause of it. The heart shadow may appear spuriously enlarged due to projectional problems or a depressed sternum (pectus excavatum), or fluid or fat around the heart. Echocardiography provides more accurate information about cardiac chamber dimensions and wall thickness, but without these potential interpretational problems and radiological risks.

The test

Patients are familiar with X-rays, and understand that they are harmless unless they are repeated many times.

The report

Chest X-rays are usually reported by a consultant radiologist, who may advise on further imaging depending on the question that is being asked.

Electrocardiography

This is the most widely used and available cardiac test, and it is now commonly performed in primary care by both GPs and practice nurses. It records the electrical activity of the heart over a period of several seconds.

Value and limitations

Electrocardiography is very helpful for excluding myocardial infarction as a cause of chest pain. However, ECG signs of infarction may develop several hours after infarction and may not be apparent on an ECG that is recorded during ischaemic chest pain. If myocardial infarction is suspected, the patient should be urgently referred to hospital.

A normal ECG has a high specificity in excluding heart failure, myocardial infarction and arrhythmia as a cause of palpitation during the test.

Indications

- Suspected myocardial infarction.
- Heart failure as a cause of breathlessness.
- Palpitation.
- Bradycardia.
- Syncope and dizzy turns.
- Screening before major surgery in patients over 50 years of age or in younger patients with a cardiac history.

The test

The patient lies down in a fairly horizontal and relaxed position. The ECG will show muscle tremor in patients who shiver, move or have muscle movement due to Parkinson's disease, and this may make the ECG uninterpretable. A high-quality ECG trace depends on good electrode contact with a hairless and greaseless skin. Accurate electrode placement is important. The skin should be wiped with alcohol and, if necessary, shaved and abraded with very fine sandpaper. No other preparations are necessary. The patient feels no discomfort other than the cold sensation of an alcohol skin wipe or hair shaving. The test carries no risk, and can be completed within a few minutes.

The report

Electrocardiographs may provide computer-interpreted reports, but these require confirmation by an experienced physician. These reports generally have a high negative predictive accuracy in excluding arrhythmia and infarction in normal individuals, but have a relatively lower accuracy in diagnosing abnormalities.

Management of abnormal test results

If there is a clinical or computer-generated report suggesting myocardial infarction, the patient should be referred for a specialist opinion, and this should be done urgently if clinically indicated.

Patients with newly diagnosed atrial fibrillation or benign ectopic beats who are clinically stable may be managed in primary care (*see* Chapter 18). Patients who feel distressed or who have significant arrhythmias, should be referred to hospital (*see* Chapter 18).

Exercise testing

This is the most widely used and useful method of investigating patients with known or suspected coronary heart disease, and it could be performed in primary care. The purpose of the test is to assess reversible myocardial ischaemia. It provides both diagnostic and prognostic information. It is performed in hospital cardiac units and is usually supervised by a technician. A doctor is available in the rare event of a complication, and to interpret the test result. Resuscitation equipment is available.

Chapter 14 includes a discussion of Bayes' theorem and the interpretation of exercise test results.

Physiological responses to exercise

During exercise, the systolic blood pressure normally increases due to increased cardiac work, the diastolic pressure normally decreases due to peripheral vasodilatation, and the patient should reach at least 70% of their age-predicted maximal heart rate (calculated as 220 minus age in years). Shortness of breath and fatigue are the usual reasons why normal individuals have to stop exercise.

An inadequate heart rate response is a sign of sinus node disease, and would support the decision for pacemaker implantation with other appropriate indications. An exaggerated systolic blood pressure response is consistent with hypertension.

Markers of a poor prognosis

Any of the following features suggest left ventricular impairment and/or significant coronary artery disease and therefore a poor prognosis:

- a poor exercise time
- failure of the systolic blood pressure or heart rate to increase during exercise
- ischaemia (angina and/or ST-segment depression) at a low heart rate and workload
- frequent ventricular ectopic beats or ventricular tachycardia during or after exercise

- ST-segment elevation in Q-wave-bearing leads after infarction
- slow resolution of ST-segment depression and heart rate after exercise.

Markers of a good prognosis

The absence of markers of a poor prognosis indicates a low probability of coronary artery disease and a good prognosis.

The test

Patients are exercised on either a cycle or a treadmill. Many patients prefer a cycle and feel more secure. Only the resistance increases on a cycle, but both the inclination and the speed of a treadmill increase and patients may feel insecure. Cycles are smaller, take up less space, are quieter and, because there is less upper body movement, the ECG quality may be superior. Cycles may not be suitable for patients who find cycling difficult.

Although anti-anginal medication, including β-blockers, may decrease the sensitivity of exercise testing, most cardiologists do not advise patients to stop these drugs before the test because of logistics and the small risk of withdrawal. Patients are usually asked to sign a consent form because of the very occasional risk of death (1 in 100 000), infarction or ventricular arrhythmia requiring treatment. A profound vagal response is also uncommon and resolves quickly when the patient lies down or, if necessary, is given atropine.

Recording the ECG

The skin preparation and electrode positions are similar to those for a resting ECG, but for exercise testing the arm leads are placed below the clavicles and the leg leads are placed above the iliac crests. To minimise noise the electrodes and cables are taped to the skin. A resting blood pressure and ECG are recorded.

Exercise end-points

The patient is then exercised, usually to their maximum tolerance. The test is stopped if the patient cannot exercise any more due to fatigue, breathlessness, claudication or dizziness, or if they develop angina, ST-segment depression or significant arrhythmias, or their heart rate or systolic blood pressure fail to increase appropriately.

They then lie down or sit down until they and their heart rate and blood pressure have recovered and the ECG changes have resolved. Glyceryl trinitrate (GTN) may be given to patients who develop angina.

Analysing the results

All exercise test variables are analysed. It is helpful for the physician to observe and talk to the patient during the test to ask them about their symptoms.

The Duke treadmill score is used in a few centres. It may improve the accuracy of an exercise test result. The formula takes into account the degree of angina, the extent of ST-segment depression and the exercise duration.

Value and limitations of the test

An appreciation of Bayesian analysis is helpful for understanding the value and limitations of the test (*see* Chapter 14). Exercise testing is of most diagnostic use in patients at intermediate risk of coronary heart disease. A 'negative' test result will probably be a false-negative result in a patient with a high probability of coronary heart disease, whereas a 'positive' test result will probably be a false-positive result in a patient with a low probability of coronary heart disease.

Exercise testing contributes no diagnostic information about the likelihood of the presence of coronary heart disease in patients with previous myocardial infarction, those with previous revascularisation or those with angina. However, it does provide prognostic information. It is commonly used to assess recurrent or new symptoms in patients who have had angioplasty or coronary artery surgery. An exercise test showing no ischaemic or haemodynamic abnormality has a high negative predictive accuracy in a patient with a low risk of having coronary heart disease.

It provides an objective assessment of fitness and exercise capacity, and is helpful in the evaluation of a patient who is complaining of undiagnosed breathlessness.

It has a lower predictive accuracy in women, and the reason for this is not clear. The ST-segment response to exercise is the objective hallmark of myocardial ischaemia, but this cannot be interpreted in patients with an abnormal ST-segment at rest. This includes patients with bundle branch block and pre-excitation syndromes. Nevertheless, exercise tolerance, vulnerability to exercise-induced arrhythmia and symptoms can be evaluated.

Indications

- Evaluation of patients at intermediate risk of having coronary artery disease.
- Prognostic evaluation of patients with known coronary artery disease and after myocardial infarction.
- Serial evaluation of patients after revascularisation.
- Evaluation of the heart rate response in patients with suspected chronotropic incompetence.
- Evaluation of the blood pressure response in patients with hypertension.
- Evaluation of the response to anti-anginal treatment.
- Evaluation of exercise capacity and response to treatment in patients with heart failure.

Contraindications

- Unstable angina.
- Physical disability that precludes exercise.
- Severe aortic stenosis.
- Uncompensated heart failure.
- Severe uncontrolled hypertension.

The report

This should provide the information described above. If the exercise test is requested for diagnostic reasons, it should state the probability of coronary heart disease (high, intermediate or low), the haemodynamic response (normal or abnormal) and the exercise duration. The details that are included should permit a prognostic assessment. Treatment and management recommendations (e.g. no treatment and no further tests *or* drugs and coronary angiography) should be included. The GP will then be in a position to discuss the findings with the patient.

Nuclear cardiac imaging

This is of limited clinical value in a small number of clinical situations, and accordingly is only available in a few hospitals in the UK. The widespread availability of open-access exercise testing to assess myocardial ischaemia, transthoracic echocardiography to assess left ventricular function and cardiac anatomy, stress echocardiography to assess myocardial ischaemia and hibernating myocardium and coronary angiography in most district general hospitals has relegated nuclear perfusion imaging to the position of a test that is largely of historical interest in the evaluation of patients with suspected coronary heart disease.

Principle of nuclear perfusion imaging

The uptake of radioactive chemical into the left ventricular muscle depends on the blood supply. No radionuclide will be taken up into dead heart muscle, and less will be taken up into an area of heart muscle that is supplied by a narrowed coronary artery compared with an area of normal heart muscle that is supplied by a normal artery. These differences only become apparent when the heart is subjected to stress induced by exercise or drugs.

The test

Most tests are performed to assess myocardial ischaemia and are similar to an exercise stress test on a cycle or treadmill. In addition, a radioactive nuclear chemical (usually thallium) is injected into an arm or hand vein at peak exercise. The patient lies down under a gamma camera and the uptake of radionuclide is imaged in different projections. Further images are taken after around 4 hours to investigate reperfusion. The report is subjective and computer enhancements are used.

Indications

Nuclear perfusion imaging may be used to investigate reversible ischaemia, in patients with resting ECG abnormalities (e.g. bundle branch block) that would make exercise-induced changes uninterpretable or in cases where stress echocardiography cannot be performed. In all other cases, the sensitivity and specificity of nuclear perfusion imaging do not differ significantly from those of an exercise test, and the technique is not superior to stress echocardiography.

Value and limitations

The accuracy of the test is affected by a large number of factors. False-negative scans may be due to inadequate stress, anti-ischaemic medication, collateral circulation, poor-quality imaging or breast attenuation. False-positive scans may occur in patients with conduction abnormalities or cardiomyopathies, or due to technical problems. Nuclear material, if used repeatedly, carries a small risk, and the test is invasive, costly and time consuming. Although the dose of radiopharmaceutical used is probably not dangerous, patients may be reluctant to receive an injection of such a substance when less dangerous, cheaper and quicker alternative tests are available.

The report

This should indicate the probability of coronary heart disease. Identifying the location of coronary artery disease is difficult and often unreliable in view of relative perfusion. For example, a patient with severe triple-vessel coronary artery disease and homogenous reduced myocardial blood supply may have no relative perfusion defect identified, and the scan may be reported as 'normal'. There is also variability in coronary arterial blood supply to the inferior wall of the left ventricle from the right and/or circumflex arteries, so attempts to localise coronary artery disease with nuclear perfusion imaging are often inaccurate. Interpretation of the scans is vulnerable to observer error.

Echocardiography

This is the most powerful diagnostic non-invasive cardiac imaging test, and it carries no risk. It is widely available, cheap and completely safe. It is now performed and reported instantaneously in primary care by visiting specialists or technicians using portable machines, as well as in hospital. Echocardiography may be combined with Doppler measurements of blood flow across diseased valves and septal defects.

Value and limitations

Echocardiography provides important anatomical and functional information about the heart muscle, the chamber sizes, ventricular wall thickness, the valves and intracardiac connections. The pericardial space and pericardium may be visualised easily, and this is useful as part of the evaluation of breathlessness in patients with chest or breast malignancy.

A normal echocardiogram virtually excludes heart failure, indicates that a heart murmur is probably due to turbulence of blood in a normal heart and not due to an underlying structural heart abnormality, and excludes pathological enlargement of the heart (cardiomegaly), a question that is commonly raised as an incidental finding on a chest X-ray.

Images may not be of diagnostic quality in obese patients and those with chronic airways disease. Interpretation of left ventricular function is subjective, but is made more objective by measurements of left ventricular end-systolic and end-diastolic dimensions.

Indications for echocardiography

- Left and right ventricular function and size in suspected heart failure of any cause.
- Diagnosis and severity of valve abnormalities and septal defects in patients with murmurs.
- Ventricular wall thickness in patients with hypertension, cardiomyopathy and aortic valve stenosis.
- Mechanical complications of acute myocardial infarction.
- Intracardiac connections in patients with congenital heart disease.

The severity of heart valve conditions is assessed by examining the anatomical appearance of the valve, the flow characteristics (with Doppler examination) and the haemodynamic consequences of the valve lesion for left ventricular function, dimensions and wall thickness. Intervention for heart valve conditions should be undertaken before left ventricular impairment occurs.

The severity of heart failure is assessed by examining right and/or left ventricular wall movement (pumping action of the ventricles) and thickening (the normal ventricular wall thickens in systole) and chamber dimensions.

The following common cardiac conditions may be diagnosed by echocardiography:

- heart failure
- aortic stenosis and gradient – significant left ventricular impairment will result in a spuriously low aortic valve peak systolic gradient
- aortic regurgitation
- mitral stenosis and valve area (which determines severity and need for intervention)
- mitral valve prolapse
- mitral regurgitation
- hypertensive heart muscle disease
- left ventricular impairment due to infarction
- dilated cardiomyopathy
- hypertrophic cardiomyopathy.

Serial echocardiography is useful for monitoring the progression of valvular heart disease in order to decide on the timing of valve surgery and its effects on left ventricular dimensions and function, to assess the effects of antihypertensive treatment on left ventricular wall thickness, and after myocardial infarction to investigate recovery and resolution of left ventricular impairment.

The test

The test is completely harmless and carries no risk in pregnant women. The investigation is performed in a darkened room so that the heart images can be seen more easily on the monitor. Patients are asked to take off their upper clothes and lie at an angle of around 45° on their left side. Ultrasound jelly is then applied to the transducer, which is pressed firmly over the chest and moved to find a satisfactory echo-window in an intercostal space. The transducer is angled and rotated to obtain several views of the heart. The patient will hear a 'whooshing' noise which represents the electronic Doppler signal denoting blood flow. The test can be completed within a few minutes depending on the question that is being asked and the echogenicity of the patient.

The report

This should provide both anatomical and physiological information. Colour-flow Doppler examination may show physiological mitral and/or tricuspid regurgitation. Heart failure is excluded if left ventricular function is normal. The management of specific valve disorders and left ventricular abnormalities is discussed in Chapter 17.

Transoesophageal echocardiography

This technique is complementary to transthoracic echocardiography. It is performed in outpatients in cardiac units, and often in very ill patients in the intensive-care unit. Transoesophageal echocardiography produces clearer images of the heart than transthoracic echocardiography because the probe is closer to the heart and the echo signals only have to pass through the posterior wall of the oesophagus, and are not attenuated by the chest wall and lungs.

The test

The procedure is similar to upper gastrointestinal endoscopy. The patient should fast for at least 4 hours before the test, and must sign a consent form. Some patients are unable to swallow the probe and find the procedure unpleasant, but with satisfactory preparation, explanation, sedation and pharyngeal anaesthesia, and in the hands of an experienced physician, most patients tolerate the procedure well. Antibiotic prophylaxis is not routinely given even in patients with prosthetic valves unless intubation is traumatic. The test is contraindicated in patients with dysphagia, oesophageal problems, respiratory disease or severe coagulopathy, and in those who are unable to co-operate. The patient's ECG, oxygen saturation and blood pressure are monitored during the procedure because probe passage down the oesophagus may cause hypertension. The procedure takes around 30 minutes.

Complications are rare, occurring in 0.3% of patients, and they include oesophageal perforation, arrhythmia, heart failure and laryngeal spasm. Mortality is reported to be 1 in 10 000, but the greatest risk is in very ill patients.

Indications for transoesophageal echocardiography

- Inadequate transthoracic echocardiography – airways disease, obesity, breast implants.
- Atrial thrombus/myxoma – prior to cardioversion, radiofrequency ablation, closure of atrial septal defect.
- Prosthetic heart valve – function, thrombus, vegetation.
- Aortic disease – suspected dissection.
- Endocarditis on a native or prosthetic valve – vegetations, abscess.
- Congenital heart disease – cardiac anatomy.
- Atrial septum – patent foramen, septal defect.
- Unexplained stroke in young people – intracardiac thrombus, patent foramen, atrial septal defect, aortic/mitral vegetations, left atrial myxoma.

Value and limitations of transoesophageal echocardiography

This technique provides very clear anatomical information about the cardiac structures, but involves oesophageal intubation, which carries a small risk of complications. It permits echocardiographic investigation in patients who are anaesthetised and unconscious in the intensive-care unit, and in those with chest wall problems or dressings which prevent adequate transthoracic study.

Stress echocardiography

This is a specialised extension of echocardiography which is performed in specialist units, not in primary care. It may be used as an alternative to an exercise test to induce myocardial ischaemia. It can distinguish viable myocardium (areas of heart muscle which may improve with revascularisation) from 'dead' muscle. Dobutamine is the most commonly used stress agent, but dipyridamole and adenosine are also used, although side-effects are more common with these drugs. Exercise may be used to stress the heart, but is less practicable and accurate because imaging is difficult if the patient is moving.

The test

A conventional echocardiogram is performed first and the images are stored as a baseline. Dobutamine, a β-agonist which increases heart rate and contractility, is then infused intravenously. In a normal heart, this results in an increase in left ventricular wall contraction and thickness. Dead heart muscle does not respond to dobutamine, whereas viable myocardium does.

Value and limitations

These are similar to those described above for echocardiography. Interpretation of the images is subjective, and the diagnostic quality of the test depends largely on the experience of the reporting physician.

The sensitivity and specificity of stress echocardiography are similar to those for exercise testing. The technique is more accurate than exercise testing in women, and in patients with an abnormal ECG at rest (left ventricular hypertrophy, bundle branch block and left ventricular hypertrophy).

Infusion of dobutamine may result in chest pain, dizziness, palpitation and arrhythmia, breathlessness and headache.

Indications

The presence or absence of viable myocardium helps to decide whether revascularisation is appropriate. Revascularising 'dead' (infarcted) heart muscle would not be expected to improve either the symptoms or the prognosis. 'Dead' myocardium is seen as an area of the left ventricular wall which does not move or thicken. Contraction or thickening of previously 'dead' myocardium during dobutamine infusion suggests viability. The rationale for revascularising these 'viable' areas of muscle is that their function might improve left ventricular function and prognosis. Viability is not an issue when considering revascularisation for patients with angina and narrowed coronary arteries supplying normal myocardium.

The main indications can be summarised as follows:

- in patients who cannot exercise
- when the ECG response to exercise cannot be interpreted
- for the evaluation of patients with known or suspected coronary artery disease
- for the evaluation of viable myocardium.

Twenty-four-hour ambulatory (Holter) ECG recording

First described by Dr Holter in 1949, this test records a patient's heart rhythm and rate, usually during a 24-hour period. It enables the effects of exercise, sleep, emotion and other day-to-day activities to be evaluated in patients who complain of intermittent palpitation, giddy turns or loss of consciousness. The commonly recorded arrhythmias are ectopic beats and atrial fibrillation. Patients are given a diary card on which to record the time, duration and nature of their symptoms so that these may be correlated with arrhythmias timed on the recorder.

Ambulatory devices also record the ST-segment, and are occasionally used in the evaluation of patients with coronary heart disease and 'silent ischaemia'.

Magnetic tapes are still used in hospitals, and are the most widely used in all patients and yield most information in individuals with frequent daily symptoms. Recently, solid-state and neural-network technology devices have allowed GPs to take and print their own recordings, and computer software provides a reliable diagnosis. For patients with less frequent symptoms, event recorders enable the patient to trigger the recorder, which is placed against the chest wall during an attack. Some patients find event recorders difficult to use. Loop recorders, which are similar in size to a small pacemaker and are implanted under the skin of the chest wall, record continuously for several months and are designed to capture arrhythmias responsible for elusive and occasional symptoms.

Arrhythmias in healthy individuals

It is important for GPs to appreciate the range of arrhythmias that may be recorded in healthy people so that they can explain and reassure patients that not all arrhythmias indicate heart disease (see Table 25.1). Bradycardia and heart block are more common

Table 25.1:   Ambulatory ECG findings in 'normal' people

Heart rate (range, beats/min)	Heart rate (sleep, beats/min)	Ectopics (% of patients)	VT (% of patients)	SVT (% of patients)	Sinus pause > 2.0 s (% of patients)	Mobitz I (% of patients)
37–180	45	10–25	2	5–30	2	2

VT, ventricular tachycardia; SVT, supraventricular tachycardia.

in young people. Ventricular ectopic beats and paroxysmal atrial fibrillation are not uncommon in older people, but may not result in symptoms.

Value and limitations

The quality of the ECG depends on good skin preparation, absence of interference due to cable movement, and correct calibration. Tape slippage is a potential problem with conventional tape recorders. Reliable computer algorithms improve the diagnostic accuracy.

Symptoms and arrhythmias

An arrhythmia coinciding with the patient's symptoms provides the diagnosis. Conversely, a cardiac arrhythmia as a cause of symptoms is excluded if symptoms occur in the absence of an arrhythmia. It is difficult to reach a conclusive diagnosis if the patient is symptom-free, particularly if symptoms are infrequent. However, patients may not always experience symptoms with ectopic beats and short runs of paroxysmal atrial fibrillation. Unsustained ventricular tachycardia is less common, but may not result in symptoms. If the history is consistent with these arrhythmias, it is likely that an arrhythmia is responsible.

Indications

- Patients who have symptoms consistent with a cardiac arrhythmia.
- Patients with palpitation, giddy turns, loss of consciousness or transient ischaemic attacks.
- To assess the response to medical treatment.
- To assess the prognosis in patients with arrhythmias after myocardial infarction.
- To assess symptoms after pacing for either bradycardia or tachycardia.

Cardiac catheterisation and angiography

The main purpose of the test is to obtain anatomical information about the location and severity of coronary artery disease, and haemodynamic data. It provides superior information to non-invasive coronary artery imaging, and also provides the opportunity to perform angioplasty at the same time. It is now widely available in district general hospitals as well as in main teaching centres, although coronary angioplasty is mainly performed in centres with on-site cardiac surgical facilities.

The test

Cardiac catheterisation and angiography is performed by cardiologists as a day case using local anaesthesia and, in some patients, light sedation. Small-lumen tubes are passed sequentially through a sheath which is most commonly inserted into the right femoral artery. The sheath is used to allow easy access to the artery, and prevents forward flow of blood through the sheath, although blood can still flow to the foot outside the sheath. The left femoral, right radial and brachial arteries are also occasionally used in patients with difficult arterial access. Different-shaped catheters are used to intubate and inject radio-opaque contrast into the left ventricle and the right and left coronary arteries, and another catheter may be used to measure pressures in the pulmonary artery and right heart chambers in patients with valvular disease or septal defects, and in the uncommon cases where cardiac transplantation is considered.

The test is most commonly performed in patients with known or suspected coronary artery disease, when only the left ventricle and coronary arteries are catheterised. Fluoroscopy is used to position the catheters, and cine-pictures are taken during contrast injection and opacification of the left ventricle and both coronary arteries (and bypass grafts in patients who are being investigated after coronary artery surgery) in multiple views to obtain an accurate three-dimensional impression of each coronary artery narrowing.

A pigtail-shaped catheter is introduced into the left ventricle under fluoroscopy, and the pressure is measured. This may be increased in patients with impaired left ventricular function. Contrast is then injected and pictures are taken to record left ventricular function. The presence of mitral regurgitation is visualised as reflux of contrast back into the left atrium. The pigtail catheter is then removed while any pressure gradient across the aortic valve (as may be seen in aortic stenosis) is recorded. Specially shaped catheters are then inserted in turn to inject the right and left coronary arteries. The catheters and the sheath are removed and digital pressure is applied over the femoral artery until the bleeding stops. This may be uncomfortable. The patient is kept supine for at least 4 hours and then gradually allowed to sit up and stand, to reduce the likelihood of bleeding. Some cardiologists use collagen-plug closure devices to shorten the period of bed rest after the angiogram. Patients are able to get up sooner if the brachial artery (usually the right) is used. This is now not commonly done, except if the femoral arteries are not suitable.

Patient information

Some patients find the test uncomfortable, but most are anxious about the implications of a result showing obstructive coronary artery disease. Injection of local anaesthetic into the skin over the femoral artery may sting, and injection of contrast into the left ventricle may cause a feeling of flushing and occasionally nausea. Passage of a catheter in the aorta is painless except if the aorta is dissected by the catheter tip, which is very rare. The patient should be warned by the operator about the recognised complications, which are more common in patients with atheromatous disease in the aorta. The result and the probable management plan should be explained to the patient before they go home, although the final management plan is often decided at a later department cardiothoracic meeting. The patient should not drive, cycle or participate in sports for at least 24 hours after the angiogram, to avoid the risk of bleeding from the femoral artery.

Indications

- Angina that is not controlled adequately with medical treatment, and in patients with mild angina and cardiovascular risk factors.
- Unstable angina.

- Important reversible ischaemia on exercise testing or other non-invasive testing.
- In patients who cannot exercise or when the test is unhelpful.
- Continuing angina, ischaemia or haemodynamic impairment after myocardial infarction.
- After successful resuscitation from cardiac arrest or ventricular tachycardia.
- Prior to aortic or mitral valve intervention in patients with angina, cardiovascular risk factors or endocarditis.
- Certain types of congenital heart disease.
- To assess the possibility of revascularisation in heart failure.

Value and limitations

Coronary angiography is the 'gold-standard' test for investigating anatomical coronary artery disease, but it does not provide physiological information.

The percentage risks of coronary angiography in low-risk patients are small. Most complications occur in older patients with atheromatous vascular disease, which is the main indication for performing the investigation.

Box 25.1: Frequency of complications of coronary angiography	
Death	0.10
Myocardial infarction	0.08
Stroke	0.08
Transient ischaemic attack	0.10
Arrhythmia	0.50
Vascular complication	0.50
Any other complication	0.50

The commonest femoral artery vascular complications occur in patients with a wide pulse pressure (e.g. in hypertension and aortic regurgitation) and include haematoma or, less commonly, a false aneurysm of the femoral artery. These present as a painful, swollen and spreading bruise over the puncture site, and are diagnosed with duplex ultrasound. All patients with a painful, swollen pulsatile mass over the puncture site should be referred back to the cardiologist for assessment. False aneurysms may close up and heal spontaneously if there is a low flow rate between the main femoral artery and the sac of the aneurysm. Closure of an occlusion of the false aneurysm sac may be achieved by injection of thrombin into the sac of the aneurysm, duplex ultrasound-guided manual compression over the neck of the false aneurysm, or (rarely) surgical repair may be required.

The report

A stenosis obstructing more than 50% of the arterial lumen would be expected to result in reduced flow down the artery and angina, whereas a short lesion less than 50% of the diameter of the lumen would not be considered flow-limiting. Stenoses are therefore graded as a percentage narrowing, or classified as mild (50–75%), moderate (75–90%), severe (91–99%) or blocked (100%) according to a visual examination ('eyeballing') of the angiogram.

The cardiologist should write back with the angiogram report, including information on left ventricular function and other relevant information (e.g. coexisting valve abnormalities). There should be a management plan with suggestions for medical and secondary prevention treatment and a decision regarding revascularisation.

Coronary artery disease and symptoms

Surprisingly, there is a poor correlation between symptoms and coronary artery disease. A patient with severe triple-vessel coronary artery disease may be symptom-free until the occurrence of a myocardial infarct. Conversely, a patient with very mild disease may have very troublesome angina. This paradox highlights the importance of treating the patient in conjunction with the angiographic result and other clinical and investigative information, rather than just the angiogram.

Possible treatment strategies

Medical treatment is advised if there is no need for revascularisation based on symptoms or coronary angiographic findings, or in the uncommon situation where revascularisation by either angioplasty or coronary artery surgery is not feasible or would be too risky.

Coronary artery bypass surgery is generally advised in patients who are unsuitable for coronary angioplasty, which is equally effective in relieving angina. Repeat revascularisation is more likely to be required in patients who have had angioplasty because of the risks of restenosis, which are lower with the use of stents and particularly coated stents. Coronary artery surgery is preferred to angioplasty in patients with severe triple-vessel coronary artery disease and left ventricular impairment, because it confers the added advantage of improving prognosis as well as symptoms. In patients in whom no prognostic benefit is expected and coronary artery surgery is considered too high a risk or refused, coronary angioplasty is considered.

All patients with coronary artery disease should have cardiovascular risk factor evaluation and treatment.

Magnetic resonance imaging

This is only available in a few centres in the UK, and is expensive. Its diagnostic role in imaging the heart, pericardium, aorta and pulmonary vessels is developing and remains unclear. It is occasionally used to obtain anatomical information that is not adequately provided by echocardiography.

The test

Magnetic resonance imaging provides information about cardiac anatomy, valve disease, intracardiac and intravascular blood flow, cardiac chamber contraction and filling, and tissue perfusion. Because of cardiac and respiratory movement, the technique is currently most appropriate for the cardiovascular structures that undergo least movement. These include the aorta, pericardium and pulmonary vessels. It is not yet as accurate as coronary angiography for imaging coronary arteries, although technological advances show promise in this area.

The patient has to lie within the magnet in a narrow, dark tunnel, and many find this experience intolerably claustrophobic, despite sedation. Open scanners are less claustrophobic. The test takes around 20 minutes.

Indications and contraindications

The test is safe, non-invasive and does not require ionising radiation. It is therefore useful in the serial assessment of patients with congenital heart disease, valvular disease, intracardiac tumours and thrombus, cardiomyopathies and pericardial disease.

Magnetic resonance imaging is contraindicated in patients with pacemakers, cardiac defibrillators, cerebral aneurysm clips and cochlear implants. It is not contraindicated in patients with metallic prosthetic heart valves, coronary artery stents or metallic sternal wires inserted after cardiac surgery.

Indications for magnetic resonance imaging

- Acute aortic dissection.
- Characterisation of cardiomyopathies.
- Imaging of the pericardium.

Answers to case studies

1   An ECG at rest may show features of left ventricular hypertrophy, which may reflect hypertensive heart disease. Repolarisation abnormalities do not reliably indicate myocardial ischaemia. If you think the patient is describing angina, exercise testing will not provide much additional diagnostic information but may provide some prognostic information. His exercise performance, the presence or absence of angina or breathlessness and the time to 1 mm of ST depression will help you to evaluate the degree of myocardial ischaemia. If severe, he should be seen urgently and possibly admitted directly to hospital. The patient should be treated for angina with aspirin 75 mg om (unless there are important contraindications) and a β-blocker. He should be advised to take GTN spray (which has a longer shelf life than tablets) and this should be taken prophylactically as well as to abort spontaneous attacks of angina. He should be referred to a cardiologist for coronary angiography and revascularisation if appropriate. All his risk factors should be attended to.

2   This lady needs a careful, considered and comprehensive assessment. Gastro-intestinal malignancy must be excluded before embarking on cardiac evaluation of her aortic valve disease. There would be no point in attempting to replace her aortic valve if she had carcinoma of the stomach. The decision is more difficult if she has severe aortic stenosis and a respectable lesion in her gut. The gastrointestinal condition must be fully diagnosed, the severity of her aortic valve disease and the state of her cardiac function quantified and her general

medical condition carefully assessed. Investigation in primary care might include haematology, thyroid function, renal and liver function, ECG, echocardiography, a chest X-ray and abdominal ultrasound. Gastrointestinal endoscopy carries a risk in patients with important aortic valve disease and this will need to be discussed with the gastroenterologist.

3   The history is important. Try to establish what she is experiencing. Is it vertigo, light headedness, breathlessness, palpitation, loss of balance, fear or what? There are several causes. It is important to exclude heart block (which may be intermittent), ventricular tachycardia, paroxysmal atrial fibrillation or other atrial tachycardias, transient cerebral ischaemic attacks, cerebral pathology or an ENT problem. Orthostatic hypotension usually results in syncope rather than dizzy turns. Pulmonary emboli are an unusual cause. Review her medication (β-blockers). Sometimes, no cause can be found. Initial investigations should include an ECG to make sure there are no conduction problems (bundle branch block) or signs of myocardial infarction. Look for unusual ECG abnormalities – long QT syndrome, pre-excitation). A negative 24-hour ECG recording during symptoms excludes a cardiac arrhythmia. Capturing an arrhythmia during an attack provides the diagnosis. An echocardiogram should be requested if there is a murmur suggesting important aortic valve disease or a third heart sound or a displaced apex beat suggesting a cardiomyopathy. These cases are difficult and the patient should be advised that she may have to have several tests and specialist referral before a diagnosis is reached. Once a cardiac cause has been excluded, patients are usually referred to a neurologist and if these tests are negative to an ENT specialist.

Further reading

- The American College of Cardiology website (www.acc.org/clinical/statements.htm) publishes clinical practice and investigation guidelines.

Index

.